KV-054-356

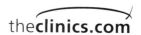

ENDOCRINOLOGY AND METABOLISM CLINICS

OF NORTH AMERICA

Type 2 Diabetes and
Cardiovascular Disease

GUEST EDITORS
Daniel Einhorn, MD, FACP, FACE
Julio Rosenstock, MD

March 2005 • Volume 34 • Number 1

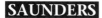
SAUNDERS
An Imprint of Elsevier, Inc.
PHILADELPHIA   LONDON   TORONTO   MONTREAL   SYDNEY   TOKYO

W.B. SAUNDERS COMPANY
A Division of Elsevier Inc.

The Curtis Center • Independence Square West • Philadelphia, Pennsylvania 19106

http://www.theclinics.com

ENDOCRINOLOGY AND METABOLISM
CLINICS OF NORTH AMERICA
March 2005
Editor: Joe Rusko

Volume 34, Number 1
ISSN 0889-8529
ISBN 1-4160-2686-X

Copyright © 2005 by Elsevier Inc. All rights reserved. No part of this publication may be reproduced or transmitted in any form or by any means, electronic or mechanical, including photocopy, recording, or any information retrieval system, without written permission from the Publisher.

Single photocopies of single articles may be made for personal use as allowed by national copyright laws. Permission of the publisher and payment of a fee is required for all other photocopying, including multiple or systematic copying, copying for advertising or promotional purposes, resale, and all forms of document delivery. Special rates are available for educational institutions that wish to make photocopies for non-profit educational classroom use. Permissions may be sought directly from Elsevier Science Rights & Permissions Department, PO Box 800, Oxford OX5 1DX, UK; phone: (+44) 1865 843830, fax: (+44) 1865 853333, e-mail: permissions@elsevier.co.uk. You may also contact Rights & Permissions directly through Elsevier's home page (http://www.elsevier.com), selecting first 'Customer Support', then 'General Information', then 'Permissions Query Form'. In the USA, users may clear permissions and make payments through the Copyright Clearance Center, Inc., 222 Rosewood Drive, Danvers, MA 01923, USA; phone: (978) 750-8400, fax: (978) 750-4744, and in the UK through the Copyright Licensing Agency Rapid Clearance Service (CLARCS), 90 Tottenham Court Road, London WIP 0LP, UK; phone: (+44) 171 436 5931; fax: (+44) 171 436 3986. Other countries may have a local reprographic rights agency for payments.

The ideas and opinions expressed in *Endocrinology and Metabolism Clinics of North America* do not necessarily reflect those of the Publisher. The Publisher does not assume any responsibility for any injury and/or damage to persons or property arising out of or related to any use of the material contained in this periodical. The reader is advised to check the appropriate medical literature and the product information currently provided by the manufacturer of each drug to be administered to verify the dosage, the method and duration of administration, or contraindications. It is the responsibility of the treating physician or other health care professional, relying on independent experience and knowledge of the patient, to determine drug dosages and the best treatment for the patient. Mention of any product in this issue should not be construed as endorsement by the contributors, editors, or the Publisher of the product or manufacturers' claims.

Endocrinology and Metabolism Clinics of North America (ISSN 0889-8529) is published quarterly by Elsevier Inc. Corporate and editorial offices: 170 S Independence Mall W 300 E, Philadelphia, PA 19106-3399. Accounting and circulation offices: 6277 Sea Harbor Drive, Orlando, FL 32887-4800. Periodicals postage paid at Orlando, FL 32862, and additional mailing offices. Subscription prices are USD 170 per year for US individuals, USD 279 per year for US institutions, USD 85 per year for US students and residents, USD 210 per year for Canadian individuals, USD 336 per year for Canadian institutions, USD 235 per year for international individuals, USD 336 per year for international institutions and USD 118 per year for Canadian and foreign students/residents. To receive student/resident rate, orders must be accompanied by name of affiliated institution, date of term, and the *signature* of program/residency coordinator on institution letterhead. Orders will be billed at individual rate until proof of status is received. Foreign air speed delivery is included in all *Clinics* subscription prices. All prices are subject to change without notice. POSTMASTER: Send address changes to *Endocrinology and Metabolism Clinics of North America*, W.B. Saunders Company, Periodicals Fulfillment, Orlando, FL 32887-4800. **Customer Service: 1-800-654-2452 (US). From outside of the US, call 1-407-345-4000. E-mail: hhspcs@harcourt.com.**

Reprints. For copies of 100 or more, of articles in this publication, please contact the Commercial Rights Department, Elsevier Inc., 360 Park Avenue South, New York, NY 10010-1710. Tel. (212) 633-3813, Fax: (212) 462-1935, e-mail: reprints@elsevier.com

Endocrinology and Metabolism Clinics of North America is covered in *Index Medicus, EMBASE/Excerpta Medica, Current Contents/Clinical Medicine, Current Contents/Life Sciences, Science Citation Index, ISI/BIOMED, BIOSIS, and Chemical Abstracts.*

Printed in the United States of America.

GUEST EDITORS

DANIEL EINHORN, MD, FACP, FACE, Diabetes and Endocrine Associates, Scripps Whittier Institute for Diabetes; and Clinical Professor, Medicine, University of California at San Diego, La Jolla, California

JULIO ROSENSTOCK, MD, Dallas Diabetes and Endocrine Center; and Clinical Professor, Medicine, University of Texas Southwestern Medical School, Dallas, Texas

CONTRIBUTORS

JOHN B. BUSE, MD, PhD, Associate Professor, Medicine, Division of Endocrinology; Chief, Division of General Medicine and Clinical Epidemiology; and Director, Diabetes Care Center, University of North Carolina School of Medicine, Chapel Hill, North Carolina

MARIA DEL PILAR SOLANO, MD, Assistant Professor, Clinical Medicine, Division of Diabetes, Endocrinology, and Metabolism, Diabetes Research Institute, University of Miami, Miami, Florida

DANIEL EINHORN, MD, FACP, FACE, Diabetes and Endocrine Associates, Scripps Whittier Institute for Diabetes; and Clinical Professor, Medicine, University of California at San Diego, La Jolla, California

VIVIAN A. FONSECA, MD, Professor, Department of Medicine and Pharmacology, Tulane University Medical Center; and Veterans Affairs Hospital, New Orleans, Louisiana

HERTZEL C. GERSTEIN, MD, MSc, Professor, Division of Endocrinology and Metabolism and the Population Health Research Institute, Department of Medicine, McMaster University and Hamilton Health Sciences, Hamilton, Ontario, Canada

RONALD B. GOLDBERG, MD, Professor, Medicine, Division of Diabetes, Endocrinology, and Metabolism; Director, Lipid Disorders Unit; and Associate Director, Diabetes Research Institute, University of Miami, Miami, Florida

IRL B. HIRSCH, MD, Division of Metabolism, Endocrinology, and Nutrition, Department of Medicine; and Medical Director, Diabetes Care Center, University of Washington Medical Center, Seattle, Washington

SILVIO E. INZUCCHI, MD, Professor, Section of Endocrinology, Department of Medicine, Yale University School of Medicine, New Haven, Connecticut

ALI JAWA, MD, Assistant Professor, Section of Endocrinology, Diabetes, and Metabolism, Tulane University and Hospital, New Orleans, Louisiana

DAVID M. KENDALL, MD, Chief, Clinical Services; Medical Director, International Diabetes Center; and Associate Professor, Medicine, University of Minnesota Medical School, Minneapolis, Minnesota

BIJU P. KUNHIRAMAN, MD, Fellow, Section of Endocrinology, Diabetes, and Metabolism, Tulane University and Hospital, New Orleans, Louisiana

ETIE S. MOGHISSI, MD, FACP, FACE, Co-Chair, Inpatient Diabetes and Metabolic Control Task Force, American Association of Clinical Endocrinologists, Inglewood, California

ROBERT E. RATNER, MD, Professor, Georgetown University College of Medicine, Washington, DC; and Attending Endocrinologist, MedStar Research Institute, Hyattsville, Maryland

GERALD M. REAVEN, MD, Professor, Medicine, Division of Cardiovascular Medicine, Falk Cardiovascular Research Center, Stanford Medical Center, Stanford, California

MATTHEW C. RIDDLE, MD, Professor, Medicine, Division of Endocrinology, Diabetes, and Clinical Nutrition, Oregon Health and Science University, Portland, Oregon

JULIO ROSENSTOCK, MD, Dallas Diabetes and Endocrine Center; and Clinical Professor, Medicine, University of Texas Southwestern Medical School, Dallas, Texas

JAMES R. SOWERS, MD, FACE, FACP, FAHA, Thomas W. and Joan F. Burns Missouri Chair in Diabetology; Director, Missouri University Diabetes and Cardiovascular Center; Associate Dean, Clinical Research; Professor, Department of Internal Medicine, University of Missouri School of Medicine; and Veterans Affairs Medical Center, Columbia, Missouri

ROBERT S. SHERWIN, MD, CNH Long Professor of Medicine, Section of Endocrinology, Department of Medicine, Yale University School of Medicine New Haven, Connecticut

GABRIEL I. UWAIFO, MD, Assistant Professor, Georgetown University College of Medicine; and Attending Endocrinologist, MedStar Research Institute, Washington, DC

ADAM WHALEY-CONNELL, DO, Chief Resident, Internal Medicine; and Fellow, Division of Nephrology, Department of Internal Medicine, University of Missouri School of Medicine, Columbia, Missouri

CONTENTS

treatment of lipid disorders beyond those of LDL-C may be necessary to significantly reduce cardiovascular risk in the diabetes mellitus population.

The ability of insulin to stimulate glucose disposal varies six- to eightfold among apparently healthy individuals. The only way that insulin-resistant persons can prevent the development of type 2 diabetes is by secreting the increased amount of insulin that is necessary to compensate for the resistance to insulin action. The greater the magnitude of muscle and adipose tissue insulin resistance, the more insulin must be secreted to maintain normal or near-normal glucose tolerance. Although compensatory hyperinsulinemia may prevent the development of fasting hyperglycemia in insulin-resistant individuals, the price paid is the untoward physiologic effects of increased circulating insulin concentrations on tissues that retain normal insulin sensitivity. This article focuses on the interplay between insulin resistance at the level of the muscle and adipose tissue and normal hepatic insulin sensitivity, which leads to the atherogenic lipoprotein profile characteristic of insulin-resistant individuals.

The Joint National Committee recently reconvened to prepare their seventh report in an attempt to help clarify the guidelines for the management of hypertension (HTN) for clinicians. This was due, in large part, to recent reports of large, multi-center outcome trials with new conclusions and the increasing recognition of widespread underuse of resources for HTN management. There is abundant evidence that combinations of two, three, or more antihypertensive agents may be required to reach goal blood pressure of 130/80 mm Hg in hypertensive patients who have diabetes. There are several important implications for diabetic patients in the new guidelines; this article attempts to clarify them and provide clinicians with a current strategy for the management of HTN in patients who have diabetes.

This article discusses glycemic management of type 2 diabetes, reviewing the characteristics, advantages, and limitations of the various treatment options. A broad strategy is proposed, with

disease. Glucose levels rise because of insufficient insulin caused by insulin resistance or insulin deficiency. Elevated glucose and insufficient insulin effects are implicated in the pathogenesis of cardiovascular disease. Emerging data suggest that glucose lowering with insulin may reduce safely the risk for cardiovascular disease and preserve beta-cell function. Large, controlled international trials are testing the hypothesis that insulin therapy may have cardiovascular benefits.

FORTHCOMING ISSUES

THE CLINICS ARE NOW AVAILABLE ONLINE!

Access your subscription at:
http://www.theclinics.com

ELSEVIER
SAUNDERS

Endocrinol Metab Clin N Am
34 (2005) xi–xii

ENDOCRINOLOGY
AND METABOLISM
CLINICS
OF NORTH AMERICA

Preface

Type 2 Diabetes and Cardiovascular Disease

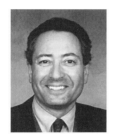   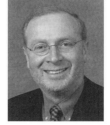

Daniel Einhorn, MD, FACP, FACE   Julio Rosenstock, MD
Guest Editors

Since the last edition of *Endocrinology and Metabolism Clinics of North America*, the distinction between type 2 diabetes (DM) and cardiovascular (CV) diseases has been blurred. The central importance of CV disease (CVD) prevention is becoming an integrated part of diabetes management. The current edition reflects this paradigm, focusing directly on CVD risk reduction strategies in type 2 DM. The solid evidence on lipid and blood pressure management is reviewed in detail and the potential impact of glycemic control and the choice of diabetes agents on the development of CVD are explored.

The first articles cover lipid issues, beginning with the outcome data supporting aggressive low density lipoprotein–cholesterol reduction and then the emerging rationale, but less robust evidence, for similar aggressive treatment of triglycerides and high density lipoprotein–cholesterol. These approaches are meant to be complementary, recognizing that we need more studies on the use of multiple lipid lowering agents in combination. The third article, written by the pioneer of insulin resistance, offers a unique, but still controversial, hypothetical construct for understanding how the atherogenic lipid profile develops. The review of blood pressure management provides the basis from the Joint National Committee on Prevention, Detection, Evaluation, and Treatment of High Blood Pressure VII for targets and treatment options specific to people who have type 2 DM.

The fifth article in this issue begins the focus on glucose control with a pragmatic review of the multiple therapeutic tools for outpatient glucose management providing simple, but effective strategies. This is followed by an article reviewing the rationale, the multiple cross-sectional studies, but

0889-8529/05/$ - see front matter © 2005 Elsevier Inc. All rights reserved.
doi:10.1016/j.ecl.2005.01.012   *endo.theclinics.com*

limited interventional evidence, for the optimal control of glucose in the hospital setting.

Attention then turns to the nonglycemic benefits from therapies traditionally ordered for glycemic control, namely the thiazolidinediones and insulin, based on hypothetical, experimental, and limited clinical data. These imply that such agents may have value in all people who have DM and possibly in those who do not have DM but who have insulin resistance or modest levels of *dysglycemia*. Finally, we close on the future of DM with a review of novel glycemic therapies that should emerge in the next few years. The last two articles thoroughly review the current evidence and the ongoing trials addressing the critical issue of prevention, not just of type 2 DM, but most notably the prevention of CVD.

There are a number of questions raised in the articles that are not yet resolvable. These include (1) should we screen asymptomatic individuals with DM for CVD; (2) how early should the diagnosis of diabetes be made; (3) how much does the glucose itself contribute to the morbidity and mortality of DM; (4) should insulin resistance be treated in and of itself as opposed to just its disease manifestations; and (5) should any level of control above *normal* for lipids, blood pressure, or plasma glucose be accepted as good enough?

We both are clinical diabetologists *at heart* and as such we have chosen the topics that are relevant to the practicing physician today with a view toward the future. We salute our contributors for their exceptional efforts, their thoughtfulness, their willingness to take a position on difficult topics, and their ability to deal with our compulsiveness. We trust that by the time the next edition comes out, this issue will have helped make careful attention to CVD a more routine practice in people who have type 2 DM.

Dedication

We dedicate this issue of the *Endocrinology and Metabolism Clinics of North America* to Eric N. Gold, MD, a consummate *endocardiologist*, who died January 1, 2005. *Endocrinology and Metabolism Clinics of North America* was his favorite publication and he would have loved this edition.

Daniel Einhorn, MD, FACP, FACE
Diabetes and Endocrine Associates
Scripps Whittier Institute for Diabetes
La Jolla, CA, USA

E-mail address: einhorn.daniel@scrippshealth.org

Julio Rosenstock, MD
Dallas Diabetes and Endocrine Center
Medical City Dallas
Dallas, TX, USA

E-mail address: juliorosenstock@dallasdiabetes.com

ELSEVIER
SAUNDERS

Endocrinol Metab Clin N Am
34 (2005) 1–25

ENDOCRINOLOGY
AND METABOLISM
CLINICS
OF NORTH AMERICA

Management of Diabetic Dyslipidemia

Maria Del Pilar Solano, MD,
Ronald B. Goldberg, MD*

*Division of Diabetes, Endocrinology, and Metabolism, Diabetes Research Institute (R77),
University of Miami, 1450 NW 10th Avenue, Miami, FL 33136, USA*

Cardiovascular disease (CVD) is a major cause of morbidity and mortality among subjects who have diabetes. It is estimated that cardiovascular complications are responsible for up to 75% of deaths among people who have type 2 diabetes [1] and constitute up to a twofold to fourfold increased risk of coronary heart disease (CHD), stroke, and peripheral vascular disease events when compared with nondiabetic individuals [2–5]; this risk is considered equivalent to that in nondiabetic subjects who have CHD [6–9]. CVD also is the leading cause of death in subjects who have type 1 diabetes. Moreover, subjects who have diabetes have a worse prognosis than their nondiabetic counterparts after an acute coronary event with a greater frequency of congestive heart failure and an increased fatality rate [10,11]. The increased CHD risk in type 2 diabetes seems to result, at least in part, from a greater burden of established cardiovascular risk factors (eg, elevated blood pressure, obesity, dyslipidemia) [12]. These factors are associated with insulin resistance and emerge early in the evolution of the diabetic state. Thus, prompt identification and management of dyslipidemia in type 2 diabetes has become a cornerstone of diabetes care. The high risk for CVD, coupled with the recognition that large numbers of diabetic subjects do not survive their first event and that their prognosis is much poorer if they do compared with nondiabetic subjects, places a responsibility on physicians to adopt a proactive approach in their therapeutic decision-making for dyslipidemia, despite incomplete clinical trial evidence.

Features of diabetic dyslipidemia

Typically, diabetic dyslipidemia is characterized by a modest elevation in triglyceride levels, reduced high-density lipoprotein cholesterol (HDL-C)

---

* Corresponding author.
E-mail address: rgoldber@med.miami.edu (R.B. Goldberg).

0889-8529/05/$ - see front matter © 2005 Elsevier Inc. All rights reserved.
doi:10.1016/j.ecl.2005.01.001

values—and although low-density lipoprotein cholesterol (LDL-C) levels generally are similar to those found in the general population—there is an increased frequency of small, dense low-density lipoprotein (LDL) particles (Table 1). National surveys indicate that 30% to 40% of patients who have diabetes have triglyceride levels that are greater than 200 mg/dL and 10% have levels that are greater than 400 mg/dL [13,14]. In the United Kingdom Prospective Diabetes Study (UKPDS), baseline HDL-C levels were 9% lower in men and 23% lower in women who had diabetes compared with controls [15]. Despite the high frequency of modestly elevated baseline triglyceride levels in the UKPDS (mean baseline 159 mg/dL), a multi-variate analysis found that triglyceride levels did not predict CHD events. LDL-C was the strongest independent predictor of CHD, followed by HDL-C [16]. In the recently reported European Diabetes Prospective Complications Study in 1864 subjects who had type 1 diabetes, lipid parameters did not predict CHD; however, age, waist-to-hip ratio, and albumin excretion rate were positive predictors of CHD [17]. Other abnormalities that were associated with diabetic dyslipidemia include increased triglyceride-rich lipoproteins in the postprandial state (postprandial lipemia), increased remnant lipoproteins, increased apolipoprotein B 100 (apo B) concentration, and an increase in small dense HDL particles [18–20], all of which have been associated with an increased risk for CHD.

Pathogenesis of diabetic dyslipidemia

An increased flux of free fatty acids to the liver that is associated with insulin resistance and abdominal obesity has been implicated in the enhanced production of large very low density lipoprotein (VLDL) particles by the liver [21], the secretion of which is not suppressed by meal-related insulin surges as it normally is in the insulin sensitive state [22]. In addition to VLDL overproduction, reduced lipoprotein lipase activity and apolipo-

Table 1
Mean plasma lipids at diagnosis of type 2 diabetes in the United Kingdom Prospective Diabetes Study

Plasma lipids	Men		Women	
	Type 2	Control	Type 2	Control
No. of patients	2139	52	1574	143
TC (mg/dL)	213	205	224	217
LDL-C (mg/dL)	139	132	151**	135
HDL-C (mg/dL)	39*	43	43**	55
TGs (mg/dL)	159**	103	159**	95

Abbreviations: TC, total cholesterol; TGs, triglycerides.
* $P < 0.02$ comparing type 2 vs. control; **$P < 0.001$.
Data from Manley SE, Frighi V, Stratton E, et al for the UK Prospective Diabetes Study Group. UK Prospective Diabetes Study 27. Plasma lipids and lipoproteins at diagnosis of NIDDM by age and sex. Diab Care 1997;20:1683–7.

protein C III enrichment of VLDL may retard VLDL and remnant clearance [23]. The accumulation of triglyceride-rich lipoproteins, coupled with the heightened action of cholesteryl ester transfer protein, leads to an increased exchange of triglyceride for cholesterol between VLDL and HDL and between VLDL and LDL particles. Hydrolysis of triglyceride-enriched LDL and HDL by hepatic lipase, also considered to be up-regulated in type 2 diabetes, results in the formation of small, cholesterol-poor HDL and LDL particles [24]. There is evidence that *diabetic HDL* is cleared more rapidly from the circulation and may be dysfunctional [24]. The small, dense LDL pattern (phenotype B) becomes common as triglyceride levels increase to greater than 132 mg/dL [25]. This is twice as frequent in diabetic individuals [20] and is considered to be atherogenic because of an increased vulnerability to oxidative modification and increased uptake by the arterial wall, effects that are aggravated by diabetes [26]. Accumulating exogenous and endogenous remnant lipoproteins are believed to be atherogenic as well [27]. Many of these abnormalities are not reflected directly in the standard lipid profile; this has given rise to several advanced lipoprotein testing methods that can identify lipoprotein size or density subfractions and particle number. The added value that these measurements have in predicting or preventing CVD in high-risk individuals who receive intensive management based on the lipid profile is unclear. They do indicate, however, that the total number of atherogenic particles is increased in type 2 diabetes.

Benefits of treatment of diabetic dyslipidemia: clinical trial evidence

Most of the available data that indicate benefit of treatment of dyslipidemia derive from subgroup analyses of intervention trials using statins and suggest that the relative cardiovascular benefits of such treatment are similar among diabetic and nondiabetic participants. Fewer studies used fibrates or niacin. All of these studies confirm the higher risk of CVD events in diabetic subjects.

Statins

Scandinavian Simvastatin Survival Study, Cholesterol and Recurrent Events Trial, and Long-Term Intervention with Pravastatin in Ischemic Disease

The first three major statin trials, namely the Scandinavian Simvastatin Survival Study (4S; simvastatin, 20–40 mg), the Cholesterol and Recurrent Events Trial (CARE; pravastatatin 40 mg) and the Long-Term Intervention with Pravastatin in Ischemic Disease (LIPID; pravastatatin 40 mg), all of which were secondary intervention studies that used different CVD end points and studied subjects with differing mean baseline LDL-C levels (136–185 mg/dL), contained small subgroups of diabetic subjects who benefited from statin treatment [28–32]. Statin therapy reduced the event rate by an average of 21% to 55% in the diabetic subgroups, although for CARE and LIPID the absolute event rate while on statin therapy remained higher than that in the nondiabetic groups who took placebo. Untested in these trials were the benefits of statin treatment in diabetic subjects who did not have overt CVD, who nevertheless have been placed in the highest risk category by the National Cholesterol Education Panel Adult Treatment Panel (NCEP ATP) III guidelines [9]. Several completed primary prevention trials did not have sufficient power or achieve sufficient LDL-C reduction to produce significant results [33–36]. The question as to whether diabetic subjects without overt heart disease benefit from statin treatment finally was resolved by the Heart Protection Study (HPS) and by the Collaborative Atorvastatin Diabetes Study (CARDS).

Heart Protection Study and Collaborative Atorvastatin Diabetes Study

HPS investigators recruited 5963 diabetic individuals with average cholesterol values (baseline LDL-C 127 mg/dL)—2912 of whom had no clinical features of CVD—and 14,573 nondiabetic individuals who had occlusive vascular disease to test the efficacy of 40 mg of simvastatin compared with placebo [37]. Treatment with simvastatin yielded an approximate 30% reduction in LDL-C and reduced the risk of the first major cardiovascular event by 33% in the diabetic subjects who did not have CVD and by 18% in those who had pre-existing CVD (no significant difference in effect size in these two groups, although placebo and statin-treated groups in those who had pre-existing CHD had major vascular event rates that were more than three times greater than those who did not have pre-existing CHD). These effects were independent of age (all subjects were > 40 years of age), gender, diabetes duration, type of diabetes (there were 600 subjects who had features of type 1 diabetes and who responded in a similar manner to the rest of the group), level of glycemic control, triglyceride, and HDL-C levels. Furthermore, the relative benefit of statin therapy in diabetic individuals whose baseline LDL-C was less than 116 mg/dL at entry was similar to that obtained in those whose LDL-C was greater than 116 mg/dL (27% versus 20% relative risk reduction [RRR] in first major CVD event) (Table 2). (It has been pointed out that because a direct LDL-C method was used in HPS, this LDL-C cut point would be ~120 mg/dL using the standard Friedewald calculation.) There was a sufficient number of individuals among the combined diabetic and nondiabetic cohorts whose baseline LDL-C was less than 100 mg/dL to show that the proportional reduction in CVD event risk by simvastatin was similar to those whose LDL-C was greater than 130 mg/dL [38]. The investigators concluded that "statin therapy should be considered routinely for diabetic patients at sufficiently high risk of major vascular events, irrespective of their initial cholesterol levels" [37]. Most would agree that almost all diabetic subjects who are older than 40 years fit this description.

Table 2
Heart Protection Study: diabetes subgroup data

Measure difference (mg/dL)	CVD event-rate (%/4.8 y)		RRR (%)
	Placebo	Simvastatin	
LDL-C < 116	20.9	15.7	↓27
LDL-C ≥ 116	27.0	23.3	↓20
HDL-C < 35	31.1	25.9	↓20
HDL-C ≥ 35	21.3	15.8	↓27
Non–HDL-C < 156	19.8	15.2	↓28
Non–HDL-C ≥ 156	27.2	22.3	↓25
TGs < 178	22.8	16.8	↓30
TGs ≥ 178	27.6	24.1	↓17

Abbreviation: RRR, relative risk ratio.

Data from Heart Protection Study Collaborative Group. MCR/BHF Heart Protection Study of Cholesterol Lowering with Simvastatin in 5963 People with Diabetes: a randomized, placebo-controlled trail. Lancet 2003;361:2005–16.

The CARDS provides strong support for the results in the cohort that had diabetes but no CVD in the HPS [39]. This was the first statin trial to be conducted exclusively in diabetic subjects. The investigators randomized 2838 men and women (mean age 62 years; mean LDL-C, 118 mg/dL) who had type 2 diabetes, but no CVD, and at least one risk factor (hypertension, smoking, micro- or macro-albuminuria, retinopathy) to treatment with placebo or atorvastatin, 10 mg per day. When the study was ended prematurely after a median follow-up of 3.9 years because of the early positive findings, mean LDL-C in the group that received active treatment had decreased to 78 mg/dL and was associated with significant reductions in acute CHD events (36%) and stroke (48%). In similar fashion to the HPS findings, there was a similar relative statin benefit for CHD in subjects who had LDL-C levels that were greater or less than 120 mg/dL.

Reversal of Atherosclerosis and Aggressive Lipid Lowering and Pravastatin or Atorvastatin Evaluation and Infection Therapy Trials

The Reversal of Atherosclerosis and Aggressive Lipid Lowering (RE-VERSAL) and Pravastatin or Atorvastatin Evaluation and Infection Therapy (PROVE-IT) trials, reported recently, are the first of a new generation of statin trials that compared the benefits of "moderate" and "intensive" statin therapy. Although neither trial was directed primarily at diabetic subjects, their findings are important for all high-risk patients, and together with HPS led to a reshaping of NECP ATP III. In REVERSAL, 634 subjects who had an identified coronary artery stenotic lesion had the plaque in this area characterized by intravascular ultrasound before and 18 months after randomization to pravastatin, 40 mg per day, or atorvastatin, 80 mg per day [40]. Despite the fact that subjects in the group that received pravastatin achieved a mean LDL-C of 110 mg/dL, plaque volume continued to expand (+2.7%) compared with those in the group that took atorvastatin, whose plaque volume remained stable (mean LDL-C, 79 mg/dL). Although the clinical meaning of these differences are not clear, the fact that more intensive statin therapy modified plaque behavior beyond that achieved by pravastatin, 40 mg per day—an intervention that demonstrated effectiveness in primary and secondary prevention trials—is provocative and raises the possibility that increased LDL-C lowering or maximized statin therapy (or both) may yield greater benefit than submaximal treatment.

PROVE-IT was a much larger clinical outcomes trial that tested the same question. In this study, 4162 subjects (18% had diabetes) who presented with an acute coronary syndrome were randomized to the same two treatments as in REVERSAL for an average period of follow-up of 30 months [41]. Subjects who took atorvastatin achieved a median LDL-C of 65 mg/dL and had a significant ($P < .005$) reduction in deaths and major cardiovascular events after 2 years compared with those who took pravastatin (median LDL-C, 99 mg/dL). This finding supports the concept that in very high-risk subjects, intensive statin therapy was more effective in reducing coronary events. Diabetic subjects who have established CVD reasonably could be included in such a group. Whether the findings from these short-duration trials might reflect so-called "pleiotropic statin effects" in addition to the lowering of LDL-C is conjectural. The results of similar long-term comparative statin trials, using conventional clinical end points, that are conducted in patients who have stable CHD are awaited eagerly.

Fibrates

There have been three clinical intervention trials that used fibrate monotherapy and included a subgroup of diabetic individuals. Neither the Helsinki Heart Study, a primary prevention study with gemfibrozil [42], nor the Bezafibrate Infarction Prevention (BIP) trial, a secondary prevention study [43], both with small diabetic subgroups, demonstrated a significant benefit of fibrate treatment in diabetic subjects; bezafibrate did not reduce CVD outcomes overall in the full cohort of the BIP trial. The Veterans Affairs Cooperative Studies Program High-Density Lipoprotein Cholesterol Intervention trial (VAHIT), however, found that treatment with gemfibrozil, 1200 mg per day, in 2531 men who had CHD—25% of whom had diabetes, low HDL-C, and a below average mean LDL-C value (LDL-C, 111 mg/dL)—reduced the risk of CHD death, nonfatal myocardial infarction (MI), or confirmed stroke by 24% in the diabetic and nondiabetic subsets [44]. The only lipid measure that predicted the CVD benefit was the increase in HDL-C (+7%) with treatment. Inclusion of previously undiagnosed diabetic subjects in the group that had established diabetes expanded and confirmed these results, and demonstrated a 37% reduction in the incidence of nonfatal MI or fatal CHD in these patients [45]. In addition, an analysis that included diabetic subjects and nondiabetic subjects who had a marker for insulin resistance demonstrated that the beneficial effect of gemfibrozil was limited to this combined group (about 50% of the total VAHIT population); this suggested that gemfibrozil was particularly effective in insulin-resistant subjects. In support of the VAHIT results were the findings in the Diabetes Atherosclerosis Intervention Study, which demonstrated an improvement in angiographic stenoses in type 2 diabetic subjects who were treated with fenofibrate [46]. These two studies suggest that gemfibrozil, and possibly, fenofibrate, are effective in reducing CHD events and stroke in diabetic (or nondiabetic insulin-resistant) subjects who had average or below average LDL-C levels and established CVD.

Niacin

The Coronary Drug Project, published in 1975, was the only study that evaluated the effect of niacin monotherapy on cardiovascular events [47]. In this study, 1119 men who had a history of MI were allocated to treatment with niacin, 1 g to 3 g per day, and 2789 participants received placebo. The mean baseline total cholesterol and triglyceride values were 250 mg/dL and 177 mg/dL, respectively. Despite a lack of benefit on total mortality, the risk of recurrent nonfatal MI was reduced by 27% with niacin. A recent reanalysis of the data showed that the benefit of niacin treatment on recurrent MI was similar at all levels of blood glucose, including patients whose fasting blood glucose was greater than 126 mg/dL [48]. Evidence for a beneficial effect from the addition of niacin therapy to statin treatment was suggested by the HDL Atherosclerosis Treatment Study (HATS) [49]. The effect of combination therapy (simvastatin plus niacin) on angiographic end points was compared with placebo in 160 individuals who had CHD and low HDL-C levels; 16% had diabetes. Simvastatin plus niacin resulted in a significant angiographic benefit with some regression of lesions, an effect that has not been documented clearly with statin therapy alone. Furthermore, despite the small sample size, treatment with niacin plus simvastatin was associated with a significant (60%) reduction in cardiovascular events (CHD death, nonfatal MI, stroke, or revascularization for worsening ischemia), which is a numerically greater effect than was demonstrated in statin monotherapy trials, with the exception of the hypercholesterolemic 4S diabetic subgroup.

National Cholesterol Education Panel Adult Treatment Panel III Guidelines

In the original NCEP ATP III guidelines [9], diabetes is considered to be a CHD equivalent. The lipid targets for individuals who have diabetes are the same as for individuals who have established CHD; the primary target is an LDL-C of less than 100 mg/dL [9]. In a recent update [50], ATP III modified the cut point for LDL-C lowering by pharmacotherapy in high-risk patients from an LDL-C of more than 130 mg/dL to an LDL-C of more than 100 mg/dL, based mainly on the HPS results. In addition, they proposed a new category of very high-risk patients, included among whom are diabetic subjects who have CVD, in which the option of an LDL-C target of 70 mg/dL for statin therapy might be expected to yield additional benefit. They did note that in diabetic subjects who did not have CHD and whose LDL-C was less than 116 mg/dL, the effect of statin treatment in HPS was only marginal (RRR 30%, $P = .05$), and thus, clinical judgement was needed to be exercised at this level. The ATP III panel pointed out that some diabetic subjects may not have a CHD risk equivalent (eg, younger patients and those who do not have other CVD risk factors, in whom an LDL-C > 130 mg/dL might be a more appropriate cut point for pharmacotherapy). They also proposed that a minimal "standard" statin dose be chosen if CVD prevention is to be successful (ie, at least 30%–40% decrease in LDL-C) (Box 1).

For individuals who have triglyceride levels of greater than 200 mg/dL, a secondary lipid target that was proposed originally by the ATP-III panel is the non–HDL-C (total cholesterol minus HDL cholesterol). Non–HDL-C correlates well with apo B and includes all atherogenic lipoproteins that contain apo B 100 (ie, LDL, lipoprotein (a), intermediate-density lipoprotein [IDL], and VLDL). The goal set for non–HDL-C is 30 mg/dL higher than the LDL target (< 130 mg/dL for diabetic subjects), although the update panel did not discuss decreased cut points or targets for non–HDL-C in those groups of subjects for whom new, lower LDL-C treatment cut points and goals are recommended. When triglyceride values are at least 500 mg/dL, the first priority is to lower triglyceride levels because of the risk of pancreatitis. HDL-C is the third lipid target and HDL-C increasing strategies may be considered in "high risk" individuals who have HDL-C levels that are less than 40 mg/dL. In the ATP III guidelines, however, HDL-C target levels were not established because of the lack of definitive information regarding the benefit of increasing HDL-C.

American Diabetes Association guidelines

The American Diabetes Association (ADA) categorizes diabetic individuals into low, intermediate, and high CHD risk based on their lipid profiles. The desirable LDL-C, HDL-C, and triglyceride levels are less than 100 mg/dL, more than 40 mg/dL in men/more than 50 mg/dL in women, and less than 150 mg/dL, respectively. The primary treatment strategy, as in NCEP ATP III, is decreasing LDL-C to less than 100 mg/dL (Table 3). The recommended LDL-C level to start pharmacologic therapy is more than 100 mg/dL in individuals who have established CHD and at least 130 mg/dL in those who do not have CHD. The 2004 recommendations also state that "statin therapy to achieve an LDL-C reduction of ~30% regardless of

Box 1. National Cholesterol Education Program Adult Treatment Panel III drug therapy targets for subjects who have coronary heart disease risk equivalents, including diabetes

1. LDL-C
- LDL-C goal < 100 mg/dL; < 70 mg/dL for very high-risk subjects (eg, those who have CVD)
- LDL-C ≥ 100 mg/dL; drug therapy beneficial in patients who have a CHD risk equivalent
- LDL-C ≥ 130 mg/dL; pharmacotherapy recommended in all subjects

2. Triglyceride/non–HDL-C
- Triglyceride 150 mg/dL to 199 mg/dL; emphasis on weight reduction and physical activity
- Triglyceride > 200 mg/dL; non–HDL-C goal < 130 mg/dL
- Non–HDL-C > 130 mg/dL; consider drug therapy

3. HDL-C
- Low HDL-C < 40 mg/dL; no goals for increasing HDL-C
- Isolated low HDL-C (triglyceride < 200 mg/dL); fibrates or niacin can be considered

Data from Grundy SM, Cleeman JI, Merz CN, et al. Cooordinating Committee of the National Cholesterol Education Program; National Heart, Lung, and Blood Institute; American College of Cardiology Foundation; American Heart Association. Implications of recent clinical trials for the National Cholesterol Education Program Adult Treatment Panel III guidelines. Circulation 2004;110:227–3; and Expert Panel on Detection, Evaluation, and Treatment of High Blood Cholesterol in Adults. Executive Summary of the Third Report of the National Cholesterol Education Program (NCEP) Expert Panel on Detection, Evaluation, and Treatment of High Blood Cholesterol in Adults (Adult Treatment Panel III). JAMA 2001;285:2486–589.

baseline LDL-C levels may be appropriate" based on the HPS results in diabetic subjects who were older than 40 years of age and who had a total cholesterol of at least 135 mg/dL. The second lipid strategy is increasing HDL-C with a target of more than 40 mg/dL for men and more than 50 mg/dL for women; the third priority is decreasing triglyceride to less than 150 mg/dL. These targets, however, are not based solely on results of clinical trials, but are arbitrary cut points that are used to separate ranges of values that are considered "acceptable" or "at increased risk." The ADA guidelines also emphasize the importance of glycemic control and lifestyle interventions, such as weight loss, exercise, and smoking cessation in the management of hypertriglyceridemia and low HDL-C levels [51].

Table 3
Treatment decisions by low-density lipoprotein cholesterol levels in adults who have diabetes

| Status | Therapy (mg/dL) | | | |
| | Medical nutrition | | Drug | |
	Initiation level	LDL-C goal	Initiation level	LDL-C goal
With CHD, PVD, or CVD	> 100	≤ 100	> 100	≤ 100
Without CHD, PVD, and CVD	> 100	≤ 100	≥ 130[a]	≤ 100

   Recent findings from the Heart Protection Study [37,38], in people with diabetes over the age of 40 years with a total cholesterol ≥ 135 mg/dL, suggest that statin therapy to achieve an LDL reduction of ~30% regardless of baseline LDL levels may be appropriate.
   Abbreviation: PVD, peripheral vascular disease.
   [a] In patients with LDL between 100 mg/dL and 129 mg/dL, a variety of treatment strategies are available, including more aggressive MNT and pharmacologic treatment with a statin.
   Data from American Diabetes Association. Dyslipidemia management in adults with diabetes. Diab Care 2004;27(Suppl 1):S68–71.

American College of Physicians guidelines

   The American College of Physicians (ACP) recently published its review and report on the management of LDL-C in type 2 diabetes [52]. Their recommendation was that all subjects who have CHD should be on lipid lowering-therapy, with statins as the primary agent of choice. For individuals who do not have CHD or those who have other CVD risk factors also are recommended for pharmacotherapy, and like ATP III and the ADA, the ACP endorsed the use of at least a moderate dosage of statin.

Therapeutic interventions

Lifestyle modification

   Nutrition therapy is essential in the management of diabetic dyslipidemia. NCEP and ADA guidelines both recommend reducing the intake of saturated fatty acids and transsaturated fatty acids to decrease LDL-C levels [9,50,53]. ATP III recommends limiting the intake of saturated fat to less than 7% of the daily calories and the intake of cholesterol to less than 200 mg/d. This diet, also known as the Step 2 diet, was shown in a meta-analysis to be associated with a 16% reduction in LDL-C [54]. Additional dietary options to decrease LDL-C include increasing the amount of soluble dietary fiber to 10 g/d to 25 g/d, adding 2 g/d of plant stanols/sterols, and including soy protein in the diet. These interventions have been associated with an additional 5% to 15% reduction in LDL-C values [55–57].
   The distribution of macronutrients in the diet is a matter of debate, particularly in individuals who have diabetic dyslipidemia. Low-fat, high-carbohydrate (> 60% of total caloric intake) diets have been associated with an increase in triglyceride and a decrease in HDL-C levels [58]. When monounsaturated fat is substituted for saturated fat in the diet, the LDL-C

lowering effect is similar to that obtained with a low-fat, high carbohydrate diet without the increase in triglyceride and the decrease in HDL-C levels [59,60]. Therefore, ATP III recommends limiting the intake of carbohydrates to less than 60% in individuals who have the metabolic syndrome, which is present in more than 80% of people who have type 2 diabetes. Furthermore, for individuals who have elevated triglyceride and low HDL-C levels, even lower carbohydrate intake (ie, < 50% of calories) could be considered. The ADA also recommends replacing saturated fat with carbohydrates or monounsaturated fat [53]. Low carbohydrate diets have been used for many years and recently have become even more popular. Although these diets may have short-term beneficial effects on serum lipids, fasting glucose, and weight reduction, these benefits have not been shown to persist over a more lengthy period [61]. Furthermore, low carbohydrate diets have not been evaluated adequately in individuals who have diabetes and hyperlipidemia; their long-term safety and efficacy remain unknown.

Exercise and pharmacologic approaches to weight loss in overweight individuals who have diabetes also are important strategies in the management of atherogenic dyslipidemia. The predominant effect of exercise is on maintaining or achieving weight reduction targets and its most consistent effect on lipids is to increase HDL-C. Lastly, supplementing the diet with omega-3 fatty acids (3–8 g/d) is another intervention that decreased triglyceride levels by 15% to 30% in diabetic subjects in short-term studies without significant adverse effects on hemoglobin A1c (HbA1c) or HDL-C, and only a slight increase in LDL-C values [62,63].

Pharmacologic treatment

Oral antihyperglycemic agents

Improved glycemic control, regardless of type of treatment, is associated with improved lipid values in individuals who have moderate to severe hyperglycemia. In the Veterans Affairs Cooperative Study in Type II Diabetes, intensive glycemic control with insulin therapy that resulted in a reduction of HbA1c from 9.3% to 7.2% was associated with a 31% decrease in triglyceride levels after 1 year, and a 23% reduction at 2 years without a significant change in LDL-C or HDL-C [64]. Beyond its effects on glycemic control, metformin was associated with a modest reduction in triglyceride levels in hyperlipidemic and hypertensive patients who did not have diabetes, as well as in some, but not all, studies of diabetic subjects who received monotherapy or in combination with sulfonylureas [65]. Changes of lesser magnitude in LDL-C and HDL-C also were reported with metformin treatment in some of these studies. Rosiglitazone and pioglitazone increased HDL-C and reduced the density of LDL particles [66–69]. Pioglitazone seemed to have a neutral effect on LDL-C concentration and a moderate reduction in triglyceride levels, whereas rosiglitazone elevated LDL-C modestly [67]. In general, pioglitazone seems to be associated with more beneficial lipid effects than rosiglitazone in published small studies. This was confirmed by a recently reported double-blind, randomized, head-to-head 24-week treatment comparision study of pioglitazone versus rosiglitazone in moderately hypertriglyceridemic type 2 diabetic subjects not receiving other antihyperglycemic or lipid-modifying agents. Pioglitazone was associated with significant triglyceride reduction whereas there was no net triglyceride change with rosiglitazone treatment. In addition, pioglitazone was associated with greater increases in HDL-C and LDL particle size, and less LDL-C increase than with rosiglitazone. Furthermore, apo C-III and LDL particle number increased with rosiglitazone therapy, but decreased with pioglitazone. These results suggest a beneficial anti-dyslipidemic effect of pioglitazone [70].

Pharmacologic lipid-modifying strategies

The NCEP and the ADA have given first priority to the achievement of LDL-C targets that recommend that many, if not most, subjects be treated with LDL-C-lowering medication if their LDL-C levels are more than 100 mg/dL and advise statin therapy for all diabetic subjects whose LDL-C levels are more than 130 mg/dL. At levels between 100 mg/dL and 129 mg/dL—where both sets of guidelines previously had deferred from making firm pharmacotherapeutic recommendations (except for the ADA in subjects who had CVD)—now both guidelines generally are supportive of statin therapy at a level that is likely to achieve at least a 30% to 40% decrease in LDL-C. Furthermore, both guidelines open the way to initiating pharmacotherapy with statins, essentially independent of the LDL-C, in subjects who are deemed to be at high or very high risk; the NCEP report set an optional goal of 70 mg/dL in the latter group of individuals. Because almost 80% of subjects who have diabetes have LDL-C levels that are more than 100 mg/dL [13], these proposals and the robustness of the clinical trial data that underpin them support the initiation of lipid-lowering pharma-cotherapy with at least a moderate dosage of statin (rosuvastatin 5–10 mg/d; atorvastatin 10–20 mg/d, simvastatin 20–40 mg/d; and pravastatin, lovastatin, and fluvastatin 40–80 mg/d) in most diabetic subjects; subjects who have CVD should be considered for maximal intensity statin and or combination therapy. Although diabetic subjects who did not have CVD and whose LDL-C levels were less than 116 mg/dL obtained only borderline benefit from simvastatin in HPS, a similar group that received atorvastatin in the CARDS trial achieved a significant 27% reduction in major events ($P = .025$). This strengthens the case for initiating statin therapy, even in subjects (> 40 years of age) who have a low LDL-C and who do not have heart disease, as long as they have at least one major risk factor.

What are the exceptions to these recommendations? One of these is the individual who has severe hypertriglyceridemia (> 400–500 mg/dL), in whom fibrates are more effective in reducing markedly elevated triglyceride values. Another exception might be in diabetic subjects whose cardiovascular risk is deemed not to be high within the forthcoming decade (eg, type 1 diabetes and recent-onset type 2 diabetes in persons who are younger than 30 years of age), especially if there are no risk factors or presence of the metabolic syndrome. Although this age-based cut point seems reasonable for type 1 diabetic subjects, based on studies of CVD incidence as a function of age [61,62], there is little information on the risks of cardiovascular disease in the increasingly important type 2 diabetic subgroup in this age category. In a recent comparison of macrovascular event rates in subjects who had newly-diagnosed type 2 diabetes who were less than 45 years of age (mean age, 38 years) and older than 45 years of age (mean age, 60 years), event rates were five-fold greater in the older age group over a 4-year period of follow-up [71]; this attests to the powerful effect of age on CVD incidence in diabetic subjects.

Near-routine prescription of a statin for diabetic patients creates a significant dilemma in regard to the place of fibrates and of niacin, both of which demonstrated CVD benefit in monotherapy trials in subjects who had established CHD. One option is to use these agents in combination with statins; it is clear that statin-treated patients continue to have CVD events, albeit at a lower rate than untreated individuals. Conversely, these drugs may interact with statins and occasionally cause serious complications. There is no evidence that combination therapy provides further benefit over effective monotherapy with statins; it is difficult to justify using these combinations routinely. Viewed in these terms, pharmacotherapeutic decision-making for diabetic dyslipidemia essentially boils down to the following questions: Which agent should be used to initiate therapy and what should be the goal be? When should statin/fibrate, statin/niacin, or other drug combinations be used? There are little to no clinical trial data to help with the answers to these questions; a pragmatic approach based on available evidence and clinical judgment is proposed.

Initiating therapy in subjects whose low-density lipoprotein cholesterol is at least 130 mg/dL

Clinical trial studies demonstrate a clear benefit of statin treatment at LDL-C levels of at least 130 mg/dL; there is little controversy about initiating statin therapy in this situation. Moreover, the VAHIT study did not test the effect of fibrates in subjects whose LDL-C values were at least 130 mg/dL. In the BIP study, bezafibrate did not show any benefit in subjects whose mean LDL-C was approximately 149 mg/dL, so there is less support for initiating therapy with fibrates in dyslipidemic subjects whose LDL-C is more than 130 mg/dL. Finally, niacin therapy alone, which reduces LDL-C by 10% to 20%, would be inadequate for reaching LDL-C targets in many of these individuals. Statins reduce LDL-C by 20% to 55% and have a good safety and tolerability profile; effects on muscle and on liver enzyme levels are the most important safety concerns. Elevation of liver enzymes to more than three times the upper limit of normal (ULN) was reported in less than 1.5% of participants, and clinical significant myopathy (creatine kinase $\geq$ 10 $\times$ ULN) was reported in less than 0.3% of participants in large clinical trials (both nonsignificantly different from placebo) [38,72]. The risk of myopathy increases with the concomitant use of medications that inhibit the metabolism of statins. Therefore, potent inhibitors of the cytochrome CPY3A4 system (eg, cyclosporine, gemfibrozil, ketoconazole, itraconazole, erythromycin, clarithromycin, indinavir, nelfinavir, nefazodone) should be avoided, particularly with simvastatin, atorvastatin and lovastatin. Pravastatin, fluvastatin, and rosuvastatin are not metabolized significantly by the cytochrome CPY3A4 enzymes and are not known to interact with the above medications. The combination of a statin with ezetemibe is likely to be effective in achieving LDL-C goals of approximately 70 mg/dL; the availability of single-tablet fixed combinations of simvastatin plus ezetemibe (Vytorin) should be helpful in this regard. A more potent statin also is more likely to achieve optimal lowering of LDL-C and non–HDL-C. When the NCEP LDL-C target is not achieved with a statin alone, or in cases in which statins are not tolerable, combination therapy with etezimibe, bile acid sequestrants, or niacin may be effective; each agent reduces LDL-C by 10% to 20%.

Initiating therapy in subjects whose low-density lipoprotein cholesterol is less than 130 mg/dL

Although for some time the ADA has recommended starting a statin when LDL-C is more than 100 mg/dL in diabetic patients who have established CHD, there have been no other firm recommendations in favor of pharmacotherapy for subjects whose LDL-C is less than 130 mg/dL until recently, although ATP III did suggest statin or fibrate therapy as options in this LDL-C range. The recent ATP III update supports statin therapy in this LDL-C range in high-risk subjects, based on the more recent statin trials, and does not specifically mention fibrates in this connection as an alternate first option (unless there is significant hypertriglyceridemia). The ADA guidelines state that statin treatment now may be considered, irrespective of the LDL-C value, in view of the positive HPS results in this group of patients. Clinical data from VAHIT, however, support the use of gemfibrozil in diabetic patients who have coronary artery disease and dyslipidemia and less than average LDL-C and minimally elevated triglyceride levels. On this basis, NCEP ATP III included statin and fibrate therapy as options for these individuals when the LDL-C is 100 mg/dL to 129 mg/dL. Thus, in this group of subjects, the clinician is faced with the dilemma of choosing between a fibrate or a statin, or for that matter, between a statin and niacin as first-line therapy. Several points need to be made in this regard.

It has been argued that gemfibrozil was more effective in reducing "hard" CHD events and strokes in dyslipidemic subjects who had below average

LDL-C values and diabetes or features of the metabolic syndrome in the VAHIT, than statins were in the CARE, LIPID, and Anglo-Scandinavian Cardiac Outcomes Trials [73]. In addition, because statin therapy does not seem to especially benefit insulin-resistant subjects, whereas gemfibrozil seemed to, it was proposed that gemfibrozil treatment should be favored over statins in dyslipidemic diabetic subjects whose LDL-C values were less than 130 mg/dL [73]. In the larger statin studies, such as HPS and now in CARDS, however, statin treatment was about as or more efficacious than gemfibrozil in VAHIT, not only in those who had CVD, but also in subjects who did not have established CVD. Only a single, positive, event-based fibrate study has been conducted in diabetic subjects; all had established CVD, which limits the evidence base in support of fibrate therapy.

It also can be argued that fibrates modify the dyslipidemia that is typical of diabetes more effectively than statins. Fibrates decrease triglyceride (25%–50%) and increase HDL-C (7%–15%) levels better than do statins, although the way in which they do this differs. Statins act principally by up-regulating the LDL receptor and enhancing clearance of apo B 100–containing lipoproteins, whereas fibrates exert their action by activating peroxisome proliferator-activated receptor–α (PPARα), which has multiple effects on triglyceride-rich lipoprotein metabolism, especially their clearance. Fibrates increase LDL particle size distribution better than statins. This may be, in part, because they reduce triglyceride levels more than statins do; however, the relationship of these changes to their CVD benefit is not known. It seems that at least within a large population of diabetic subjects, the LDL-C level is the most powerful predictor of CVD; fibrates do not decrease LDL-C significantly in dyslipidemic subjects. The tendency to recommend statin therapy for reduction of elevated LDL-C levels, and fibrate therapy for hypertriglyceridemia, is no longer tenable following the recognition that LDL-C levels below average may continue to exert atherogenic effects, and that intensive statin therapy decreased triglyceride, VLDL levels, and remnant lipoproteins significantly. Conversely, the benefit that was attributed to gemfibrozil in VAHIT was demonstrated in subjects who did not have definitive hypertriglyceridemia and was not related to decreases in triglyceride. It also was pointed out that although most of the CVD benefit in statin trials can be related to their major effect on lipids (ie, decreasing of LDL-C), the effect of gemfibrozil on the lipid profile cannot explain much more than 25% of the CVD benefit [73]. Presumably, the bulk of the benefit would be explained by other cardioprotective PPARα effects of gemfibrozil, related to its actions on inflammatory processes and the vascular wall; not understanding the mechanisms that are involved adds to the difficulty in resolving this issue. Fibrates and statins rarely are reported to cause rhabdomyolysis.

The case for niacin is weaker, by virtue of the fact that a significant number of individuals are not able to tolerate an effective dosage, notwithstanding the recent data that demonstrated the usefulness of niacin preparations in the treatment of dyslipidemia in diabetic subjects. Furthermore, the evidence base for CVD benefit in diabetic subjects is limited. Until a direct comparative intervention trial is completed (not until 2009), the question as to whether combination therapy has significant clinical benefits over monotherapy will remain unresolved. On balance, the robustness of the clinical trial data, the extensive clinical experience with statins, and the wealth of data that support their antiatherogenic activity tends to support initiation of therapy with statin drugs, rather than fibrates or niacin, in subjects whose LDL-C is less than 130 mg/dL, except in those who have severe hyper-triglyceridemia. One of the more potent statins is preferred to make it more likely that effective decreases in LDL-C and non–HDL-C triglyceride is achieved.

Secondary targets: beyond decreasing low-density lipoprotein cholesterol

Non–HDL-C is the focus of the secondary therapeutic strategy that was proposed by ATP III in the management of dyslipidemia, after the LDL-C goal is achieved and when triglyceride levels are at least 200 mg/dL. There is now evidence in diabetic subjects that non–HDL-C values are more predictive of CHD rates than are LDL-C levels [74]. The ADA guidelines recommend decreasing triglyceride levels to low-risk targets (ie, < 150 mg/dL), although it is not known whether decreasing non–HDL-C or triglyceride levels are correlated independently with CVD benefit. Although gemfibrozil decreased triglyceride levels significantly in the VAHIT study in the absence of a change in LDL-C and in which the baseline triglyceride was less than 200 mg/dL, this did not correlate with the CVD benefit. Fibrates do not change non–HDL-C significantly unless the triglyceride level exceeds 250 mg/dL to 300 mg/dL; therefore, this ATP III measure has little practical value as a cut point or target for fibrate therapy in the average patient who has diabetes. Statins are the most effective agents for decreasing levels of non–HDL-C. In addition to statins' LDL lowering effects, they also reduce VLDL cholesterol and IDL cholesterol, probably by enhancing their removal rates by way of the LDL-receptor, although it was suggested that at high dosages, statins may reduce VLDL secretion as well [75]. Therefore, even if LDL-C levels are decreased to target levels on statin therapy, increasing the dosage of statin, switching to a more potent statin, or adding ezetemibe would achieve greater non–HDL-C and triglyceride lowering and help to achieve secondary lipid lowering goals. Furthermore, if significant triglyceride lowering is achieved with high-dose statins, an increase in LDL particle size may be achieved [76]. In addition, treatment with statins also results in a greater reduction of the total number of LDL particles and apo B concentration than other agents. It has been argued that apo B may be a better marker of dyslipidemia than non–HDL-C [77–79]; in either case, statin therapy seems to be a first choice in pharmacotherapy. These considerations tend to marginalize fibrates for the most part to combination therapy. Finally, on the issue of increasing HDL, ATP III indicates that in high-risk subjects whose HDL-C levels that are less than 40 mg/dL, as a third priority, consideration should be given to the use of niacin and fibrates, although no goal for HDL-C is defined. Similarly, the ADA indicates that increasing HDL-C may be considered in subjects who have high-risk levels of HDL-C (ie, HDL-C values of < 40 mg/dL in men and < 50 mg/dL in women), without defining targets. Although there is widespread interest in increasing HDL-C, the current limitations in being able to increase HDL-C significantly, as well as the gaps in the understanding of the consequences of HDL-increasing interventions on atherogenesis, make it premature to construct formal recommendations. This does not imply that fibrates and niacin, the two agents that are recommended most commonly for increasing HDL, do not have value in the treatment of dyslipidemia.

Combination therapy

The concept that underlies the addition of a second or third agent is to optimize improvements in the lipid profile that is achieved by initial statin therapy. That further CVD prevention methods are needed is without doubt, in view of evidence such as that in the HPS, which noted an almost 20% 10-year event rate in the simvastatin-treated cohort that had diabetes and no baseline evidence of CVD [37]. In terms of the NCEP and ADA guidelines, this means decreasing LDL-C at least to less than 100 mg/dL, reducing non–HDL-C values to less than 130 mg/dL and triglyceride values to less than 150 mg/dL, and increasing HDL-C levels to more than 40 mg/dL (or > 50 mg/dL in women, according to ADA). This strategy is based on the empiric assumption that further improvement in the lipid profile, beyond that which was achieved initially with monotherapy, will yield additional CVD benefit. There are no data from a controlled clinical trial that compared monotherapy with combination treatment. It was shown clearly that the addition of ezetimibe to a statin will decrease LDL-C and non–HDL-C to NCEP goals in more individuals than a statin alone will do [80]. Ezetimibe, an intestinal inhibitor of cholesterol absorption, was associated with an additional 15% to 20% reduction in LDL-C levels among individuals who had hypercholesterolemia, had modest beneficial effects on triglycerides and HDL-C, and was well-tolerated [80]. Bile acid sequestrants also may help to decrease LDL-C but should be used with caution because they increase triglyceride levels in hypertriglyceridemic subjects [81].

It also is clear that achievement of all three lipid goals is more likely with statin plus fibrate or statin plus niacin combinations [82–84]. The added complexity and risks of combination therapy, in the absence of persuasive clinical trial evidence for additional CVD benefit, however, must place some limitations on the use of these combinations. The presence of CVD or severe metabolic syndrome seems to be a strong indication for combined therapy in patients who have diabetes, as perhaps should be the presence of hypertension, albuminuria, smoking, and a increased serum creatinine.

Statin-niacin combination therapy

The addition of niacin to statin therapy has a significant lipid-modifying benefit because niacin decreases triglycerides by 20% to 50% (upper limit requires high dosages of niacin), reduces LDL-C by 5% to 25%, increases HDL-C by 15% to 35%, and decreases non–HDL-C moderately. Thus, addition of niacin to a statin may be helpful in achieving LDL-C and non–HDL-C goals. Niacin increases HDL-C to a greater extent than any other agent. Although the benefits of increasing HDL-C levels are not well-understood and pharmacologic agents that affect HDL-C values also have effects on other lipoproteins, the VAHIT and HATS studies are supportive of this strategy. At high dosages, niacin decreases lipoprotein (a) values up to 30% [85]. Triglyceride decreases result in a shift in LDL and HDL particle density from small dense to larger, more buoyant particles [86]. Moreover, the HATS trial demonstrated that the combination of simvastatin and niacin was effective in reducing CVD events [49]. Niacin has significant adverse effects, however. The most common is an unpleasant flushing or tingling, particularly at higher dosages, and stepped titration of the dose is required, thus increasing the time and effort that is required from the medical team. Hepatotoxicity is the most important of the side effects, particularly with "long-acting" or "sustained release" niacin preparations that use dosages of more than 2000 mg daily [87]. The extended release once-a-day preparation of niacin (Niaspan) has been found to be effective and safe with a low incidence of hepatotoxicity [88]. Rare cases of myopathy were reported with the combined use of niacin and lovastatin [89], but have not been described in studies of Niaspan and lovastin in a single tablet formulation [84]. The incidence of myopathy that is associated with the combination of niacin and statins seems to be significantly less than with statins and gemfibrozil [92]; this supports the case for greater safety with the former combination. Past use of niacin in diabetic patients has been limited because of concerns that this agent may lead to deterioration in glucose control. Recent studies showed only modest increases in HbA1c values in patients whose diabetes was well-controlled and who received up to 3000 mg of immediate-release niacin [91] and up to 1500 mg of Niaspan [88]. Dosages as small as 1000 mg per day may increase HDL-C moderately. Nevertheless care should be exercised when using this agent in diabetic subjects; it probably is wise to delay niacin therapy until glycemic control is improved if the HbA1c level is more than 8.0%.

Statin-fibrate combination therapy

The addition of a fibrate to statin treatment achieved ADA goals in most diabetic subjects who received it [82,83]. Combination treatment with a statin and a fibrate should be used with caution because the risk of myopathy is increased, particularly in individuals who have predisposing conditions like renal failure [90]. Myopathy and rhabdomyolysis were reported in the published literature with simvastatin, cerivastatin, lovastatin, atorvastatin plus gemfibrozil, and pravastatin plus fenofibrate [93–97]. Several short-to-medium term studies (N = 81–420) that evaluated the efficacy and safety of different statin-fibrate combinations in patients who had combined hyperlipidemia showed additive effects on lipids and lipoproteins, a low incidence of clinically significant myopathy, and no case of rhabdomyolysis [98–102]. The absence of severe myositis in these studies is not surprising in view of its selective and low incidence, even in combination therapy. Recently, it was demonstrated that gemfibrozil and fenofibrate differ in their effects on statin pharmacokinetics. Gemfibrozil significantly inhibited the glucuronidation of statins—an important but previously unrecognized metabolic pathway of statin catabolism—whereas fenofibrate had little effect [103,104]. This probably explains why plasma statin levels are increased significantly with gemfibrozil treatment and not with fenofibrate. Thus, fenofibrate is preferred to gemfibrozil for use in combination therapy with statins, despite the fact that clinical trial data that support its use are less robust It also should be pointed out that several cases of fenofibrate monotherapy–associated rhabdomyolysis have been reported in the literature [105]. Thus, a risk of rhabdomyolysis is associated with fenofibrate therapy. A recently reported national survey of the prevalence of rhabdomyolysis associated with statin-fibrate combination therapy estimated that the prevalence of rhabdomyolysis was approximately 10 times more frequent with statin plus fenofibrate treatment than statin monotherapy and about a 100 times more likely with statin plus gemfibrozil treatment compared with statin monotherapy [106]. Whether combination with statin drugs increases this risk, as apparently is true for gemfibrozil, is unknown. In the ATP III update, wider use of the statin-fenofibrate combination is mentioned based on the supposition that fenofibrate will be less likely to cause rhabdomyolysis, in combination with statin treatment, than gemfibrozil. Finally, fenofibrate is more likely to increase serum creatinine levels than is gemfibrozil and should be avoided in patients who have renal disease; in these patients, the combination of statin and niacin probably is safer than a statin-fibrate regimen.

References

[1] Harris MI, Entmacher PS. Mortality from diabetes. In: Harris MI, Hamman RF, editors. Diabetes in America. Washington, DC: US Government Printing Office; 1985. Publication #NIH85–1468. p. 1–48.
[2] Stamler J, Vaccaro O, Neaton JD, et al. Diabetes, other risk factors, and 12-yr cardiovascular mortality for men screened in the Multiple Risk Factor Intervention Trial. Diabetes Care 1993;16:434–44.
[3] Kannel WB, McGee DL. Diabetes and cardiovascular risk factors: the Framingham study. Circulation 1979;59:8–13.
[4] Savage P. Cardiovascular complications of diabetes mellitus: what we know and what we need to know about their prevention. Ann Intern Med 1996;1241:123–6.
[5] Pyorala K, Laakso M, Uusitupa M. Diabetes and atherosclerosis: an epidemiologic view. Diabetes Metab Rev 1987;3:463–524.

[6] Haffner SM, Lehto S, Ronnemaa T, et al. Mortality from coronary heart disease in subjects
     with type 2 diabetes and in nondiabetic subjects with and without prior myocardial
     infarction. N Engl J Med 1998;339:229–34.
[7] Hu FB, Stampfer MJ, Solomon C, et al. Diabetes mellitus and mortality from all causes
     and coronary heart disease in women: 20 years of follow-up. Diabetes 2000;49(Suppl 1):
     A20.
[8] Malmberg K, Yusuf S, Gerstein HC, et al for the OASIS Registry Investigators. Impact
     of diabetes on long term prognosis in patients with unstable angina and non-Q-wave
     myocardial infarction. Results of the OASIS (Organization to Assess Strategies for
     Ischemic Syndromes) Registry. Circulation 2000;102:1014–9.
[9] Expert Panel on Detection, Evaluation, and Treatment of High Blood Cholesterol in
     Adults. Executive Summary of the Third Report of the National Cholesterol Education
     Program (NCEP) Expert Panel on Detection, Evaluation, and Treatment of High Blood
     Cholesterol in Adults (Adult Treatment Panel III). JAMA 2001;285:2486–589.
[10] Abbott RD, Donahue RP, Kannel WB, et al. The impact of diabetes on survival following
     myocardial infarction in men vs. women: the Framingham Study. JAMA 1988;260:
     3456–60.
[11] Miettinem H, Lehto S, Salomaa V, et al for the FINMONICA Myocardial Infarction
     Register Study Group. Impact of diabetes on mortality after the first myocardial infarction.
     Diabetes Care 1998;21:69–75.
[12] Grundy SM, Benjamin IJ, Burke GL, et al. Diabetes and cardiovascular disease:
     a statement for healthcare professionals from the American Heart Association. Circulation
     1999;100:1134.
[13] Cowie CC, Harris ML. In: Harris MI, editor. Physical and metabolic characteristics of
     persons with diabetes. Diabetes in America. 2nd edition. Washington, DC: National
     Institutes of Health; 1995. p. 117–64.
[14] Alexander CM, Landsman PB, Teutsch SM, et al. NCEP-defined metabolic syndrome,
     diabetes, and prevalence of coronary heart disease among NHANES III participants age 50
     years and older. Diabetes 2003;52:1210–4.
[15] Manley SE, Frighi V, Stratton E, et al for the UK Prospective Diabetes Study Group. UK
     Prospective Diabetes Study 27. Plasma lipids and lipoproteins at diagnosis of NIDDM by
     age and sex. Diabetes Care 1997;20:1683–7.
[16] Turner RC, Millns H, Neil HAW, et al for the UK Prospective Diabetes Study Group. Risk
     factors for coronary artery disease in non-insulin dependent diabetes mellitus: United
     Kingdom Prospective Diabetes Study (UKPDS 23). BMJ 1998;316:823–8.
[17] Soedamah-Muthu SS, Chaturvedi N, Toeller M. Risk factors for coronary heart disease in
     type 1 diabetic patients in Europe: the EURODIAB Prospective Complications Study.
     Diabetes Care 2004;27:530–7.
[18] Kreisberg R. Diabetic dyslipidemia. Am J Cardiol 1998;82:67U–73U.
[19] Sniderman AD, Scantlebury T, Clanfone K. Hypertriglyceridemic hyperapoB: the
     unappreciated atherogenic dyslipoproteinemia in type 2 diabetes mellitus. Diabetes Care
     2002;25:579–82.
[20] Feingold KR, Grunfeld C, Pang M, et al. LDL subclass phenotypes and triglyceride
     metabolism in non-insulin dependent diabetes. Arterioscler Thromb Vasc Biol 1992;12:
     1496–502.
[21] Sniderman AD, Cianflone K. Substrate delivery as a determinant of hepatic apoB secretion.
     Arterioscler Thromb 1993;13:629–36.
[22] Taskinen MR. Triglyceride is the major atherogenic lipid in NIDDM. Diabetes Metab Rev
     1997;13:93–8.
[23] Duvillard L, Pont F, Florentin E, et al. Metabolic abnormalities of apolipoprotein B-
     containing lipoproteins in non-insulin-dependent diabetes: a stable isotope kinetic study.
     Eur J Clin Invest 2000;30:685–94.

[24] Rashid S, Uffelman KD, Lewis GF. The mechanism of HDL lowering in hyper-triglyceridemic, insulin-resistant states. J Diabetes Complications 2002;16:24–8.
[25] Demacker PN, Veerkamp MJ, Bredie SJ, et al. Comparison of the measurements of lipids and lipoproteins versus assay for apolipoprotein B for estimation of coronary heart disease risk: a study in familial combined hyperlipidemia. Atherosclerosis 2000;153: 483–90.
[26] Tribble DL, Holl LG, Wood PD, et al. Variations in oxidative susceptibility among six low-density lipoprotein subfractions of differing density and particle size. Atherosclerosis 1992; 93:189–99.
[27] Havel R. Triglyceride-rich lipoproteins and atherosclerosis-new perspectives. Am J Clin Nutr 1994;59:795–9.
[28] Garvey WT, Kwon S, Zheng D, et al. Effects of insulin resistance and type 2 diabetes on lipoprotein subclass particle size and concentration determined by nuclear magnetic resonance. Diabetes 2003;52:453–62.
[29] Keech A, Colquhoun D, Best J, et al. Secondary prevention of cardiovascular events with long-term pravastatin in patients with diabetes or impaired fasting glucose. Results from the LIPID trial. Diabetes Care 2003;26:2713–21.
[30] Pyorala K, Pedersen TR, Kjekshus J, et al. Cholesterol lowering with simvastatin improves prognosis of diabetic patients with coronary heart disease. A subgroup analysis of the Scandinavian Simvastatin Survival Study (4S). Diabetes Care 1997;20: 614–20.
[31] Haffner SM, Alexander CM, Cook TJ, et al. Reduced coronary events in simvastatin treated patients with coronary heart disease and diabetes or impaired fasting glucose levels. Arch Intern Med 1999;159:2661–7.
[32] Goldberg RB, Mellies MJ, Sacks FM, et al. Cardiovascular events and their reduction with pravastatin in diabetic and glucose-intolerant myocardial infarction survivors with average cholesterol levels. Subgroup analysis in the Cholesterol And Recurrent Events (CARE) trial. Circulation 1998;98:2513–9.
[33] Shepherd J, Cobbe SM, Ford I, et al for the West of Scotland Coronary Prevention study Group. Prevention of coronary heart disease with pravastatin in men with hypercholes-terolemia. N Engl J Med 1995;333:1301–7.
[34] Downs JR, Clearfield M, Weis S, et al for the AFCAPS/TexCAPS Research Group. Primary prevention of acute coronary events with lovastatin in men and women with average cholesterol levels: results of AFCAPS/TexCAPS. JAMA 1998;279: 1615–22.
[35] The ALLHAT officers and coordinators for the ALLHAT Collaborative Research Group. Major outcomes in moderately hypercholesterolemic, hypertensive patients randomized to pravastatin vs usual care: the Antihypertensive and Lipid-Lowering Treatment to prevent Heart Attack Trial (ALLHAT-LLT). JAMA 2002;288:2998–3007.
[36] Sever PS, Dahlof B, Poulter NR, et al for the ASCOT investigators. Prevention of coronary and stroke events with atorvastatin in hypertensive subjects who have average or lower-than-average cholesterol concentratons, in the Anglo-Scandinavian Cardiac Outcome Trial-Lipid Lowering Arm (ASCOT-LLA): a multicentre randomized controlled trial. Lancet 2003;361:1149–58.
[37] Heart Protection Study Collaborative Group. MCR/BHF Heart Protection Study of Cholesterol Lowering with Simvastatin in 5963 People with Diabetes: a randomized placebo-controlled trial. Lancet 2003;361:2005–16.
[38] Heart Protection Study Collaborative Group. MCR/BHF Heart Protection Study of Cholesterol Lowering with Simvastatin in 20,536 High-risk Individuals: a randomized placebo-controlled trial. Lancet 2002;360:7–22.
[39] Colhoun HM, Betteridge DJ, Durrington PN, et al. Primary prevention of cardiovascular disease with atorvastatin in type 2 diabetes in the Collaborative Atorvastatin Diabetes

Study (CARDS): multicentre randomised placebo-controlled trial. Lancet 2004;364: 685–96.

[40] Nissen SE, Tuzcu EM, Schoenhagen P, et al REVERSAL Investigators. Effect of intensive compared with moderate lipid-lowering therapy on progression of coronary atherosclerosis: a randomized controlled trial. JAMA 2004;291:1071–80.

[41] For the Pravastatin or Atorvastatin Evaluation Infection Therapy-Thrombolysis in Myocardial Infarction. Comparison of intensive and moderate lipid lowering with statins after acute coronary symptoms. Obstet Gynecol Surv 2004;59(7):522–4.

[42] Koskinen P, Manttari M, Manniven V, et al. Coronary heart disease incidence in NIDDM patients in the Helsinki Heart Study. Diabetes Care 1992;15:820–5.

[43] The BIP Study Group. Secondary prevention by raising HDL cholesterol and reducing triglycerides in patients with coronary artery disease. The Bezafibrate Infarction Prevention (BIP) Study. Circulation 2000;102:21–7.

[44] Rubins HB, Robins SJ, Collins D, et al. Gemfibrozil for the secondary prevention of coronary heart disease in men with low levels of high-density lipoprotein cholesterol. N Engl J Med 1999;341:410–8.

[45] Rubins HB, Robins SJ, Collins D, et al. Diabetes, plasma insulin, and cardiovascular disease. Subgroup analysis from the Department of Veterans Affairs High-Density Lipoprotein Intervention Trial (VA-HIT). Arch Intern Med 2002;162: 2597–604.

[46] Diabetes Atherosclerosis Intervention Study Investigators. Effect of fenofibrate on progression of coronary-artery disease in type 2 diabetes: the Diabetes Atherosclerosis Intervention Study, a randomized study. Lancet 2001;357:905–10.

[47] The Coronary Drug Project Research Group. Clofibrate and niacin in coronary heart disease. JAMA 1975;231:360–81.

[48] Canner PL, Furberg CD, Terrin ML, et al. Benefits of niacin by glycemic status in patients with healed myocardial infarction (from the Coronary Drug Project). Am J Cardiol 2005; 95:254–7.

[49] Brown BG, Zhao XQ, Chait A, et al. Simvastatin and niacin, antioxidant vitamins, or the combination for prevent of coronary disease. N Engl J Med 2001;345: 1583–92.

[50] Grundy SM, Cleeman JI, Merz CN, et al. Cooordinating Committee of the National Cholesterol Education Program; National Heart, Lung, and Blood Institute; American College of Cardiology Foundation; American Heart Association. Implications of recent clinical trials for the National Cholesterol Education Program Adult Treatment Panel III guidelines. Circulation 2004;110:227–39.

[51] American Diabetes Association. Dyslipidemia management in adults with diabetes. Diabetes Care 2004;27(Suppl 1):S68–71.

[52] Snow V, Aronson MD, Hornbake ER, et al. Lipid control in the management of type 2 diabetes mellitus: a clinical practice guideline from the American College of Physicians. Ann Intern Med 2004;140:644–9.

[53] American Diabetes association. Evidence-based nutrition principles and recommendations for the treatment and prevention of diabetes and related complications. Diabetes Care 2003;26:S51–61.

[54] Yu-Poth S, Zhao G, Etherton T, et al. Effects of the National Cholesterol Education Program's step I and II dietary intervention program on cardiovascular disease risk factors: a meta-analysis. Am J Clin Nutr 1999;69:632–46.

[55] Temme EH, Van Hoydonck PG, Schouten EG, et al. Effects of a plant sterol-enriched spread on serum lipids and lipoproteins in mildly hypercholesterolemic subjects. Acta Cardiol 2002;57:111–5.

[56] Gylling H, Miettinen TA. Serum cholesterol and cholesterol and lipoprotein metabolism in hypercholesterolemic NIDDM patients before and during sitostanol ester-margarine treatment. Diabetol 1994;37:773–80.

[57] Chandalia M, Garg A, Lutjohann D, et al. Beneficial effects of high dietary fiber intake in patients with type 2 diabetes mellitus. N Engl J Med 2000;342:1392–8.

[58] Anderson JW, Allgood LD, Turner J, et al. Effects of Psyllium on glucose and serum lipid responses in men with type 2 diabetes and hypercholesterolemia. Am J Clin Nutr 1999;70: 466–73.

[59] Turley ML, Skeaff CM, Mann JI, et al. The effect of a low-fat, high-carbohydrate diet on serum high density lipoprotein cholesterol and triglyceride. Eur J Clin Nutr 1998;52: 728–32.

[60] Garg A. High-monounsaturated-fat diets for patients with diabetes mellitus: a meta-analysis. Am J Clin Nutr 1998;67:577S–82S.

[61] Bravata DM, Sanders L, Huang J, et al. Efficacy and safety of low-carbohydrate diets. A systematic review. JAMA 2003;289:1837–50.

[62] Friedberg CE, Janssen MJFM, Heine R, et al. Fish oil and glycemic control in diabetes. A meta-analysis. Diabetes Care 1998;21:494–500.

[63] Woodman RJ, Mori TA, Burke V, et al. Effects of purified eicosapentaenoic and docosahexaenoic acids on glycemic control, blood pressure, and serum lipids in type 2 diabetic patients with treated hypertension. Am J Clin Nutr 2002;76:1007–15.

[64] Emanuele N, Azad N, Abraira C, et al. Effect of intensive glycemic control on fibrinogen, lipids, and lipoproteins: Veterans Affairs Cooperative Study in Type II Diabetes Mellitus. Arch Intern Med 1998;18:2485–90.

[65] Palumbo PJ. Metformin: effects on cardiovascular risk factors in patients with non-insulin-dependent diabetes mellitus. J Diabetes Complications 1998;12:110–9.

[66] Winkler K, Konrad T, Fullert S, et al. Pioglitazone reduces atherogenic dense LDL particles in nondiabetic patients with arterial hypertension: a double-blind, placebo-controlled study. Diabetes Care 2003;26:2588–94.

[67] Freed MI, Ratner R, Marcovina SM. Effects of rosiglitazone alone and in combination with atorvastatin on the metabolic abnormalities in type 2 diabetes mellitus. Am J Cardiol 2002; 90:947–52.

[68] van Wijk JPH, de Koning EJP, Martens EP, et al. Thiazolidinediones and blood lipids in type 2 diabetes. Arterioscler Thromb Vasc Biol 2003;23:1744–9.

[69] Chiquette E, Ramirez G, DeFronzo R. A meta-analysis comparing the effect of thiazolidinediones on cardiovascular risk factors. Arch Int Med 2004;164:2097–104.

[70] Goldberg RB, Kendall DM, Deeg MA, et al. Comparison of lipid and glycemic effects of pioglitazone and rosiglitazone in type 2 diabetic patients and dyslipidemia. Presented at the American Heart Association Scientific Sessions, New Orleans, Louisiana, November 2004.

[71] Hillier TA, Pedula KL. Complications in young adults with early-onset type 2 diabetes: losing the relative protection of youth. Diabetes Care 2003;26:2999–3005.

[72] Pfeffer MA, Keech A, Sacks FM, et al. Safety and tolerability of pravastatin in long-term clinical trials: prospective Pravastatin Pooling Project (PPP). Circulation 2002;105:2341–6.

[73] Robins SJ. Cardiovascular disease with diabetes or the metabolic syndrome: should statins or fibrates be first line therapy? Curr Opin Lipidol 2003;14:575–83.

[74] Lu W, Resnick HE, Jablonski KA, et al. Non-HDL cholesterol as a predictor of cardiovascular disease in type 2 diabetes. The Strong Heart Study. Diabetes Care 2003;26: 16–23.

[75] Scharnagl H, Schinker R, Gierens H, et al. Effect of atorvastatin, simvastatin, and lovastatin on the metabolism of cholesterol and triacylglycerides in HepG2 cells. Biochem Pharmacol 2001;62:1545–55.

[76] Pontrelli L, Parris W, Adeli K, et al. Atorvastatin treatment beneficially alters the lipoprotein profile and increases low-density lipoprotein particle diameter in patients with combined dyslipidemia and impaired fasting glucose/type 2 diabetes. Metabolism 2002;51: 334–42.

[77] Wagner AM, Perez A, Zapico E, et al. Non-HDl cholesterol and apolipoprotein B in the dyslipidemic classification of type 2 diabetic patients. Diabetes Care 2003;26:2048–51.

[78] Sniderman AD, Lamarche B, Tilley J, et al. Hypertriglyceridemic hyperapoB in type 2 diabetes. Diabetes Care 2002;25:579–82.

[79] Wagner AM, Perez A, Calvo F, et al. Apolipoprotein (B) identifies dyslipidemic phenotypes associated with cardiovascular risk in normocholesterolemic type 2 diabetic patients. Diabetes Care 1999;22:812–7.

[80] Gagne C, Bays HE, Weiss SR, et al. Efficacy and safety of ezetimibe added to ongoing statin therapy for treatment of patients with primary hypercholesterolemia. Am J Cardiol 2002; 90:1084–91.

[81] Crouse JR III. Hypertriglyceridemia: a contraindication to the use of bile acid binding resins. Am J Med 1987;83:243–8.

[82] Wagner AM, Jorba O, Bonet R, et al. Efficacy of atorvastatin and gemfibrozil, alone and in low dose combination, in the treatment of diabetic dyslipidemia. J Clin Endocrinol Metab 2003;88:3212–7.

[83] Athyros VG, Papageorgiou AA, Athyrou VV, et al. Atorvastatin and micronized fenofibrate alone and in combination in type 2 diabetes with combined hyperlipidemia. Diabetes Care 2002;25:1198–202.

[84] Kashyap ML, McGovern ME, Berra K, et al. Long-term safety and efficacy of a once-daily niacin/lovastatin formulation for patients with dyslipidemia. Am J Cardiol 2002;89:672–8.

[85] Carlson LA, Hamsten A, Asplaund A. Pronounced lowering of serum levels of lipoprotein Lp(a) in hyperlipidemic subjects treated with nicotinic acid. J Intern Med 1989;226:271–6.

[86] Superko HR, Krauss RM. Differential effects of nicotinic acid in subjects with different LDL subclass patterns. Atherosclerosis 1992;95:69–76.

[87] McKenney JM, Proctor JD, Harris S, et al. A comparison of the efficacy and toxic effects of sustained –vs immediate-release niacin in hypercholesterolemic patients. JAMA 1994;271: 672–7.

[88] Grundy SM, Vega GL, McGovern ME, et al. Efficacy, safety, and tolerability of once-daily niacin for the treatment of dyslipidemia associated with type 2 diabetes. Arch Intern Med 2002;162:1568–76.

[89] Reaven P, Witztum JL. Lovastatin, nicotinic acid, and rhabdomyolysis. Ann Intern Med 1988;109:597–8.

[90] Omar MA, Wilson JP, Cox TS. Rhabdomyolysis and HMG-CoA reductase inhibitors. Ann Pharmacother 2001;35:1096–107.

[91] Elam MB, Hunninghake DB, Davis KB, et al. Effect of niacin on lipid and lipoprotein levels and glycemic control in patients with diabetes and peripheral arterial disease: the ADMIT study. A randomized trial. JAMA 2000;284:1263–70.

[92] Shepherd J. Fibrates and statins in the treatment of hyperlipidemia: an appraisal of their efficacy and safety. Eur Heart J 1995;16:5–13.

[93] Pierce LR, Wysowski DK, Gross TP. Myopathy and rhabdomyolysis associated with lovastatin-gemfibrozil combination therapy. JAMA 1990;264:71–5.

[94] Tal A, Rajeshawari M, Isley W. Rhabdomyolysis associated with simvastatin-gemfibrozil therapy. South Med J 1997;90:546–7.

[95] Pogson G, Kindred L, Carper B. Rhabdomyolysis and renal failure associated with cerivastatin-gemfibrozil combination therapy. Am J Card 1999;83:1146.

[96] Duell PB, Connor WE, Illingworth DR. Rhabdomyolysis after taking atorvastatin with gemfibrozil. Am J Cardiol 1998;81:368–9.

[97] Raimondeau J, Le Marec H, Chevallier JC, et al. [Biological myolysis during combined fenofibrate-pravastatin therapy]. Presse Med 1992;21:663–4.

[98] Ellen RL, McPherson R. Long term efficacy and safety of fenofibrate and a statin in the treatment of combined hyperlipidemia. Am J Cardiol 1998;81:60B–5B.

[99] Athyros V, Papageorgiou AA, Hatzikonstandinou HA, et al. Safety and efficacy of long-term statin-fibrate combinations in patients with refractory familial combined hyperlipidemia. Am J Cardiol 1997;80:608–13.

[100] Iliadis EA, Rosenson RS. Long-term safety of pravastatin-gemfibrozil therapy in mixed hyperlipidemia. Clin Cardiol 1999;22:25–8.
[101] Murdock DK, Murdock AK, Murdock RW. Long-term safety and efficacy of combination gemfibrozil and HMG-CoA reductase inhibitors for the treatment of mixed lipid disorders. Am Heart J 1999;138:151–5.
[102] Vega GL, Ma PT, Cater NB, et al. Effects of adding fenofibrate (200 mg/day) to simvastatin (10 mg/day) in patients with combined hyperlipidemia and metabolic syndrome. Am J Cardiol 2003;91:956–60.
[103] Prueksaritanont T, Zhao JJ, Ma B, et al. Mechanistic studies on metabolic interactions between gemfibrozil and statins. Pharmacol Exp Ther 2002;301:1042–51.
[104] Prueksaritanont T, Tang C, Qiu Y, et al. Effects of fibrates on metabolism of statins in human hepatocytes. Drug Metab Dispos 2002;30:1280–7.
[105] Barker BJ, Goodenough RR, Falko JM. Fenofibrate monotherapy induced rhabdomyolysis. Diabetes Care 2003;26:2482.
[106] Jones PH, Davidson MH. Reporting rate of rhabdomyolysis with fenofibrate + statin versus gemfibrozil + any statin. Am J Cardiol 2005;95:120–2.

ELSEVIER
SAUNDERS

Endocrinol Metab Clin N Am
34 (2005) 27–48

ENDOCRINOLOGY
AND METABOLISM
CLINICS
OF NORTH AMERICA

The Dyslipidemia of Diabetes Mellitus: Giving Triglycerides and High-Density Lipoprotein Cholesterol a Higher Priority?

David M. Kendall, MD[a,b,*]

[a]International Diabetes Center, 3800 Park Nicollet Boulevard,
Minneapolis, MN 55416-2699, USA
[b]University of Minnesota, 420 Delaware Street SE, Minneapolis, MN 55455, USA

Cardiovascular diseases (CVD) currently account for much of the morbidity and mortality associated with diabetes mellitus [1–3]. CVD accounts for nearly three fourths of deaths in patients who have diabetes mellitus, and cardiovascular events such as myocardial infarction (MI), stroke, and coronary artery bypass are associated with substantial morbidity [4]. Overall, individuals who have type 2 diabetes mellitus are two to four times more likely to suffer a CVD event than non-diabetic individuals [4,5]. Indeed, diabetes mellitus patients with no prior history of CVD have a risk for CVD similar to that of patients who have established CVD [1].

Although lipid management focusing on the treatment of elevated low-density lipoprotein cholesterol (LDL-C) is crucial and of benefit (see prior article by Del Pilar Solano and Goldberg in this issue), the increase in CVD risk observed in patients who have type 2 diabetes mellitus results from more than elevated LDL-C levels. A common cluster of CVD risk factors including dyslipidemia, hypertension, hyperglycemia, insulin resistance, and a prothrombotic, proinflammatory state likely are responsible for this enormous risk for vascular disease [6,7] and the management of many—if not all—of these risk factors likely will be of substantial benefit for diabetes mellitus patients [7–10].

Given the higher cardiovascular risk for those who have diabetes mellitus at any level of LDL-C [11], current guidelines recommend broader use of

---
* International Diabetes Center, 3800 Park Nicollet Boulevard, Minneapolis, MN 55416-2699.
E-mail address: kendad@parknicollet.com

0889-8529/05/$ - see front matter © 2005 Elsevier Inc. All rights reserved.
doi:10.1016/j.ecl.2004.11.004

pharmacologic therapy to manage and lower LDL-C levels [12,13]. Although LDL-C reduction in patients who have diabetes mellitus is an essential component of care, diabetes mellitus patients have LDL-C levels that are on average no higher than those observed in nondiabetic individuals, but have more low-density lipoprotein (LDL) particles, with many small, dense LDL particles that increase CVD risk substantially [12]. LDL-C reduction alone does not eliminate much of the excess risk for CVD in diabetes mellitus. Patients who have diabetes mellitus treated with statin therapy have a residual risk for CVD events comparable to or higher than nondiabetic patients who do not receive such treatment.

These observations underscore the importance of other CVD risk factors in patients who have diabetes mellitus. Specifically, disorders of high-density lipoprotein cholesterol (HDL-C) and triglycerides (TGs) likely play an important role [12,14–17]. Low levels of HDL-C are common in patients who have diabetes mellitus and are a strong determinant of CVD risk independent of the level of LDL-C. Also, increased levels of very low-density lipoproteins (VLDL) and TGs can be associated with endothelial dysfunction, impaired microcirculatory flow, and an increased thrombotic risk [18]. The atherogenic dyslipidemia of diabetes mellitus is associated with other prothrombotic changes, including an increase in activity of coagulation factor VII, and in the synthesis and secretion of plasminogen activator inhibitor–1. These additional risk determinants, whether directly or indirectly related to dyslipidemia, have been correlated with an increased risk of MI and sudden coronary death in patients who have diabetes mellitus [19].

Recent epidemiologic and clinical trials support that lipid-altering therapy that targets low HDL-C and elevated TGs may reduce significantly CVD risk in patients who have diabetes mellitus. These findings suggest that focusing on the so-called "atherogenic dyslipidemia" of diabetes mellitus is advisable and likely of significant benefit in diabetes mellitus patients [20–22]. Specifically, the findings of recent controlled clinical trials have demonstrated substantial reduction in CVD morbidity and a decline in CVD-related mortality in patients with low HDL-C or elevated TGs when treated with either fibric-acid derivatives (fibrates) or niacin therapy [23–32].

This article focuses on the importance of management of these "other" lipid disorders in diabetes mellitus, particularly HDL-C and TGs. The use of fibric-acid derivatives and niacin as well as combination statin-fibrate therapy and statin-niacin therapy is reviewed. The potential role of glucose-lowering therapies in patients who have the dyslipidemia of diabetes mellitus is discussed.

Pathogenesis of dyslipidemia in diabetes mellitus: lipoprotein metabolism and the role of insulin resistance

Low levels of HDL-C, elevated TG concentrations [16], and the development of small, dense LDL particles [17] are common in patients who have diabetes mellitus and each is associated with a significant increase in CVD risk [20–22]. The origins of the dyslipidemia of diabetes are complex but derive from specific abnormalities in lipoprotein metabolism and abnormalities in insulin action [26,33]. High concentrations of VLDL and elevated levels of serum TGs result from overproduction of TG-rich VLDL particles, reduced clearance of these particles, or both. High TGs are even more common in patients who have poorly controlled diabetes mellitus—from a combination of increased substrate (free fatty acid [FFA]) flux to the liver and from reduced clearance of VLDL particles (a process facilitated by the action of insulin) (Fig. 1) [26]. In addition, low levels of HDL-C can occur from reduced production of nascent HDL particles, increased clearance of these particles, or as a result of transfer of cholesterol ester from HDL particles to larger VLDL particles (through the action of cholesterol ester transfer protein [CETP]). As a result of this latter pathway, low levels of HDL-C generally are observed in any patient with high TGs, a finding more common in those with characteristics of insulin resistance (see Fig. 1) [26].

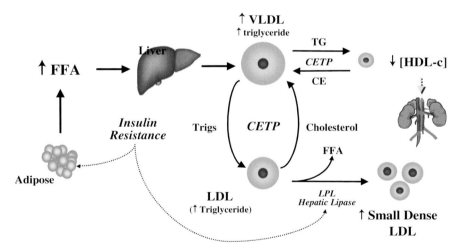

Fig. 1. The role of insulin resistance (IR) in the development of dyslipidemia in diabetes mellitus. IR at the adipocyte results in increased FFA flux and increased FFA concentration in the peripheral circulation. Accumulation of FFA also could arise from defects in fatty acid transporters or intracellular binding proteins. Increased FFA stimulates the assembly and secretion of VLDL, resulting in excess circulating TG concentration. VLDL stimulates the exchange of cholesterol ester (CE) from HDLs and LDLs, reducing concentrations of HDL-C. In addition, apolipoprotein A-I (ApoA-I) may dissociate from TG-enriched HDL. Free ApoA-I is cleared rapidly from plasma by excretion through the kidney, further reducing the availability of HDL for reverse cholesterol transport. TG-enriched LDL also may undergo lipolysis, increasing small, dense LDL particles. CETP, cholesterol ester transfer protein. (*Adapted from* Ginsberg HN. Insulin resistance and cardiovascular disease. J Clin Invest 2000;106:453–8; with permission.)

The finding of high TG and low HDL-C levels is characteristic of the classic dyslipidemia of diabetes mellitus [13].

The characteristic dyslipidemia of type 2 diabetes mellitus is thought to be linked to the generalized metabolic disorder of insulin resistance (IR) (see Fig. 1) [26]. IR is accepted generally to be a core metabolic defect of type 2 diabetes mellitus. It is estimated that up to 90% of individuals who have type 2 diabetes mellitus have some degree of IR. IR, when coupled with an inadequate pancreatic insulin response, gives rise to the hyperglycemia characteristic of this disease. In addition, IR is associated with a significantly higher risk for CVD, which may be in part result from the development of other CVD risk factors (including hypertension, atherogenic dyslipidemia, microalbuminuria, and a proinflammatory, prothrombotic vascular environment). IR may alter directly the production and clearance of VLDL particles (see Fig. 1 [26]. Resistance to the actions of insulin increases intracellular hydrolysis of TGs in adipose tissue. The ensuing increase in circulating FFAs promotes the hepatic assembly and secretion of VLDL, further increasing serum TG levels. These same VLDL particles interact with other lipoproteins as described above, exchanging TGs for cholesterol esters contained within HDL and LDL. In addition, the hydrolysis of TGs ultimately leads to HDL degradation and a reduction in HDL-C concentration, and favors the conversion of LDL particles to small, dense (and more atherogenic) LDL particles [26,34]. This role of IR is supported further by the observation that this same lipid disorder is seen commonly in patients who have pre–diabetes mellitus and the metabolic syndrome [13,35,36].

Managing high-density lipoprotein cholesterol and triglycerides in diabetes mellitus: a review of outcome trials

Many clinicians still struggle with whether management of HDL-C or TGs is of benefit for the patient who has diabetes mellitus. Many large clinical trials have underscored the potential benefit of therapies targeting this atherogenic dyslipidemia in diabetes mellitus, specifically focusing on therapies targeting high TGs, low HDL-C, or both. Although only some of these trials have been designed to assess rates of cardiovascular morbidity and mortality, they provide substantial support for the hypothesis that treating HDL-C or TGs will have significant potential benefit for diabetes mellitus patients. Table 1 summarizes the results of the largest of these major studies [23–25,27–32,37,38].

Although lowering LDL-C levels (with statin therapy) in patients who have diabetes mellitus is of unquestioned benefit, this treatment does not eliminate CVD risk. This observation has led several groups of investigators to determine whether specific lipid-altering therapy—with statins, fibrates, or niacin—may reduce CVD risk further. One large study of statin therapy for patients with lower levels of HDL-C has been performed. In the Air Force Coronary Atherosclerosis Prevention Study–Texas Coronary

Table 1
Summary of trials targeting high-density lipoprotein cholesterol and triglycerides

Study (no. of participants) [Ref.]	Therapy	Baseline lipid measures (mg/dL)	% change in lipid measures	Endpoint	Relative risk	
					Diabetes subgroup	Nondiabetic or total population
AFCAPS–TexCAPS (N = 155) [37]	Lovastatin 20–40 mg	LDL-C 150, HDL-C 36(m)/40(w), TG 158	↓ 25, ↑ 6, ↓ 15	CHD death, NFMI, unstable angina, or sudden cardiac death	0.45 ($P =$ NS)	0.63 ($P < 0.001$)
HHS (N = 135) [28,29]	Gemfibrozil 600 mg/2×d	LDL-C 201, HDL-C 46, TG 238	↓ 10, ↑ 6, ↓ 26	CHD death or NFMI	0.32 ($P =$ NS)	0.66 ($P < 0.02$)
CDP[a] (N = 251) [24,25,38]	Niacin 3 g/d	TC 250, TG 177	↓ 10, ↓ 26	NFMI, Total mortality	0.42, 0.71	0.75 ($P < 0.05$), 0.89 ($P < 0.05$)
VA-HIT[a] (N = 769) [23,27]	Gemfibrozil 1200 mg/d	LDL-C 112, HDL-C 32, TG 161	↓ 2, ↑ 6, ↓ 31	CHD death, NFMI, or stroke	0.68 ($P = 0.04$)	0.82 ($P =$ NS)
DAIS (N = 418) [30]	Fenofibrate (micronized) 200 mg/d	LDL-C 130, HDL-C 39, TG 229	↓ 6, ↑ 7, ↓ 28	Death, NFMI, angioplasty, or coronary revascularization	0.77 ($P =$ NS)	—
HATS (N = 34)[b] [31,32]	Simvastatin 10–40 mg + niacin 2–4 g	LDL-C 130, HDL-C 31, TG 214	↓ 35, ↑ 26, ↓ 34	CHD death, NFMI, stroke, or revascularization	0.52 (NS)	0.35 ($P < 0.01$)

Abbreviations: AFCAPS-TexCAPS, Air Force/Texas Coronary Atherosclerosis Prevention Study; CDP, Coronary Drug Project; CHD, coronary heart disease; DAIS, Diabetes Atherosclerosis Intervention Study; HATS, HDL-Atherosclerosis Treatment Study; HDL-C, high-density lipoprotein cholesterol; HHS, Helsinki Heart Study; LDL-C, low-density lipoprotein cholesterol; NFMI, nonfatal myocardial infarction; NFMI, nonfatal myocardial infarction; NS, not significant; TC, total cholesterol; TG, triglyceride level; VA-HIT, Veterans Affairs-High-density lipoprotein Intervention Trial.
[a] Baseline lipids and percent change are based on total treatment population.
[b] Included patients with both impaired fasting glucose plus diabetes.

Atherosclerosis Prevention (AFCAPS–TexCAPS) trial, lovastatin therapy resulted in a 27% reduction in LDL-C levels and a concomitant 6% increase in HDL-C levels [37]. In subjects who had diabetes mellitus and in the study cohort as a whole, statin therapy significantly reduced the risk for CVD events. Unfortunately, the study included only a few patients who had diabetes mellitus and, perhaps more important, the CVD event rates observed in this trial (approximately 1% per year) were significantly lower than those generally seen in a higher-risk diabetes mellitus population. As such, it is difficult to generalize these findings to the diabetes mellitus population as a whole. Recent data [39,40], however, support the use of LDL-C–lowering therapy in many patients who have diabetes mellitus. Undoubtedly, these data and the prior results of AFCAPS support broad use of statin therapy for lowering LDL-C in patients who have diabetes mellitus, particularly those with lower levels of HDL-C.

Fibrate therapy long has been advocated for the treatment of patients who have dyslipidemia in diabetes mellitus, and these agents remain the treatment of choice for patients with high serum TGs (>400 mg/dL). Fibrates increase HDL-C, albeit modestly (by an average of approximately 5%–15%) [23,30,41]. Given the capacity of fibrates to alter levels of TGs and HDL-C, several outcome trials using fibrate therapy in diabetes mellitus have been performed. The earliest of these studies is a larger primary prevention trial, the Helsinki Heart Study (HHS) [28,29]. In HHS, gemfibrozil therapy for treatment of elevated total cholesterol resulted in a significant reduction in coronary events. Gemfibrozil-treated subjects did not have a reduction in overall mortality, however, leading many to question the potential benefit of such therapy. Subsequent post-hoc analysis of these data [42] suggested that the population most likely to benefit from fibrate therapy was the population that had diabetes mellitus or those with markers of the metabolic syndrome (such as central obesity and high TG and low HDL-C levels). This observation is unsurprising given that this population most likely was affected by the characteristic lipid disorder responsive to fibrates, and that these populations are also at substantially higher risk for CVD.

More recently, the Veterans Affairs–High-density lipoprotein Intervention Trial (VA-HIT) demonstrated a significant reduction in combined CVD endpoints with the use of gemfibrozil in patients who had established CVD, low levels of HDL-C, and minimal elevations of LDL-C (see Table 1) [23–25,27–32,37,38]. In VA-HIT, the benefit of gemfibrozil treatment on CVD death, MI, or stroke was most evident in patients who had diabetes mellitus and in those with hyperinsulinemia [27]. The Diabetes Atherosclerosis Intervention Study (DAIS) included only patients who had diabetes mellitus with and without established CVD [30]. In this study, treatment with fenofibrate was associated with a significantly smaller increase in the extent of stenosis compared with placebo therapy (change in diameter, 2.11% versus 3.65%; $P = .02$). These changes were associated with a nonsignificant

24% reduction in the combined clinical endpoint of death, MI, angioplasty, or coronary revascularization [30].

In addition to the benefits of fibrate and statin therapy, a recent preliminary analysis of data from the Coronary Drug Project (CDP) suggested that niacin therapy, like other lipid-altering therapies targeting HDL-C and TGs, may be associated with a reduced rate of CVD events, and that this response was observed irrespective of baseline blood glucose level of the treated subjects (see Table 1) [23–25,27–32,37,38]. More recently, the HDL-Atherosclerosis Treatment Study (HATS) assessed the effect of combination therapy with simvastatin and niacin in 160 patients who had established CVD and low levels of HDL-C [31]. HATS included a few patients (n = 34) who had diabetes mellitus or impaired fasting glucose [32]. The preliminary results in this subgroup, however, were similar in magnitude to those of the entire cohort and demonstrated lower rates of atherosclerotic progression with the use of combination statin-niacin therapy [32]. In addition to the angiographic findings, combination therapy was associated with a nonsignificant 48% reduction in the risk for the combined clinical endpoint of death, MI, stroke, or revascularization compared with placebo (P = not significant), suggesting that intensive combination therapy may provide greater clinical benefit than therapy with statin alone [32]. This hypothesis, however, remains to be proven with a larger interventional study.

In each of these trials, the absolute risk reduction for CVD events (range 3%–8%) in patients who have diabetes mellitus was generally as great or greater than that seen in subjects without diabetes mellitus—a finding not surprising given the higher baseline risk for CVD events in the diabetes mellitus population [23–25,27–30,38]. In addition, the use of fibrates and niacin in these trials resulted in absolute risk reductions comparable to those observed in the statin trials for lowering of LDL-C levels. Specifically, data from the Scandinavian Simvastatin Survival Study, Long-Term Intervention with Pravastatin in Ischaemic Disease, and Cholesterol and Recurrent Events studies as well as from the Heart Protection Study (HPS), Anglo-Scandinavian Cardiac Outcomes Trial, and Collaborative Atorvastatin Diabetes Study (CARDS) demonstrated absolute and relative risk reductions of 4% to 10% and 25% to 40%, respectively, from statin treatment in diabetes mellitus patients [40,43–47].

Although these studies establish the efficacy of drug therapy in patients who have diabetes mellitus, many questions regarding lipid treatment remain. Lowering of LDL-C levels is clearly beneficial, yet many patients receiving statin therapy suffer subsequent coronary events. Also, despite recommendations for more aggressive LDL-C lowering, it is unknown whether LDL-C lowering is more important than therapy designed to treat low HDL-C or high TG levels. The data from HPS suggest that a benefit from LDL-C lowering exists irrespective of baseline LDL-C level in patients with and without diabetes mellitus [46,48]. In addition, the recent

Pravastatin or Atorvastatin Evaluation and Infection Therapy (PROVE-IT) trial confirmed the benefit of aggressive LDL-C lowering in high-risk patients [39]. Similarly, although fibrate therapy in patients who had diabetes mellitus and low HDL-C levels was of clear benefit in VA-HIT and the Diabetes Atherosclerosis Intervention Study (DAIS), it is unknown whether treatment of HDL-C or TGs is of additional benefit in patients who receive statin therapy, particularly if LDL-C is treated to ever-lower targets.

Nonetheless, these clinical trials support the current recommendation that treating all components of the dyslipidemia of diabetes mellitus will be of great benefit in the clinicianu efforts to reduce CVD risk in diabetes mellitus. Continuing studies, including the National Institutes of Health Action to Control Cardiovascular Risk in Diabetes (ACCORD) trial, are underway to define further the role of combination therapy in the patient who has diabetes mellitus [49]. When these studies are completed, more will be known about the need for combined treatment of LDL-C, HDL-C, and TG levels. At present, prioritizing care while keeping an open mind about the other components of lipid disorders, such as HDL-C and TGs, is important and permits the clinician to treat the individual patient based on current evidence and guidelines.

Managing high-density lipoprotein cholesterol and triglycerides in diabetes mellitus: a practical clinical approach

Based on the evidence from these clinical trials, treatment of dyslipidemia will remain a critical component of comprehensive diabetes mellitus care. Care of diabetic patients includes the periodic assessment of lipid levels. Treatment approaches will vary based on current and emerging evidence. Box 1 [50], Table 2, and Fig. 2 [50] outline a practical clinical approach to the management of lipid disorders in these potentially complex patients.

Measurement of lipids

Annual evaluation of lipid levels beginning at 20 years of age is recommended for patients who have diabetes mellitus. Earlier screening is suggested in those with higher CVD risk (such as those with a family history of heart disease) or in those who have multiple features of the metabolic syndrome. Aggressive and targeted treatment of lipid disorders should be considered for any patient whose lipid measures are not within the recommended target ranges.

Treatment targets for high-density lipoprotein cholesterol and triglycerides in diabetes mellitus

Given that the risks for CVD are elevated markedly in patients who have diabetes mellitus and are comparable to the risks seen in patients who have

Box 1. Treatment targets and recommendations for treating dyslipidemia in diabetes

LDL-C target < 70 mg/dL if at high risk; LDL-C target < 100 for all diabetes mellitus patients
   If LDL-C > 100 mg/dL
   • Drug therapy (statin preferred) if at high risk or with established CVD
      1st choice: statin
      2nd choice: add ezetimibe if not to target. Use if intolerant of statin
      3rd choice: niacin; add if low HDL-C, high TGs
   • Optimize glycemic control
   • Initiate medical nutrition therapy/therapeutic lifestyle changes for any with LDL-C > 100 mg/dL

HDL-C target > 40 mg/dL (if low HDL = target LDL-C < 100 mg/dL and TGs < 150 mg/dL as initial approach)
   If LDL-C and/or TGs to target with HDL-C < 40 mg/dL
   • Fibrate if established CVD
   • Niacin if clinically appropriate
   • Glitazone therapy for glycemic control

TG target < 150 mg/dL
   TGs = 150–250 mg/dL
   • Optimize glycemic control
   • Initiate medical nutrition therapy/therapeutic lifestyle changes for all individuals with TGs > 150 mg/dL
   • Consider pioglitazone for glucose-lowering therapy
   TGs > 250 mg/dL
   • Consider fibrate—especially if low HDL-C
   • Utilize high dose statin if appropriate
   • Consider addition of niacin
   • Consider pioglitazone for glucose-lowering therapy
   TGs > 350 mg/dL
   • Fibrate ± statin
   • Avoid resin, use of oral estrogen
   TGs > 500 mg/dL
   • Fibrate Rx usually essential
   • Consider insulin therapy
   • Further medical nutrition therapy with registered dietitian

   Courtesy of and *adapted from* International Diabetes Center, Minneapolis, MN; with permission. Available at: http://www.parknicollet.com/diabetes. Accessed August 3, 2004.

Table 2
A practical approach to the pharmacologic treatment of lipid disorders in diabetes

Lipid disorder	Therapy		Other considerations
	Primary	Alternate or add-on	
High LDL-C level	Statin	Ezetimibe	Niacin
Low HDL-C level	Fibrate	Niacin	Statin therapy. Consider TZDs as glucose-lowering therapy
High TG level	Fibrate	High-dose statin	Niacin: consider use of pioglitazone and/or insulin as components of glucose-lowering therapy
Atherogenic profile: Low HDL level High TG level Small, dense LDL	Statin or fibrate	Statin + fibrate or niacin	Use of metformin (obese) or TZDs (if low HDL level) as initial diabetes therapy can be considered (see text)

Abbreviations: LDL, Low-density lipoprotein; HDL, high-density lipoprotein; TG, triglyceride; TZDs, thiazolidinediones.

CVD, the lipid treatment targets for individuals who have diabetes mellitus are aggressive. Although the ideal levels of LDL-C, HDL-C, TGs, and other lipid components remain under debate, the current thresholds and goals are based on substantial clinical trial evidence, clinical expertise, and broad consensus [12,13]. Despite minor differences in the published recommendations, any approach to management of lipid disorders in patients who have diabetes mellitus should focus on more aggressive treatment targets for all components of the lipid profile.

Box 1 summarizes the current treatment recommendations used at the author's institution [50] and the current recommendations from the American Diabetes Association (ADA), the National Cholesterol Education Program (NCEP), and the American Heart Association. Although these recommendations differ somewhat from various national standards, they are based on clinical experience and the practical aspects of care encountered by practitioners, diabetes education teams, and patients.

In all current guidelines, LDL-C is the primary treatment target for diabetes mellitus patients, a recommendation well supported by epidemiologic and clinical outcome trial data outlining the benefit of LDL-C–lowering therapies [12,13]. Following the recent publication of HPS [46] and CARDS [40], the recommended treatment target for the highest-risk diabetes mellitus patients was lowered to less than 70 mg/dL. Although values less than 100 mg/dL are desirable, either the empiric use of statin therapy or targeting lower LDL-C values may be of significant benefit in the highest-risk patients (such as those with recent CVD events). Therapeutic lifestyle changes (TLC) serve as background therapy for patients who have

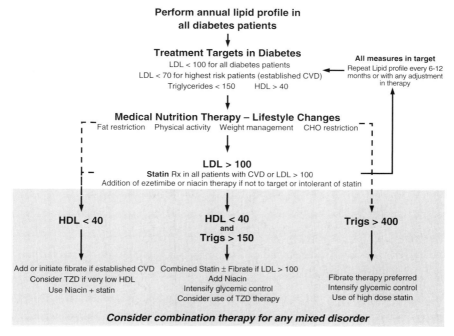

Fig. 2. A practical approach to the diagnosis and treatment of lipid disorders in diabetes mellitus. CHO, carbohydrate; Trigs, triglycerides; TZD, thiazolidinedione. (Courtesy of International Diabetes Center, Minneapolis, MN; with permission.)

diabetes mellitus and elevated LDL-C levels. Pharmacotherapy (specifically with statin agents) should be considered for any patient who has diabetes mellitus, particularly those with LDL-C levels greater than 100 mg/dL [12,13].

ADA and NCEP guidelines differ modestly with respect to specific HDL-C and TG targets [12,13]. Epidemiologic data and recent clinical trials show that these lipid parameters are important risk determinants and potential targets for therapy [20,21,23–25,27–32,37,38]. HDL-C levels less than 40 mg/dL are undesirable in men and women who have diabetes mellitus.

Although TG and HDL-C levels are established risk factors for CVD in diabetes mellitus, it is unclear which measure of the atherogenic profile (TGs, HDL, or another variable) provides the best measure of risk. Nor is it clear that such a distinction can be made easily, because levels of HDL-C and TGs are related closely metabolically. Framingham data support that HDL-C levels strongly predict CVD events. The relative risk for CVD in those with low LDL-C and low HDL-C levels is substantially higher than in those with high LDL-C and HDL-C levels [51]. In a recent multivariate post-hoc analysis of over 2500 men enrolled in VA-HIT, HDL-C ($P = .02$), but not TGs ($P = .48$) was predictive of CVD mortality and nonfatal MI in the patients receiving treatment [52]. Regardless of the priority assigned to the lipid measures, current guidelines suggest that therapy for patients with low HDL-C or high TG levels be considered, particularly if CVD is established [12,13].

The role of therapeutic lifestyle changes

Nonpharmacologic or therapeutic lifestyle changes should be considered as primary therapy for patients who have diabetes mellitus and lipid disorders (Fig. 2) [50]. Such changes emphasize dietary fat restriction, weight management, and an increase in physical activity [12]. These interventions not only benefit glycemic control, but also reduce TG concentration, increase HDL-C levels, and in certain individuals, lower LDL-C levels [53,54]. In clinical practice, the use of TLC is a challenge, because many patients either will not sustain such changes or will not achieve treatment targets for one or more lipid measure.

Most studies demonstrate that most patients will require pharmacotherapy to achieve the intensive lipid treatment targets established for diabetes mellitus; thus, the emphasis on drug treatment in this section [55,56]. Given the limited potential of nondrug therapies to achieve the specified targets in patients who have diabetes mellitus—combined with the established benefit of specific pharmacotherapies—drug therapy should be considered strongly for most patients who have dyslipidemia and diabetes mellitus. Therapies should be tailored to the patient's specific lipid abnormalities and should be used in the setting of optimized nondrug therapies for maximum effect.

Treating low high-density lipoprotein cholesterol

Low HDL-C levels (<40 mg/dL) are common in individuals who have diabetes mellitus. Based on current evidence, patients who have diabetes mellitus and HDL-C levels less than 40 mg/dL should be counseled on TLC that help raise HDL-C. Nonpharmacologic approaches, including weight loss and increased physical activity, can produce modest increases in HDL-C levels (average increase <10%) [57]. If such lifestyle measures cannot achieve recommended HDL-C targets, pharmacotherapy is indicated specifically in those who have established CVD.

Pharmacologic options for raising HDL-C levels include statins, fibric-acid derivatives, and niacin. Each vary in their capacity to increase HDL-C levels. Increases from statin therapy are generally 5% to 10%. Fibrates may increase HDL-C levels up to 15%, although in most clinical trials HDL-C increases averaged 6% to 7% with gemfibrozil or fenofibrate therapy [27,28,30]. Niacin is believed to be the most potent agent for raising HDL-C levels, with increases of up to 35% reported [13]. Fibrates and niacin also are associated with a shift in LDL-particle distribution to the larger, less atherogenic, less dense subfraction.

Based on the findings of VA-HIT, fibrates should be considered for diabetes mellitus patients who have low HDL-C levels, normal LDL-C levels, and a history of CVD. Although fibrate therapy in this trial increased HDL-C levels only modestly, CVD risk was reduced substantially in patients who had diabetes mellitus [27]. Fibrates remain the preferred therapy for patients with elevated TG levels (see later discussion). Niacin is the most effective pharmacologic agent for raising HDL-C levels and has other favorable effects on lipid profiles. Niacin can lower TG levels (by 20%–50%) and reduces LDL-C and lipoprotein-(a) levels [13,58,59]. In clinical use, niacin treatment has been associated with a 27% relative reduction in MI and an 11% reduction in long-term mortality [24,38].

For many years, niacin use in patients who have diabetes mellitus was discouraged because of its capacity to reduce insulin sensitivity and increase blood glucose levels [60,61]. Recent studies have suggested, however, that niacin is tolerated well in patients who have type 2 diabetes mellitus, assuming that adjustments in glucose-lowering therapy are possible [62,63]. The Arterial Disease Multiple Intervention Trial demonstrated a 29% increase in HDL-C levels, a 23% reduction in TG levels, and an 8% reduction in LDL-C levels in patients who had diabetes mellitus [62]. Glucose levels increased transiently but returned to baseline with continued niacin therapy. Hemoglobin A1c (HbA1c) levels and glycemic therapy were not changed significantly after 1 year of niacin treatment.

Similarly, in the Assessment of Diabetes Control and Evaluation of the Efficacy of Niaspan Trial, extended-release niacin (niacin ER) produced a dose-dependent increase in HDL-C levels of 19% to 24% and a reduction in TG levels of 13% to 28% in patients who had diabetes mellitus [63]. Fasting blood glucose levels rose transiently but returned to baseline by week 16. At the higher dose (1500 mg), there was a small but significant increase in HbA1c levels of 0.29% (P = .048 versus placebo) and a nonsignificant increase in antidiabetic pharmacotherapy [63]. Given these results, niacin therapy should be considered for patients who have low levels of HDL-C where further reductions in TG or LDL-C levels may be beneficial. In general, niacin can be used in patients who have well-controlled diabetes mellitus or in those where some flexibility with glucose-lowering therapy is available. Glucose levels should be monitored regularly and glycemic therapy adjusted as needed.

Treating elevated triglyceride levels

Although the specific contributions of TG elevations (independent of HDL-C or LDL-C levels) as a predictor of CVD risk is somewhat controversial [12,13,21,64], most practitioners recognize this disorder as common and warranting specific treatment, particularly if TG levels are greater than 400 mg/dL. Similarly, the optimal approach to clinically managing elevated TG levels is not well standardized. Some data show that diabetes mellitus patients with higher TG levels are at higher risk for CVD events, particularly following bypass surgery [65]. A rational clinical approach assumes that low HDL-C and elevated TG levels identify patients at risk for the "atherogenic" profile, and pharmacotherapy should be considered for patients who have TG levels above 200 mg/dL, despite the use of lifestyle changes [12].

Ideally, TG levels should be reduced to less than 150 mg/dL in diabetes mellitus patients. Initial therapy for hypertriglyceridemia also should focus on lifestyle modification and emphasize glucose control [12,14,35]. In one study, a 17% reduction in fasting blood glucose levels was associated with a 32% reduction in TG levels [66]. If lifestyle modification or glucose control fails to yield target TG levels, fibrate therapy is the treatment of choice because it can lower TG levels more than 50% [13]. In particular, in individuals with TG levels over 400 mg/dL, fibrate therapy is first-line pharmacologic treatment.

In the HHS, gemfibrozil reduced TG levels by 26%, lowered LDL-C levels by 10%, and increased HDL-C levels by 6% in patients who had diabetes mellitus [28]. In the more recent DAIS study, fenofibrate lowered TG levels 29% and LDL-C 6%, whereas HDL-C levels increased 7% [30]. Similarly, for diabetes mellitus patients in VA-HIT, gemfibrozil reduced TG levels 20% and increased HDL-C levels 5% [27]. Again, niacin therapy also can be considered for patients with elevated TG levels who either are intolerant of fibrate therapy or fail to achieve targets with these agents. In addition, use of high-dose statin therapy may be used to lower TG levels, although this therapy should not be considered as first-line therapy.

Using combination therapy in patients who have diabetes mellitus

Lipid abnormalities in patients who have type 2 diabetes mellitus are not confined to one lipid measure. Because mixed lipid disorders are the most common abnormality in patients who have diabetes mellitus, practitioners often face the clinical challenge of controlling several components of the lipid profile. Unsurprisingly, this is accomplished rarely with either medical nutritional changes or single-drug therapy, because most current therapies are suited best for one aspect of lipid metabolism.

Several studies have evaluated the safety and effectiveness of combined statin-fibrate therapy. In 40 patients who had type 2 diabetes mellitus and combined hyperlipidemia, atorvastatin and fenofibrate reduced LDL-C levels 46%, reduced TG levels 50%, and increased HDL-C levels 22% at 6 months [67]. Although combination therapy increased creatinine kinase (CPK) more than either monotherapy, mean CPK levels remained within normal limits. In a separate study, simvastatin plus bezafibrate reduced TG levels by 42%, significantly more than the reduction seen with the use of either drug alone ($P < .01$) [68]. This combination also reduced LDL-C levels 29%, significantly more than statin monotherapy ($P < .01$), and increased HDL-C levels 25%, significantly more than statin therapy alone ($P < .01$). In addition, cardiovascular events were reduced from 9.5% during the 6-month period of monotherapy to less than 2% during the 1-year period of combination therapy, with no clinically significant side effects [68].

Combined statin-fibrate therapy may be associated with an increased risk for drug-induced myopathy [69]. Despite reluctance by many clinicians to use combined statin-fibrate therapy, clinical studies support the safety of using these agents in combination. More recent data demonstrate that fenofibrate (perhaps because of its differing drug metabolism) may be associated with a lower rate of drug-associated changes in CPK compared with gemfibrozil when these agents are used in combination with statins [70]. Studies of combined statin-fibrate use are underway, including the ACCORD trial, which will assess the impact of combined simvastatin-fenofibrate therapy on CVD risk in high-risk patients who have type 2 diabetes mellitus [49].

Statin-niacin combination therapy also is safe and effective in patients who have diabetes mellitus. In the recent HATS trial, combination simvastatin-niacin therapy reduced LDL-C levels 31%, reduced TG levels 40%, and increased HDL-C levels 30% in patients who had diabetes mellitus or impaired fasting glucose [32]. This combination was safe and well tolerated [71]. In a separate short-term study, atorvastatin plus niacin ER was compared with each individual therapy in 53 patients who had diabetic dyslipidemia, defined by small LDL particles, low HDL_2 levels, or both [72]. In patients with small, dense LDL particles, combination therapy decreased LDL-C levels significantly more than niacin alone, and increased LDL-particle size significantly more than atorvastatin alone. In patients with reduced HDL_2 concentrations, combination therapy increased HDL-C levels and HDL_2 mass significantly more than atorvastatin. Combination therapy also reduced TG levels more effectively compared with monotherapy. A daily formulation of niacin ER plus lovastatin, 2000/40 mg, reduced LDL-C levels by 45%, lowered TG levels by 42%, and increased HDL-C levels by 41% [73].

Cholesterol-absorption inhibitors are the newest entry in the pharmacologic armamentarium for dyslipidemia. In women with a history of CVD, the addition of stanol ester margarine to statin treatment reduced LDL-C levels an additional 15% [74]. Cholesterol-binding resins have been used for years, but use has been limited by gastrointestinal side effects. More recently, colesevolam was introduced as an alternative to resin use. This bile acid–binding polymer provides additional LDL-C lowering as an adjunct to either dietary changes or other therapies such as statins. Ezetimibe is among the new cholesterol-absorption inhibitors available. In a study of patients who had familial hypercholesterolemia, the addition of ezetimibe to a maximum statin dose decreased LDL-C levels an additional 20% [75]. The effectiveness of these combinations in patients who have diabetes mellitus is untested. The main effect of ezetimibe seems to be on LDL-C levels, with minimal effects reported on TGs or HDL-C [76].

Although combination therapy has significant appeal as an effective means of controlling the complex lipid abnormalities of diabetes mellitus by combining the beneficial effects of each therapy, the results of continuing clinical trials are needed to assess the efficacy and safety of these combinations in managing the dyslipidemia of diabetes mellitus. These trials will shed more light on the role managing the atherogenic lipid triad in diabetes mellitus patients. Specifically, determining whether combinations of therapy result in greater risk reduction compared with monotherapy and can be used with acceptable risk will help clinicians better determine therapeutic needs for diabetes mellitus patients. Given the current understanding of the specific benefit of treating LDL-C elevations and targeting low levels of HDL-C and high levels of TGs in patients who have diabetes mellitus, combination therapy should be considered when necessary to achieve lipid goals. With the wide variety of agents available, the specific combination must be tailored to the patient's lipid abnormalities, with a clear understanding of the risks and benefits of each therapy and proposed combination.

Other considerations

Some clinicians have suggested that specific glucose-lowering therapies may be of additional benefit in patients who have type 2 diabetes mellitus and CVD. Results from the UKPDS showed that obese subjects who had type 2 diabetes mellitus had lower rates of CVD when metformin was used as initial therapy [77]. The possible mechanisms by which metformin therapy lowered rates of CVD are unknown.

Perhaps more germane to a discussion of lipid management in diabetes mellitus is that specific medications also may affect favorably the lipid profile in patients who have type 2 diabetes mellitus. Glucose lowering alone may lower TG concentrations, likely through the action of insulin on FFA production (see Fig. 1) [26]. Insulin therapy itself, through its direct effect on the adipocyte and the liver, can lower TG concentrations significantly but have minimal impact on HDL-C levels [78]. Insulin action promotes uptake of FFAs through the fat cell, thereby reducing substrate for VLDL production, the likely mechanism by which insulin exerts its beneficial effect on TG concentrations. Similarly, insulin may limit production of VLDL directly or enhance TG clearance, particularly in those with significant insulin deficiency or with markedly abnormal blood glucose levels. Metformin therapy is associated with only modest changes in lipids.

Recently, there has been substantial interest in the role of insulin-sensitizing medications, specifically thiazolidinediones (TZD), for the treatment of patients who have diabetes mellitus and associated dyslipidemia. TZD therapy may increase significantly HDL-C levels, with some studies demonstrating increases of more than 20% [78,79]. Data from the registration trials and smaller comparative trials suggest that TZD therapy also may lower TG levels and reduce the fraction of small, dense LDL particles [78–82]. These studies also suggest that the available TZDs may differ in their ability to affect lipid profiles. Although both available TZDs, rosiglitazone and pioglitazone, increase concentrations of HDL-C and reduce the fraction of small, dense LDL particles, retrospective analyses, nonrandomized trials, and smaller randomized but unblended trials [78–82] have suggested that pioglitazone therapy may have the most consistent beneficial effect on TGs (with reductions of 10%–30%) and miminal effect on LDL-C concentrations. In contrast, rosiglitazone has not lowered TG concentrations consistently and may be associated with a significant increase in LDL-C concentration. The clinical relevance of these lipid differences is unknown in today's clinical environment, however, because increasing numbers of diabetes mellitus patients likely will be candidates for statin therapy. Importantly, one study of combination therapy with rosiglitazone and atorvastatin was associated with significant reductions in LDL-C and apolipoprotein-B levels, and these changes were unaffected by concomitant TZD therapy [83].

A clinical trial comparing the effects of rosiglitazone and pioglitazone has recently been completed and presented in abstract form [84]. These data suggest that in a population with type 2 diabetes and dyslipidemia, pioglitazone lowers triglycerides approximately 12% from baseline while rosiglitazone therapy resulted in a 15% increase in triglycerides from baseline. In addition, pioglitazone therapy was associated with a significantly greater increase in HDL-c and a smaller increase in LDL-c. Pioglitazone was also associated with a reduction in LDL particle concentration while rosiglitazone increased LDL particle concentration. Both compounds reduced LDL particle size and had similar effects on A1C levels.

Whether this potential difference results from changes in lipoprotein production, clearance of lipid particles, or other effects of these agents is unknown, but some studies suggest that pioglitazone may favorably affect VLDL clearance. No convincing data exist to support a PPARα-like effect of either agent.

Although TZDs are not approved for use specifically as lipid-altering therapy, the use of these agents for glycemic control (see Table 2) should be considered in patients with low levels of HDL-C or high TG levels when additional diabetes mellitus medication is needed. Given the increasing attention directed at the role of insulin resistance in the development of CVD and its putative role in the development of metabolic abnormalities associated with diabetes mellitus, further research will be needed to understand better the role of diabetes mellitus therapies in managing multiple risk factors. Clinical trials will be needed to assess the impact of specific diabetes mellitus therapy, including the use of TZDs, on CVD event rates. Several such trials are underway in the United States and Europe.

Summary

CVD is the primary cause of morbidity and mortality in patients who have diabetes mellitus. Most such patients have at least one lipid abnormality. Managing these complex lipid disorders is a crucial component of comprehensive diabetes mellitus care and limits the risk for cardiovascular morbidity and mortality. With the high prevalence of mixed lipid disorders, management must focus on all components of the lipid profile. Lowering LDL-C levels remains the first priority, but abnormalities in HDL-C and TG levels also should be treated aggressively. Statins, fibrates, and niacin, along with newer therapies such as ezetimibe, can improve significantly components of the lipid profile. Alone or in combination, these agents can treat the dyslipidemia of diabetes mellitus effectively and safely.

References

[1] Haffner SM, Lehto S, Rönnemaa T, et al. Mortality from coronary heart disease in subjects with type 2 diabetes and in nondiabetic subjects with and without prior myocardial infarction. N Engl J Med 1998;339:229–34.

[2] Kannel WB, McGee DL. Diabetes and cardiovascular disease: the Framingham study. JAMA 1979;241:2035–8.

[3] Miettinen H, Lehto S, Salomaa V, et al, for the FINMONICA Myocardial Infarction Register Study Group. Impact of diabetes on mortality after the first myocardial infarction. Diabetes Care 1998;21:69–75.

[4] American Diabetes Association. National Diabetes Fact Sheet. General Information 2002. Available at: http://www.diabetes.org/diabetes-statistics/national-diabetes-fact-sheet.jsp. Accessed August 3, 2004.

[5] Grundy SM, Benjamin IJ, Burke GL, et al. Diabetes and cardiovascular disease: a statement for healthcare professionals from the American Heart Association. Circulation 1999;100: 1134–46.

[6] Reaven GM. Multiple CHD risk factors in type 2 diabetes: beyond hyperglycaemia. Diabetes Obes Metab 2002;4(Suppl 1):S13–8.

[7] Pyörälä K, Laakso M, Uusitupa M. Diabetes and atherosclerosis: an epidemiologic view. Diabetes Metab Rev 1987;3:463–524.

[8] Bierman EL. George Lyman Duff Memorial Lecture. Atherogenesis in diabetes. Arterioscler Thromb 1992;12:647–56.

[9] Haffner SM, Mykkänen L, Festa A, et al. Insulin-resistant prediabetic subjects have more atherogenic risk factors than insulin-sensitive prediabetic subjects: implications for preventing coronary heart disease during the prediabetic state. Circulation 2000;101:975–80.

[10] Stratton IM, Adler AI, Neil HA, et al, on behalf of the UK Prospective Diabetes Study Group. Association of glycaemia with macrovascular and microvascular complications of type 2 diabetes (UKPDS 35): prospective observational study. BMJ 2000;321:405–12.

[11] Garg A, Grundy SM. Management of dyslipidemia in NIDDM. Diabetes Care 1990;13: 153–69.

[12] American Diabetes Association. Dyslipidemia management in adults with diabetes. Diabetes Care 2004;27(Suppl 1):S68–71.

[13] Expert Panel on Detection, Evaluation, and Treatment of High Blood Cholesterol in Adults (Adult Treatment Panel III). Third Report of the National Cholesterol Education Program (NCEP) Expert Panel on Detection, Evaluation, and Treatment of High Blood Cholesterol in Adults (Adult Treatment Panel III) final report. Circulation 2002;106:3143–421.

[14] Kendall DM, Bergenstal RM. Comprehensive management of patients with type 2 diabetes: establishing priorities of care. Am J Manag Care 2001;7(10 Suppl):S327–43.
[15] Cowie CC, Howard BV, Harris MI. Serum lipoproteins in African Americans and whites with non-insulin-dependent diabetes in the US population. Circulation 1994;90:1185–93.
[16] Wilson PW, Kannel WB, Anderson KM. Lipids, glucose intolerance and vascular disease: the Framingham Study. Monogr Atheroscler 1985;13:1–11.
[17] Siegel RD, Cupples A, Schaefer EJ, et al. Lipoproteins, apolipoproteins, and low-density lipoprotein size among diabetics in the Framingham offspring study. Metabolism 1996;45: 1267–72.
[18] Rosenson RS, Shott S, Lu L, et al. Hypertriglyceridemia and other factors associated with plasma viscosity. Am J Med 2001;110:488–92.
[19] Juhan-Vague I, Pyke SD, Alessi MC, et al, on behalf of the ECAT Study Group. Fibrinolytic factors and the risk of myocardial infarction or sudden death in patients with angina pectoris. Circulation 1996;94:2057–63.
[20] Gordon DJ, Probstfield JL, Garrison RJ, et al. High-density lipoprotein cholesterol and cardiovascular disease: four prospective American studies. Circulation 1989;79:8–15.
[21] Hokanson JE, Austin MA. Plasma triglyceride level is a risk factor for cardiovascular disease independent of high-density lipoprotein cholesterol level: a meta-analysis of population-based prospective studies. J Cardiovasc Risk 1996;3:213–9.
[22] Lamarche B, Tchernof A, Moorjani S, et al. Small, dense low-density lipoprotein particles as a predictor of the risk of ischemic heart disease in men. Prospective results from the Quebec Cardiovascular Study. Circulation 1997;95:69–75.
[23] Rubins HB, Robins SJ, Collins D, et al, for the Veterans Affairs High-Density Lipoprotein Cholesterol Intervention Trial Study Group. Gemfibrozil for the secondary prevention of coronary heart disease in men with low levels of high-density lipoprotein cholesterol. N Engl J Med 1999;341:410–8.
[24] Canner PL, Berge KG, Wenger NK, et al, for the Coronary Drug Project Research Group. Fifteen year mortality in Coronary Drug Project patients: long-term benefit with niacin. J Am Coll Cardiol 1986;8:1245–55.
[25] Canner PL, Furberg CD, McGovern ME. Niacin decreases myocardial infarction and total mortality in patients with impaired fasting glucose or glucose intolerance: results from the Coronary Drug Project [abstract 3138]. Circulation 2002;106(Suppl II):636.
[26] Ginsberg HN. Insulin resistance and cardiovascular disease. J Clin Invest 2000;106: 453–8.
[27] Rubins HB, Robins SJ, Collins D, et al, for the VA-HIT Study Group. Diabetes, plasma insulin, and cardiovascular disease: subgroup analysis from the Department of Veterans Affairs High-Density Lipoprotein Intervention Trial (VA-HIT). Arch Intern Med 2002;162: 2597–604.
[28] Koskinen P, Mänttäri M, Manninen V, et al. Coronary heart disease incidence in NIDDM patients in the Helsinki Heart Study. Diabetes Care 1992;15:820–5.
[29] Frick MH, Elo O, Haapa K, et al. Helsinki Heart Study: primary-prevention trial with gemfibrozil in middle-aged men with dyslipidemia. Safety of treatment, changes in risk factors, and incidence of coronary heart disease. N Engl J Med 1987;317: 1237–45.
[30] Diabetes Atherosclerosis Intervention Study Investigators. Effect of fenofibrate on progression of coronary-artery disease in type 2 diabetes: the Diabetes Atherosclerosis Intervention Study, a randomised study. Lancet 2001;357:905–10.
[31] Brown BG, Zhao XQ, Chait A, et al. Simvastatin and niacin, antioxidant vitamins, or the combination for the prevention of coronary disease. N Engl J Med 2001;345:1583–92.
[32] Morse JS, Brown BG, Zhao X-Q, et al. Niacin plus simvastatin protect against atherosclerosis progression and clinical events in CAD patients with low HDLc and diabetes mellitus or impaired fasting glucose [abstract 842–3]. J Am Coll Cardiol 2001; 37(Suppl A):262A.

[33] Gotto AM Jr, Pownall HJ. Manual of lipid disorders: reducing the risk of coronary heart disease. 2nd edition. Baltimore (MD): Williams & Wilkins; 1999.

[34] Ginsberg HN. Diabetic dyslipidemia: basic mechanisms underlying the common hyper-triglyceridemia and low HDL cholesterol levels. Diabetes 1996;45(Suppl 3):S27–30.

[35] Haffner SM. Management of dyslipidemia in adults with diabetes. Diabetes Care 1998;21: 160–78.

[36] UK Prospective Diabetes Study Group. UK Prospective Diabetes Study 27: plasma lipids and lipoproteins at diagnosis of NIDDM by age and sex. Diabetes Care 1997;20: 1683–7.

[37] Downs JR, Clearfield M, Weis S, et al, for the Air Force/Texas Coronary Atherosclerosis Prevention Study. Primary prevention of acute coronary events with lovastatin in men and women with average cholesterol levels: results of AFCAPS/TexCAPS. JAMA 1998;279: 1615–22.

[38] The Coronary Drug Project Research Group. Clofibrate and niacin in coronary heart disease. JAMA 1975;231:360–81.

[39] Cannon CP, Braunwald E, McCabe CH, et al, for the Pravastatin or Atorvastatin Evaluation and Infection Therapy–Thrombolysis in Myocardial Infarction 22 Investigators. Intensive versus moderate lipid lowering with statins after acute coronary syndromes. N Engl J Med 2004;350:1495–504.

[40] Colhoun HM, Betteridge DJ, Durrington PN, et al. The Collaborative Atorvastatin Diabetes Study (CARDS). Effectiveness of lipid lowering for the primary prevention of major cardiovascular events in diabetes [abstract 15-LB]. Presented at: 64th Scientific Session of the American Diabetic Association, Orlando, June 4–8, 2004.

[41] BIP Study Group. Secondary prevention by raising HDL cholesterol and reducing triglycerides in patients with coronary artery disease: the Bezafibrate Infarction Prevention (BIP) study. Circulation 2000;102:21–7.

[42] Tenkanen L, Mänttäri M, Manninen V. Some coronary risk factors related to the insulin resistance syndrome and treatment with gemfibrozil. Experience from the Helsinki Heart Study. Circulation 1995;92:1779–85.

[43] Haffner SM, Alexander CM, Cook TJ, et al, for the Scandinavian Simvastatin Sur-vival Study Group. Reduced coronary events in simvastatin-treated patients with coro-nary heart disease and diabetes or impaired fasting glucose levels: subgroup analyses in the Scandinavian Simvastatin Survival Study. Arch Intern Med 1999;159:2661–7.

[44] Keech A, Colquhoun D, Baker J, et al, for the LIPID Group. Benefits of long term cholesterol lowering therapy using pravastatin among patients with diabetes in the lipid study [abstract]. Aust NZ J Med 2000;30:172.

[45] Goldberg RB, Mellies MJ, Sacks FM, et al, for the CARE Investigators. Cardiovascular events and their reduction with pravastatin in diabetic and glucose-intolerant myocardial infarction survivors with average cholesterol levels: subgroup analyses in the cholesterol and recurrent events (CARE) trial. Circulation 1998;98:2513–9.

[46] Heart Protection Study Collaborative Group. MRC/BHF Heart Protection Study of cholesterol-lowering with simvastatin in 5963 people with diabetes: a randomised placebo-controlled trial. Lancet 2003;361:2005–16.

[47] Sever PS, Dahlöf B, Poulter NR, et al, for the ASCOT investigators. Prevention of coronary and stroke events with atorvastatin in hypertensive patients who have average or lower-than-average cholesterol concentrations, in the Anglo-Scandinavian Cardiac Outcomes Trial—Lipid Lowering Arm (ASCOT-LLA): a multicentre randomised controlled trial. Lancet 2003;361:1149–58.

[48] Heart Protection Study Collaborative Group. MRC/BHF Heart Protection Study of cholesterol lowering with simvastatin in 20 536 high-risk individuals: a randomised placebo-controlled trial. Lancet 2002;360:7–22.

[49] ACCORD trial. Protocol abstract November 14, 2002. Available at: http://www.accordtrial.org/public/frames.cfm. Accessed April 9, 2004.

[50] International Diabetes Center. Available at: http://www.parknicollet.com/diabetes. Accessed August 3, 2004.

[51] Castelli WP. Cholesterol and lipids in the risk of coronary artery disease—the Framingham Heart Study. Can J Cardiol 1988;4(Suppl A):5A–10A.

[52] Robins SJ, Collins D, Wittes JT, et al, for the VA-HIT study group. Relation of gemfibrozil treatment and lipid levels with major coronary events. VA-HIT: a randomized controlled trial. JAMA 2001;285:1585–91.

[53] Markovic TP, Campbell LV, Balasubramanian S, et al. Beneficial effect on average lipid levels from energy restriction and fat loss in obese individuals with or without type 2 diabetes. Diabetes Care 1998;21:695–700.

[54] Obarzanek E, Sacks FM, Vollmer WM, et al, on behalf of the DASH Research Group. Effects on blood lipids of a blood pressure–lowering diet: the Dietary Approaches to Stop Hypertension (DASH) Trial. Am J Clin Nutr 2001;74:80–9.

[55] Grant RW, Cagliero E, Murphy-Sheehy P, et al. Comparison of hyperglycemia, hypertension, and hypercholesterolemia management in patients with type 2 diabetes. Am J Med 2002;112:603–9.

[56] McFarlane SI, Jacober SJ, Winer N, et al. Control of cardiovascular risk factors in patients with diabetes and hypertension at urban academic medical centers. Diabetes Care 2002;25: 718–23.

[57] Ginsberg HN. Nonpharmacologic management of low levels of high-density lipoprotein cholesterol. Am J Cardiol 2000;86:41L–5L.

[58] Pan J, Lin M, Kesala R, et al. Niacin treatment of the atherogenic lipid profile and Lp(a) in diabetes. Diabetes Obes Metab 2002;4:255–61.

[59] Pan J, Van JT, Chan E, et al. Extended-release niacin treatment of the atherogenic lipid profile and lipoprotein(a) in diabetes. Metabolism 2002;51:1120–7.

[60] American Diabetes Association. Management of dyslipidemia in adults with diabetes. Diabetes Care 2002;25(Suppl 1):S74–7.

[61] Garg A, Grundy SM. Nicotinic acid as therapy for dyslipidemia in non–insulin-dependent diabetes mellitus. JAMA 1990;264:723–6.

[62] Elam MB, Hunninghake DB, Davis KB, et al, for the ADMIT Investigators. Effect of niacin on lipid and lipoprotein levels and glycemic control in patients with diabetes and peripheral arterial disease. The ADMIT study: a randomized trial. JAMA 2000;284:1263–70.

[63] Grundy SM, Vega GL, McGovern ME, et al, for the Diabetes Multicenter Research Group. Efficacy, safety, and tolerability of once-daily niacin for the treatment of dyslipidemia associated with type 2 diabetes: results of the Assessment of Diabetes Control and Evaluation of the Efficacy of Niaspan Trial. Arch Intern Med 2002;162:1568–76.

[64] Miller M, Seidler A, Moalemi A, et al. Normal triglyceride levels and coronary artery disease events: the Baltimore Coronary Observational Long-Term Study. J Am Coll Cardiol 1998; 31:1252–7.

[65] Sprecher DL, Pearce GL, Park EM, et al. Preoperative triglycerides predict post-coronary artery bypass graft survival in diabetic patients: a sex analysis. Diabetes Care 2000;23: 1648–53.

[66] Ghazzi MN, Perez JE, Antonucci TK, et al, and the Troglitazone Study Group. Cardiac and glycemic benefits of troglitazone treatment in NIDDM. Diabetes 1997;46:433–9.

[67] Athyros VG, Papageorgiou AA, Athyrou VV, et al. Atorvastatin and micronized fenofibrate alone and in combination in type 2 diabetes with combined hyperlipidemia. Diabetes Care 2002;25:1198–202.

[68] Gavish D, Leibovitz E, Shapira I, et al. Bezafibrate and simvastatin combination therapy for diabetic dyslipidaemia: efficacy and safety. J Intern Med 2000;247:563–9.

[69] Pasternak RC, Smith SC Jr, Bairey-Merz CN, et al. ACC/AHA/NHLBI clinical advisory on the use and safety of statins. J Am Coll Cardiol 2002;40:567–72.

[70] Davidson MH. Combination therapy for dyslipidemia: safety and regulatory considerations. Am J Cardiol 2002;90(Suppl):50K–60K.

[71] Zhao X-Q, Morse JS, Dowdy AA, et al. Safety and tolerability of simvastatin plus niacin in patients with coronary artery disease and low high-density lipoprotein cholesterol (The HDL Atherosclerosis Treatment Study). Am J Cardiol 2004;93:307–12.

[72] Van JT, Pan J, Wasty T, et al. Comparison of extended-release niacin and atorvastatin monotherapies and combination treatment of the atherogenic lipid profile in diabetes mellitus. Am J Cardiol 2002;89:1306–8.

[73] Kashyap ML, McGovern ME, Berra K, et al. Long-term safety and efficacy of a once-daily niacin/lovastatin formulation in patients with dyslipidemia. Am J Cardiol 2002;89:672–8.

[74] Miettinen TA. Cholesterol absorption inhibition: a strategy for cholesterol-lowering therapy. Int J Clin Pract 2001;55:710–6.

[75] Gagné C, Gaudet D, Bruckert E, for the Ezetimibe Study Group. Efficacy and safety of ezetimibe coadministered with atorvastatin or simvastatin in patients with homozygous familial hypercholesterolemia. Circulation 2002;105:2469–75.

[76] Bays HE, Moore PB, Drehobl MA, et al, for the Ezetimibe Study Group. Effectiveness and tolerability of ezetimibe in patients with primary hypercholesterolemia: pooled analysis of two phase II studies. Clin Ther 2001;23:1209–30.

[77] Prospective Diabetes Study UK. (UKPDS) Group. Effect of intensive blood-glucose control with metformin on complications in overweight patients with type 2 diabetes (UKPDS 34). Lancet 1998;352:854–65.

[78] Emanuele N, Azad N, Abraira C, et al. Effect of intensive glycemic control on fibrinogen, lipids, and lipoproteins: Veterans Affairs Cooperative Study in Type II Diabetes Mellitus. Arch Intern Med 1998;158(22):2485–90.

[79] King AB, Armstrong DU. Lipid response to pioglitazone in diabetic patients: clinical observations from a retrospective chart review. Diabetes Technol Ther 2002;4:145–51.

[80] van Wijk JPH, de Koning EJP, Martens EP, et al. Thiazolidinediones and blood lipids in type 2 diabetes. Arterioscler Thromb Vasc Biol 2003;23:1744–9.

[81] Buse JB, Tan MH, Prince MJ, et al. The effects of oral anti-hyperglycaemic medications on serum lipid profiles in patients with type 2 diabetes. Diabetes Obes Metab 2004;6:133–56.

[82] Khan MA, St Pete JV, Xue JL. A prospective, randomized comparison of the metabolic effects of pioglitazone or rosiglitazone in patients with type 2 diabetes who were previously treated with troglitazone. Diabetes Care 2002;25:708–11.

[83] Freed MI, Ratner R, Marcovina SM, et al. Rosiglitazone Study 108 investigators. Effects of rosiglitazone alone and in combination with atorvastatin on the metabolic abnormalities in type 2 diabetes mellitus. Am J Cardiol 2002;90:947–52.

[84] Goldberg RB, et al. Late breaking clinical trials. American Heart Association Annual Meetings. New Orleans, Louisiana, 2004.

ELSEVIER
SAUNDERS

Endocrinol Metab Clin N Am
34 (2005) 49–62

ENDOCRINOLOGY
AND METABOLISM
CLINICS
OF NORTH AMERICA

Compensatory Hyperinsulinemia and the Development of an Atherogenic Lipoprotein Profile: The Price Paid to Maintain Glucose Homeostasis in Insulin-Resistant Individuals

Gerald M. Reaven, MD

Division of Cardiovascular Medicine, Falk Cardiovascular Research Center,
Stanford Medical Center, 300 Pasteur Drive, Stanford, CA 94305, USA

The ability of insulin to mediate glucose disposal varies severalfold among apparently healthy individuals. An example of this variability is seen in Fig. 1, which depicts the frequency distribution of steady-state plasma glucose (SSPG) concentrations in 490 healthy persons, who did not have known disease, after a 180-minute infusion of somatostatin, insulin, and glucose [1]. Under the conditions of this study—designated as the insulin suppression test (IST)—endogenous insulin secretion is inhibited, similar steady-state plasma insulin (SSPI) concentrations are achieved in all subjects, and the SSPG concentration provides a direct measure of the ability of insulin to dispose of a glucose load; the higher the SSPG concentration, the more insulin resistant the individual. Despite the dramatic differences in the ability of insulin to accomplish its most basic biologic function—the efficient use of glucose—none of the volunteers in this study had diabetes mellitus. Normal, or near-normal, glucose tolerance was achieved by the ability of the pancreatic β cell to secrete the amount of insulin that was needed to overcome whatever degree of tissue insulin resistance existed.

Reliance on the β cell to compensate for the variability in insulin sensitivity suggests that the maintenance of glucose homeostasis received considerable priority in the evolutionary process. Although the prevention of frank hyperglycemia by maintaining a state of compensatory hyperinsulinemia may have been a useful adaptive response at one time, it is now

E-mail address: greaven@cvmed.stanford.edu

0889-8529/05/$ - see front matter © 2005 Elsevier Inc. All rights reserved.
doi:10.1016/j.ecl.2004.12.001
endo.theclinics.com

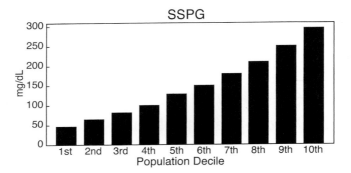

Fig. 1. Mean SSPG concentrations in 490 nondiabetic, apparently healthy volunteers divided into deciles on the basis of their SSPG concentrations determined during the insulin suppression test. The higher the SSPG, the more insulin resistant is the individual. (*Adapted from* Yeni-Komshian H, Carantoni M, Abbasi F, et al. Relationship between several surrogate estimates of insulin resistance and quantification of insulin-mediated glucose disposal in 490 healthy nondiabetic volunteers. Diabetes Care 2000;23:171–5; with permission.)

evident that this philanthropic gesture on the part of the pancreas is not without its cost. For example, Box 1 lists clinical syndromes that occur with increased prevalence in nondiabetic, insulin-resistant, hyperinsulinemic persons [2–12].

The importance of insulin resistance as a major risk factor for cardiovascular disease (CVD) was emphasized in the most recent report from the National Cholesterol Education Program, the Adult Treatment Panel III [13]. Substantial evidence indicates that the dyslipidemia that is characteristic of insulin-resistant/hyperinsulinemic individuals—increased plasma triglyceride (TG) concentrations and decreased levels of high-density lipoprotein cholesterol (HDL-C) [2,14]—increases CVD risk [15–18]. Less clear is the relative importance of insulin resistance, as opposed to compensatory hyperinsulinemia, in the development of these changes in lipoprotein metabolism. This article reviews the pathophysiology of the atherogenic lipoprotein profile that occurs commonly in insulin-resistant/hyperinsulinemic individuals, with particular focus on defining the relative roles of insulin resistance versus compensatory hyperinsulinemia in the development of these abnormalities.

Differential tissue insulin sensitivity

The term "insulin resistance" is used almost always to indicate a relative defect in the ability of a specific level of physiologic hyperinsulinemia to stimulate muscle glucose disposal. Although the ability of insulin to inhibit adipose tissue lipolysis closely parallels the defect in insulin stimulation of muscle glucose disposal, most other tissues remain normally responsive to the action of insulin. Even in this instance, however, muscle tissue and

---

Box 1. Clinical syndromes that are associated with insulin resistance

Type 2 diabetes mellitus
Cardiovascular disease
Essential hypertension
Polycystic ovary syndrome
Nonalcoholic fatty liver disease
Certain forms of cancer
Sleep apnea

---

adipose tissue differ in the nature of their dose response to insulin. Adipose tissue is much more insulin sensitive, and plasma free fatty acid (FFA) concentrations are suppressed half-maximally at a plasma insulin concentration of approximately 20 $\mu U/mL$ [19]; this level of insulin has minor effects on muscle glucose uptake. Parenthetically, these differences in the insulin dose-response curve of the two tissues are essential for normal energy metabolism. When insulin levels are decreased after an overnight fast, the antilipolytic effect of insulin is minimal, FFA release from adipose tissue stores is accentuated, and little glucose is taken up by muscle. After food is consumed, plasma insulin concentrations increase, muscle glucose uptake is maximized, and the effect of insulin on adipose tissue is to enhance glucose disposal and inhibit further breakdown of stored TG to FFA.

Although muscle and adipose tissue may differ in their relative degree of insulin sensitivity, they are similar in that when muscle is resistant to regulation by insulin, so is adipose tissue [20]. In contrast, most, if not all, of the other tissues in the body retain normal insulin sensitivity in the face of muscle and adipose tissue insulin resistance. Therefore, they can become innocent victims of the effort by pancreatic β cells to maintain euglycemia by secreting the large amounts of insulin that is needed to compensate for the muscle and adipose tissue insulin resistance. For example, compensatory hyperinsulinemia that is aimed at maintaining normal glucose tolerance will act on a normally insulin-sensitive kidney to decrease uric acid clearance and increase sodium retention. This results in the increase in uric acid concentration and salt sensitivity that occurs in insulin-resistant individuals [21,22]. Another obvious example of differential tissue insulin sensitivity is the increase in ovarian androgen secretion, secondary to compensatory hyperinsulinemia, that results in polycystic ovary syndrome [6]. Perhaps the most relevant organ in this context is the liver; by remaining normally insulin sensitive, the liver is responsible for the development of nonalcoholic fatty liver disease [7], as well as the atherogenic lipoprotein profile that serves as the major established link between insulin resistance and CVD [2,14–18].

Insulin resistance, hyperinsulinemia, and the atherogenic lipoprotein profile

It has been known for approximately 40 years that there is a highly significant relationship between insulin resistance, compensatory hyperinsulinemia, and hypertriglyceridemia [23,24]. It is now apparent that the link between insulin resistance and dyslipidemia is a much broader one, and is not limited to an increase in plasma TG concentrations. Because the additional abnormalities in lipoprotein metabolism that are associated with insulin resistance are related closely to changes in very low-density lipoprotein (VLDL) metabolism, the link among insulin resistance, compensatory hyperinsulinemia, and VLDL metabolism is the initial focus of this discussion. After this framework has been constructed, the development of the other components of the atherogenic lipoprotein profile characteristic of insulin-resistant/hyperinsulinemic individuals can be placed in the context of the changes in VLDL metabolism.

Hypertriglyceridemia

Insulin resistance at the level of the muscle leads to daylong increases in plasma insulin concentrations that are associated with elevated plasma FFA levels because of the parallel loss of normal insulin regulation of adipose tissue. Evidence of these changes can be seen in Fig. 2, which shows daylong plasma TG, insulin, and FFA concentrations in individuals of similar age, weight, and gender distribution. These subjects were selected because they were either insulin sensitive, with normal TG concentrations, or insulin resistant, with elevated plasma TG levels [25]. Fasting plasma TG concentrations were significantly greater in the insulin-resistant individuals, and the difference between the two groups widened considerably in response to breakfast at 8 AM and lunch at noon. It also can be seen that daylong plasma

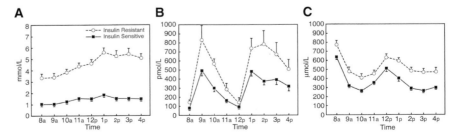

Fig. 2. Mean (± SEM) plasma TG (*A*), insulin (*B*), and FFA (*C*) concentrations measured hourly from 8 AM to 4 PM in apparently healthy volunteers. The daylong differences between the two groups were statistically significant ($P < .001$) for each variable by two-way analysis of variance. (*Adapted from* Jeng C-Y, Fuh MM-T, Sheu WH-H, et al. Hormone and substrate modulation of plasma triglyceride concentration in primary hypertriglyceridemia. Endocrinol Metab 1994;1:15–21; with permission.)

insulin concentrations were higher and FFA levels were lower in the insulin-resistant individuals.

Based on studies in animals and human beings, it seems that circulating plasma insulin concentrations determine the shape of the hepatic FFA-VLDL-TG dose-response curve [26]; the higher the ambient insulin levels, the greater the degree to which the FFAs that enter the liver are converted to hepatic TG synthesis. Looked at differently, at any given portal vein insulin concentration, the more FFA that enters the liver, the greater the resultant increase in hepatic TG synthesis and secretion.

The data in Box 2 summarize the relationships between insulin resistance (SSPG concentration as assessed with the IST), compensatory hyper-insulinemia, hepatic VLDL-TG synthesis and secretion, and plasma TG concentrations that were observed in two studies that were performed in nondiabetic individuals [24,27]. The first study involved measurements in persons whose plasma TG concentrations ranged from 69 mg/dL to 546 mg/dL [24], whereas the second study enrolled individuals who had plasma TG concentrations that were considered to be in the normal range (< 175 mg/dL) [27]. Highly significant relationships among the four variables were observed in both groups. Based on these findings, it was postulated that the major cause of hypertriglyceridemia in nondiabetic individuals is increased hepatic VLDL-TG secretion, secondary to muscle and adipose tissue insulin resistance, and maintenance of normal hepatic sensitivity to the stimulating effect on hepatic TG synthesis of the resultant elevation in plasma FFA and insulin concentrations.

Box 2. Correlation coefficients (r values[a]) between steady-state plasma glucose concentration, plasma insulin concentration, very low-density lipoprotein triglyceride secretion rate, and plasma triglyceride concentration

Fasting plasma triglyceride concentrations between 69 mg/dL and 546 mg/dL [24]
SSPG concentration→plasma insulin concentration (r = 0.74)→VLDL-TG secretion rate (r = 0.74)→plasma TG concentration (r = 0.88)

Fasting plasma insulin concentration between 37 mg/dL and 174 mg/dL [27]
SSPG concentration→plasma insulin concentration (r = 0.81)→VLDL-TG secretion rate (r = 0.68)→plasma TG concentration (r = 0.87)

---

[a] All r values were statistically significant (P < .001).

Although there is widespread agreement as to the validity of the relationships shown in Box 2, controversy exists regarding the causal relationships among insulin resistance, hyperinsulinemia, hepatic VLDL-TG secretion, and plasma TG concentration. One view is that resistance to insulin regulation of muscle and adipose tissue leads to higher ambient levels of insulin and FFA and that these two changes stimulate hepatic VLDL-TG secretion, which leads to the increase in plasma TG concentration [23–27].

Alternatively, evidence has been presented that hypertriglyceridemia occurs in insulin-resistant, nondiabetic individuals because the "normal" ability of insulin to inhibit hepatic VLDL-TG synthesis and secretion is deficient (ie, the liver is insulin resistant) [28]. It is suggested that, in the absence of this postulated normal inhibition of hepatic VLDL-TG secretion by insulin, the increase in plasma FFA concentrations in insulin-resistant individuals stimulates hepatic VLDL-TG synthesis and secretion. Evidence in support of this latter hypothesis is derived primarily from acute experiments [28]. For example, insulin acutely inhibits VLDL-TG secretion from cultured rat and human hepatocytes and HepG2 cells. The acute infusion of insulin also suppressed hepatic VLDL-TG secretion in humans, in association with a substantial decrease in plasma FFA concentration. An obvious explanation for the ability of an acute insulin infusion to decrease VLDL-TG secretion is the profound decrease in adipose tissue lipolysis that occurs secondary to even modest increases in plasma insulin concentrations [19]. Highly relevant in this context are the findings of Aarsland et al [29], who measured VLDL-TG secretion rates 1 and 4 days after subjects began a high-carbohydrate, hypercaloric diet. The dietary intervention resulted in a six-fold elevation of plasma insulin concentration that persisted throughout the study. The VLDL-TG secretion rate was, if anything, lower after 1 day of hyperinsulinemia without any change in plasma TG secretion. By Day 4, however, there were significant increases in hepatic VLDL-TG secretion and plasma TG concentrations. These data strongly suggest that the acute effects of exogenous hyperinsulinemia may not reflect the chronic effects of endogenous hyperinsulinemia. Furthermore, the importance of FFA in stimulating hepatic VLDL-TG secretion was supported by the observation that the difference between 1 and 4 days of endogenous hyperinsulinemia was the increase in hepatic secretion of preformed fatty acids into VLDL-TG [29].

Further evidence that the liver is not insulin resistant and that long-term elevations of endogenous insulin stimulate, not inhibit, hepatic VLDL-TG synthesis and secretion can be derived from the fact that high-carbohydrate diets increase plasma insulin and TG concentrations [30]. There also is evidence that these diets are associated with enhanced insulin sensitivity [31]. If hypertriglyceridemia is due to the inability of insulin to inhibit hepatic VLDL-TG secretion because of hepatic insulin resistance, high-carbohydrate diets—by increasing insulin levels and sensitivity—should lead to a decrease, not an increase, in hepatic VLDL-TG secretion and plasma TG concentration. The data in Fig. 3 demonstrate that the opposite results are observed when the hypothesis is tested. In this study [30], dietary carbohydrate intake was increased from 40% to 60% of daily caloric intake, with a reciprocal decrease in dietary fat consumption from 45% to 25% of daily calories. This dietary change resulted in an increase in fasting and daylong plasma TG concentrations (Fig. 3A). It also can be seen that the diet that contained 60% carbohydrate resulted in higher daylong plasma insulin concentrations (see Fig 3B) and lower plasma FFA levels (see Fig. 3C). The fact that elevated circulating insulin concentrations in subjects who ate the higher carbohydrate diet increased plasma TG concentrations, despite even lower plasma FFA concentrations, is not compatible with the notion that the liver is insulin resistant, nor with the view that the effect of insulin on the liver is to decrease hepatic TG secretion.

Perhaps the most compelling evidence that hypertriglyceridemia is not the consequence of an inability of insulin to overcome hepatic insulin resistance is the effect of insulin deficiency on FFA and TG metabolism [26]. If the physiologic role of insulin is to inhibit VLDL-TG secretion, the combination of low levels of insulin and extremely high plasma FFA concentrations should lead to a massive increase in hepatic VLDL-TG secretion; however, the opposite is seen (ie, a dramatic decrease in hepatic VLDL-TG secretion) [26].

In summary, there is substantial evidence that circulating insulin levels play a central role in the modulation of hepatic TG synthesis and secretion. In nondiabetic persons, muscle and adipose tissue insulin resistance results in increased daylong plasma insulin and FFA concentrations. The hyper-insulinemia that acts on an insulin-sensitive liver stimulates the incorporation of FFA into hepatic TG synthesis; this development, in turn, results in the hypertriglyceridemia that occurs so frequently in insulin-resistant individuals.

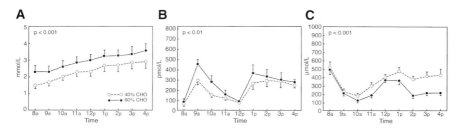

Fig. 3. Mean (± SEM) plasma TG (*A*), insulin (*B*), and FFA (*C*) concentrations measured hourly from 8 AM to 4 PM in apparently healthy volunteers following dietary periods in which they consumed diets that contained 40% (○) or 60% (●) of total calories as carbohydrate, with reciprocal changes in dietary fat intake. Breakfast was given at 8 AM and lunch was given at noon. (*Adapted from* McLaughlin T, Abbasi F, Lamendola C, et al. Carbohydrate-induced hypertriglyceridemia: an insight into the link between plasma insulin and triglyceride concentrations. J Clin Endocrinol Metab 2000;85:3085–8; with permission.)

Combined dyslipidemia

Although plasma low-density lipoprotein cholesterol (LDL-C) concentrations are not regulated by insulin resistance/compensatory hyperinsulinemia, insulin-resistant individuals are not protected from developing elevated levels of LDL-C. When a hypertriglyceridemic person also has elevated LDL-C, the resultant combined dyslipidemia increases the CVD risk of either abnormality alone [17,32]. The original Fredrickson classification of abnormalities of lipoprotein metabolism differentiated between type IIA (increase in LDL-C concentration only), type IIB (increase in TG and LDL-C concentrations), and type IV (increase in TG concentration only) hyperlipoproteinemias, which implied a metabolic similarity between types IIA and IIB. If insulin resistance/hyperinsulinemia is taken into consideration, it is types IIB and IV dyslipidemia that are most similar [33].

Fig. 4 illustrates that, although daylong plasma glucose concentrations (Fig. 4A) were similar in normal glucose-tolerant volunteers and patients who had types IIA, IIB, or IV hyperlipoproteinemias, plasma insulin concentrations (Fig. 4B) were elevated significantly throughout the day in persons who had types IIB or IV dyslipidemia [33]. These results suggest that individuals who have types IIB or IV dyslipidemia are insulin resistant; the results of the IST that is shown (Fig. 5) provide direct evidence of this. Thus, the compensatory hyperinsulinemia that is able to overcome muscle and adipose tissue insulin resistance in patients who have combined dyslipidemia also acts on the liver in these persons to increase hepatic VLDL-TG synthesis and secretion. This leads to increased plasma TG concentrations

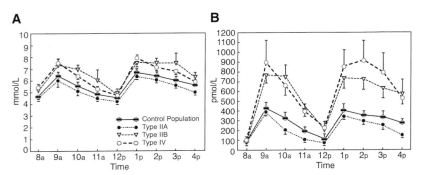

Fig. 4. Mean (± SEM) plasma glucose (*A*) and insulin (*B*) concentrations measured hourly from 8 AM to 4 PM in a control population (θ) and in patients with type IIA (●), type IIB (∇), or type IV (○) hyperlipoproteinemia. Breakfast was given at 8 AM and lunch was given at noon. Patients who had type IIB or type IV hyperlipoproteinemia had significantly ($P < .001$) higher daylong plasma insulin concentrations compared with the control group or patients who had type IIA dyslipidemia. (*Adapted from* Sheu WH-H, Shieh S-M, Fuh MM-T, et al. Insulin resistance, glucose intolerance, and hyperinsulinemia: hypertriglyceridemia versus hypercholesterolemia. Arterioscler Thromb 1993;13:367–70; with permission.)

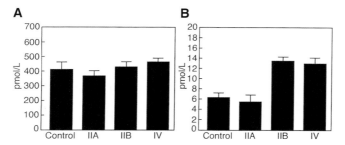

Fig. 5. Mean (± SEM) steady-state plasma insulin (SSPI; *A*) and glucose (SSP; *B*) concentrations determined during the IST in a control population and patients who had type IIA, type IIB, or type IV hyperlipoproteinemia. The SSPI concentrations were not different in the four groups, whereas the SSPG concentrations were significantly higher in persons who had type IIB or type IV dyslipidemia. (*Adapted from* Sheu WH-H, Shieh S-M, Fuh MM-T, et al. Insulin resistance, glucose intolerance, and hyperinsulinemia: hypertriglyceridemia versus hypercholesterolemia. Arterioscler Thromb 1993;13:367–70; with permission.)

and almost certainly contributes to the accentuated CVD risk that is seen in patients who have this form of abnormal lipoprotein metabolism.

Postprandial lipemia

As is evident from Fig. 2, in nondiabetic individuals, the higher the fasting TG concentration, the greater the postprandial accumulation of TG-rich lipoproteins (VLDL, VLDL remnants, chylomicrons, and chylomicron remnants). The postprandial accumulation of TG-rich lipoproteins was recognized to increase the risk for CVD [34,35], and the increased magnitude of postprandial lipemia that is observed in insulin-resistant, hyperinsulinemic individuals almost certainly contributes to their increased CVD risk. In addition to the relationship between fasting TG concentration and postprandial lipemia, in nondiabetic persons, the daylong increase in TG-rich remnant lipoproteins (RLPs) is correlated significantly with the magnitude of their insulin resistance/compensatory hyperinsulinemia [36,37]. Although the postprandial elevation of TG-rich lipoproteins is related to the fasting TG concentration, it was shown that postprandial lipemia is enhanced when insulin-resistant/hyperinsulinemic individuals are matched for degree of fasting hypertriglyceridemia with an insulin-sensitive population [38]. These observations suggest that increases in postprandial lipemia are secondary to an increase in the fasting plasma TG pool size and a decrease in the rate at which RLPs are removed from plasma following meals.

The importance of elevated plasma insulin concentrations, separate from insulin resistance, in modulating the removal of RLPs from plasma is less clear, but there is evidence that hyperinsulinemia also may act independently in this context. For example, the plasma insulin response to an oral glucose challenge was correlated significantly with RLP concentrations in patients who had impaired glucose tolerance; the decrease in RLP levels following weight loss and increased physical activity was related significantly to the concomitant decrease in the insulin response to glucose [39]. Of greater relevance was the finding that the plasma RLP response to an oral fat load was significantly greater in patients who had newly-diagnosed type 2 diabetes, defined as being hyperinsulinemic, than with either a control group or with equally hyperglycemic patients who had type 2 diabetes and a significantly lower insulin response [40]. Thus, it seems that the absolute level of plasma insulin also plays a vital role in determining the magnitude of the postprandial accumulation of RLPs in insulin-resistant individuals.

It should be emphasized that the hepatic low-density lipoprotein (LDL) receptor plays an important role in the catabolism of RLPs. The increased activity of hepatic LDL receptors following administration of 3-hydroxy-3-methylglutaryl coenzyme A reductase inhibitors (statins) decreases LDL-C and results in a significant increase in the removal of RLPs from plasma [41]. The beneficial effects of statin treatment on CVD that seem to be above and beyond the decreasing of LDL-C may result from their ability to increase hepatic uptake of TG-rich RLPs. For example, although gemfibrozil decreases fasting plasma TG concentrations much more than do statins in patients who have type 2 diabetes and combined dyslipidemia, the decreases in postprandial RLP concentration were similar following the use of these two different classes of drugs [41]. In this context, we presented preliminary evidence that treatment of nondiabetic, insulin-resistant individuals who had combined dyslipidemia with gemfibrozil or rosuvastatin resulted in similar decreases in fasting plasma TG concentrations; however, because rosuvastatin also increases the activity of hepatic LDL receptors, the decline in RLP concentrations was much greater than that following administration of gemfibrozil [42]. Whether insulin resistance or hyperinsulinemia can modulate the activity of hepatic LDL receptors directly remains to be evaluated.

Low-density lipoprotein particle diameter

Analysis of LDL particle size distribution [43] identified multiple distinct LDL subclasses, and it seems that LDL in most persons can be characterized by a predominance of either larger (diameter > 255 Å, pattern A) or smaller (diameter < 255 Å, pattern B) particles. Healthy volunteers who had small, dense LDL particles (pattern B) were insulin resistant, hyperinsulinemic, hypertriglyceridemic, and had decreased HDL-C concentrations [43]. Persons who have pattern B also are at increased risk of CVD [44].

The presence of the pattern B LDL-particle phenotype is linked closely to the fasting plasma TG concentration; the prevalence of small, dense LDL particles increases substantially as fasting plasma TG levels increase to more than 150 mg/dL [45]. Because fasting hypertriglyceridemia is secondary to the ability of hyperinsulinemia to stimulate hepatic TG synthesis and secretion, it is evident that the appearance of small, dense LDL particles is another manifestation of insulin resistance at the level of muscle and adipose tissue in the presence of normal hepatic insulin sensitivity.

High-density lipoprotein cholesterol

The importance of decreased levels of HDL-C is well-established as a risk factor for CVD [15,18], as is the observation that decreases in HDL-C concentrations occur commonly in hypertriglyceridemic persons [14]. Although frequently seen together, the two changes—an increased TG and a decreased HDL-C—can occur as isolated events, and they are associated independently with insulin resistance/hyperinsulinemia [14]. At least two explanations may account for the association between insulin resistance, hyperinsulinemia, and low HDL-C concentrations; both provide further evidence of the importance of an elevated plasma insulin concentration in the genesis of the atherogenic lipoprotein profile of the insulin resistance syndrome.

The most direct reason why HDL-C concentrations often are decreased in hypertriglyceridemic individuals is the transfer—catalyzed by cholesteryl ester transfer protein—of cholesterol from HDL to VLDL in exchange for TG [46]. The larger the VLDL pool, the greater the transfer rate, and the lower the ensuing HDL-C and higher the HDL-TG concentration. Thus, the greater the ability of insulin to stimulate the liver to synthesize and secrete VLDL-TG, the more likely it is that the HDL-C concentration will decline. There also is evidence that the fractional catabolic rate (FCR) of apoprotein A-I is increased in patients who have primary hypertriglyceridemia [47], essential hypertension [48], and type 2 diabetes [49]. In patients who have type 2 diabetes, the higher the plasma insulin concentration, the greater the increase in the FCR of apoprotein A-I and the lower the HDL-C concentration [49]. It also was demonstrated in nondiabetic individuals that the higher the apoprotein A-I FCR, the lower the HDL-C concentration; in this instance, there also is an association between higher insulin concentrations and an increased apoprotein A-I FCR [50]. Thus, it seems that the decreased HDL-C concentrations that are seen in insulin-resistant individuals is another example of compensatory hyperinsulinemia that acts on tissues that retain normal insulin sensitivity and results in changes in lipoprotein metabolism that increase the risk of CVD.

Summary

The ability of insulin to stimulate glucose disposal varies sixfold to eightfold among apparently healthy individuals. The only way that insulin-resistant persons can prevent the development of type 2 diabetes is by secreting the increased amount of insulin that is necessary to compensate for the resistance to insulin action. The greater the magnitude of muscle and adipose tissue insulin resistance, the more insulin must be secreted to maintain normal or near-normal glucose tolerance. Although compensatory hyperinsulinemia may prevent the development of fasting hyperglycemia in insulin-resistant individuals, the price paid is the untoward physiologic effects of increased circulating insulin concentrations on tissues that retain normal insulin sensitivity. This article focused on the interplay between insulin resistance at the level of the muscle and adipose tissue and normal hepatic insulin sensitivity; this leads to the atherogenic lipoprotein profile that is characteristic of insulin-resistant individuals.

It would be inappropriate to minimize the importance of differential insulin sensitivity in the genesis of the changes in lipoprotein metabolism that increase CVD risk in insulin-resistant persons. It would be equally remiss not to emphasize that differential tissue insulin resistance also is necessary to explain why insulin-resistant/hyperinsulinemic individuals are more likely to develop the clinical syndromes (with the exception of type 2 diabetes mellitus) that are listed in Box 1.

References

[1] Yeni-Komshian H, Carantoni M, Abbasi F, et al. Relationship between several surrogate estimates of insulin resistance and quantification of insulin-mediated glucose disposal in 490 healthy nondiabetic volunteers. Diabetes Care 2000;23:171–5.
[2] Reaven GM. Role of insulin resistance in human disease. Diabetes 1988;37:1595–607.
[3] Lillioja S, Mott DM, Spraul M, et al. Insulin resistance and insulin secretory dysfunction as precursors of non-insulin-dependent diabetes mellitus: prospective studies of Pima Indians. N Engl J Med 1993;329:1988–92.
[4] Yip J, Facchini FS, Reaven GM. Resistance to insulin-mediated glucose disposal as a predictor of cardiovascular disease. J Clin Endocrinol Metab 1998;83:2773–6.
[5] Reaven GM. Insulin resistance/compensatory hyperinsulinemia, essential hypertension, and cardiovascular disease. J Clin Endocrinol Metab 2003;88:2399–403.
[6] Dunaiff A. Insulin resistance and the polycystic ovary syndrome: mechanism and implications for pathogenesis. Endocr Rev 1997;18:774–800.
[7] Sanyal AJ, Campbell-Sargent C, Mirashi F, et al. Nonalcoholic steatohepatitis: association of insulin resistance and mitochondrial abnormalities. Gastroenterology 2001;120:1183–92.
[8] Argiles JM, Lopez-Soriano FJ. Insulin and cancer. Int J Oncol 2001;18:683–7.
[9] Goodwin PJ, Ennis M, Pritchard KI, et al. Fasting insulin and outcome in early-stage breast cancer: results of a prospective cohort study. J Clin Oncol 2001;20:42–51.
[10] Hu FB, Manson JE, Hunter D, et al. Prospective study of diabetes mellitus (type 2) and risk of colorectal cancer in women. J Natl Cancer Inst 1999;91:542–7.
[11] Rodriguez C, Patel AV, Calle EE, et al. Body mass index, height, and prostate cancer mortality in two large cohorts of adult men in the United States. Cancer Epidemiol Biomarkers Prev 2001;10:345–53.
[12] Vgontzas AN, Bixler EO, Chrousos GP. Metabolic disturbances in obesity versus sleep apnea: the importance of visceral obesity and insulin resistance. J Int Med 2003;254:32–44.
[13] The Expert Panel. The Third Report of the National Education Program (NCEP) Expert Panel on Detection, Evaluation, and Treatment of High Blood Cholesterol in Adults (Adult Treatment Panel III). Final report. Circulation 2002;106:3143–421.

[14] Laws A, Reaven GM. Evidence for an independent relationship between insulin resistance and fasting plasma HDL-cholesterol, triglyceride and insulin concentrations. J Int Med 1992;231:25–30.

[15] Castelli WP, Garrison RJ, Wilson PWF, et al. Incidence of coronary heart disease and lipoprotein cholesterol levels: the Framingham Study. JAMA 1986;256:2835–8.

[16] Austin MA, Hokanson JE, Edwards KI. Hypertriglyceridemia as a cardiovascular risk factor. Am J Cardiol 1998;81(Suppl 4A):7B–12B.

[17] Manninen V, Tenkanen L, Koskinen P, et al. Joint effects of serum triglyceride and LDL and HDL cholesterol concentrations on coronary heart disease risk in the Helsinki Heart Study: implications for treatment. Circulation 1992;85:37–45.

[18] Robins SJ, Rubins HB, Fass FH, et al. Insulin resistance and cardiovascular events with low HDL cholesterol: the Veterans Affairs HDL Intervention Trial (VA-HIT). Diabetes Care 2003;26:1513–7.

[19] Swislocki ALM, Chen Y-DI, Golay A, et al. Insulin suppression of plasma-free fatty acid concentration in normal individuals and patients with type 2 (non-insulin-dependent) diabetes. Diabetologia 1987;30:622–6.

[20] Abbasi F, McLaughlin T, Lamendola C, et al. The relationship between glucose disposal in response to physiological hyperinsulinemia and basal glucose and free fatty acid concentrations in healthy volunteers. J Clin Endocrinol Metab 2000;85:1251–4.

[21] Facchini F, Chen YD-I, Hollenbeck C, et al. Relationship between resistance to insulin-mediated glucose uptake, urinary uric acid clearance, and plasma uric acid concentration. JAMA 1991;266:3008–11.

[22] Facchini FS, DoNascimento C, Reaven GM, et al. Blood pressure, sodium intake, insulin resistance, and urinary nitrate excretion. Hypertension 1999;33:1008–12.

[23] Reaven GM, Lerner RL, Stern MP, et al. Role of insulin in endogenous hypertriglyceridemia. J Clin Invest 1967;46:1756–67.

[24] Olefsky JM, Farquhar JW, Reaven GM. Reappraisal of the role of insulin in hypertriglyceridemia. Am J Med 1974;57:551–60.

[25] Jeng C-Y, Fuh MM-T, Sheu WH-H, et al. Hormone and substrate modulation of plasma triglyceride concentration in primary hypertriglyceridemia. Endocrinology and Metabolism 1994;1:15–21.

[26] Reaven GM, Greenfield MS. Diabetic hypertriglyceridemia: evidence for three clinical syndromes. Diabetes 1981;30(Suppl 2):66–75.

[27] Tobey TA, Greenfield M, Kraemer F, et al. Relationship between insulin resistance, insulin secretion, very low density lipoprotein kinetics, and plasma triglyceride levels in normo-triglyceridemic man. Metabolism 1981;30:165–71.

[28] Lewis GF. Fatty acid regulation of very low-density lipoprotein production. Curr Opin Lipidol 1997;8:146–53.

[29] Aarsland A, Chinkes D, Wolfe RR. Contributions of de novo synthesis of fatty acids to total VLDL-triglyceride secretion during prolonged hyperglycemia/hyperinsulinemia in normal man. J Clin Invest 1996;98:2008–17.

[30] McLaughlin T, Abbasi F, Lamendola C, et al. Carbohydrate-induced hypertriglyceridemia: an insight into the link between plasma insulin and triglyceride concentrations. J Clin Endocrinol Metab 2000;85:3085–8.

[31] Kolterman OG, Greenfield M, Reaven GM, et al. Effect of a high carbohydrate diet on insulin binding to adipocytes and on insulin action in vivo in man. Diabetes 1979;28:731–6.

[32] Assmann G, Schulte H. Relation of high-density lipoprotein cholesterol and triglycerides to incidence of atherosclerotic coronary artery disease (the PROCAM experience). Am J Cardiol 1992;70:733–7.

[33] Sheu WH-H, Shieh S-M, Fuh MM-T, et al. Insulin resistance, glucose intolerance, and hyperinsulinemia: hypertriglyceridemia versus hypercholesterolemia. Arterioscler Thromb 1993;13:367–70.

[34] Patsch JR, Miesenbock G, Hopferwieser T, et al. Relation of triglyceride metabolism and coronary artery disease: studies in the postprandial state. Arterioscler Thromb 1992;12: 1336–45.

[35] Karpe F, Bard JM, Steiner G, et al. HDLs and alimentary lipemia: studies in men with previous myocardial infarction at young age. Arterioscler Thromb 1993;13:11–22.

[36] Jeppesen J, Hollenbeck CB, Zhou M-Y, et al. Relation between insulin resistance, hyperinsulinemia, postheparin plasma lipoprotein lipase activity, and postprandial lipemia. Arterioscler Thromb Vasc Biol 1995;15:320–4.

[37] Kim H-S, Abbasi F, Lamendola C, et al. Effect of insulin resistance on postprandial elevations of remnant lipoprotein concentrations in postmenopausal women. Am J Clin Nutr 2001;74:592–5.

[38] Chen Y-DI, Swami S, Skowronski R, et al. Differences in postprandial lipemia between patients with normal glucose tolerance and noninsulin-dependent diabetes mellitus. J Clin Endocrinol Metab 1993;76:172–7.

[39] Ai M, Tanaka A, Ogita K, et al. Relationship between hyperinsulinemia and remnant lipoprotein concentrations in patients with impaired glucose tolerance. J Clin Endocrinol Metab 2000;85:3557–60.

[40] Ai M, Tanaka A, Ogita K, et al. Relationship between plasma insulin concentration and plasma remnant lipoprotein response to an oral fat load in patients with type 2 diabetes. J Am Coll Cardiol 2001;38:1628–32.

[41] McLaughlin T, Abbasi F, Lamendola C, et al. Comparison in patients with type 2 diabetes of fibric acid versus hepatic hydroxymethyl glutaryl-coenzyme A reductase inhibitor treatment of combined dyslipidemia. Metabolism 2002;51:1355–9.

[42] Abbasi F, Chu JW, Lamendola C, et al. Rosuvastatin is efficacious as monotherapy in patients with combined dyslipidemia. J Am Coll Cardiol 2004;43.

[43] Reaven GM, Chen Y-DI, Jeppesen J, et al. Insulin resistance and hyperinsulinemia in individuals with small, dense, low density lipoprotein particles. J Clin Invest 1993;92:141–6.

[44] Austin MA, Breslow JL, Hennekens CH, et al. Low-density lipoprotein subclass patterns and risk of myocardial infarction. JAMA 1988;260:1917–21.

[45] Austin MA, King MC, Vranizan KM, et al. Atherogenic lipoprotein phenotype: a proposed genetic marker for coronary heart disease risk. Circulation 1990;82:495–506.

[46] Swenson TL. The role of the cholesteryl ester transfer protein in lipoprotein metabolism. Diabetes Metab Rev 1991;7:139–53.

[47] Fidge N, Nestel P, Toshitsugu I, et al. Turnover of apoproteins A-I and A-II of high density lipoprotein and the relationship to other lipoproteins in normal and hyperlipidemic individuals. Metabolism 1980;29:643–53.

[48] Chen Y-DI, Sheu WH-H, Swislocki ALM, et al. High density lipoprotein turnover in patients with hypertension. Hypertension 1991;17:386–93.

[49] Golay A, Zech L, Shi M-Z, et al. High density lipoprotein (HDL) metabolism in noninsulin-dependent diabetes mellitus: measurement of HDL turnover using tritiated HDL. J Clin Endocrinol Metab 1987;65:512–8.

[50] Brinton EA, Eisenberg S, Breslow JL. Human HDL cholesterol levels are determined by apoA-I fractional catabolic rate, which correlates inversely with estimates of HDL particle size: effects of gender, hepatic and lipoprotein lipases, triglyceride and insulin levels, and body fat distribution. Arterioscler Thromb 1994;14:707–20.

ELSEVIER
SAUNDERS

Endocrinol Metab Clin N Am
34 (2005) 63–75

ENDOCRINOLOGY
AND METABOLISM
CLINICS
OF NORTH AMERICA

Hypertension Management in Type 2 Diabetes Mellitus: Recommendations of the Joint National Committee VII

Adam Whaley-Connell, DO[a],
James R. Sowers, MD, FACE, FACP, FAHA[a,b,*]

[a]*Department of Internal Medicine, Health Sciences Center,
University of Missouri School of Medicine, MA410,
DC043.00, Columbia, MO 65212, USA*
[b]*Veterans Affairs Medical Center, Columbia, MO 65212, USA*

Type 2 diabetes mellitus (diabetes) is present in epidemic proportions. More than 18 million Americans currently are diagnosed; approximately 73% have concomitant hypertension (HTN) [1]. At the time of diagnosis of diabetes, HTN is present in 50% of diabetic patients [2]. HTN among diabetic patients accelerates progression to renal and cardiovascular disease (CVD); this has spurred intense interest in early and aggressive management of HTN in this population. Recent literature has emphasized that adequate HTN management seldom is achieved; less than 30% of diabetic patients have their blood pressure (BP) controlled at less than 130/80 mm Hg [3,4]. According to the American Diabetes Association (ADA) Clinical Practice Recommendations, as many as 8 million diabetics have undiagnosed HTN [5]. With known underdiagnosis and treatment of HTN in patients who have diabetes, the Joint National Committee on Prevention, Diagnosis, Evaluation, and Treatment of High Blood Pressure (JNC-VII) convened to incorporate this new literature into a simpler, clearer set of guidelines, including those for diabetic patients.

Modifying CVD risk factors has become a major goal in the management of diabetes. HTN contributes substantially to the high CVD morbidity and

Dr. Sowers' research is supported by a Grant from the National Institutes of Health (R01 HL73101-01A1 NIH/NHLBI) and a grant from the Veterans Affairs Research Service (VA Merit Review).

* Corresponding author. Department of Internal Medicine, Health Sciences Center, University of Missouri, MA410, DC043.00, Columbia, MO 65212.

E-mail address: sowersj@health.missouri.edu (J.R. Sowers).

0889-8529/05/$ - see front matter © 2005 Elsevier Inc. All rights reserved.
doi:10.1016/j.ecl.2004.11.007 *endo.theclinics.com*

mortality in patients who have diabetes [2,4,6]. In a recent prospective study that included 12,550 participants, persons who had HTN were almost 2.5 times more likely to develop diabetes than their normotensive counterparts [7]. Early aggressive BP management was shown to decrease CVD mortality in diabetic patients when combined with optimization of the other components of the metabolic syndrome and insulin resistance, such as dyslipidemia (triglycerides > 150 mg/dL, high-density lipoprotein < 40–50 mg/dL), obesity, and hyperglycemia [2,4,6]. The JNC-VII, the National Kidney Foundation, and the ADA all recommend a goal BP of less than 130/80 mm Hg [5,8–10]. The risk for CVD events doubles for each incremental increase of 20 mm Hg in systolic BP and 10 mm Hg of diastolic BP, starting at 115/75 mm Hg [10–12]. The benefits of lowering BP were demonstrated in the United Kingdom Prospective Diabetes Study, which showed that each reduction of systolic BP by 10 mm Hg reduced diabetic complications by 12%, myocardial infarction by 11%, and microvascular complications by 13% [9].

In an effort to lower BP, initial therapy traditionally has been a combination of lifestyle measures and single antihypertensive agent medical therapy. An angiotensin-converting enzyme inhibitor (ACEI) or an angiotensin receptor blocker (ARB) combined with a thiazide diuretic was shown to have significant reno- and cardio-protective properties and has become common for first-line therapy in diabetic patients [4]. Furthermore, studies showed that multiple medications, often three or more, are required to achieve the goal BP of less than 130/80 mm Hg in this patient population [2,4,6,13–15]. In a chart review of patients in Detroit and New York academic medical centers, an average of 3.1 antihypertensive agents was required to reach a goal BP of less than 130/85 mm Hg [2]. This required number of antihypertensives is similar to results of other trials of HTN treatment in type 2 diabetic patients [13–15]. Other medications that have proven to be beneficial in diabetic patients include calcium antagonists and β-blockers (BB), which are considered second-line therapy and are given in addition to the aforementioned agents.

Clinicians should not be deterred from achieving goal BP in their diabetic patients who have HTN, despite the fact that many challenges exist (eg, poor patient adherence, cost of medications, development of comorbidities). It is essential that regular monitoring of BP be done in the supine and the upright positions to recognize under- or overtreatment and to adjust medications. Managing HTN in diabetic persons is challenging, especially with increasing duration of diabetes and the development of kidney disease [16].

Pathophysiology

Diabetes is the leading cause of end stage renal disease and the requirement of dialysis in the United States [16]. Diabetic renal disease, in turn, plays an important role in the pathogenesis of HTN in types 1 and 2 diabetic patients. In diabetic renal disease, hyperglycemia and insulin resistance with dyslipidemia create a state of enhanced oxidative stress that causes endothelial dysfunction and contributes to the pathogenesis of HTN in diabetic patients [4].

The rennin–angiotensin–aldosterone system (RAAS) may play a role in the central adipocytes and in adipocyte differentiation [17]. Agents that induce blockade of the RAAS (Fig. 1) may reduce cardiovascular risk by way of their direct effects on the adipocytes and on the vasculature and reduction of BP [17]. In addition, factors, such as angiotensin-II, endothelin, vasopressin, other growth factors, and oxidative stress, potentiate anatomic and functional abnormalities in the vasculature and extracellular matrix which may be especially important in diabetes [4,17]. For these reasons, RAAS blockade is now considered an important strategy to lessen CVD and renal disease in diabetic patients [4].

In the course of diabetes and HTN, one prominent pathologic consequence is the development of chronic kidney disease (CKD). Stages 1–5 exist for the progression of kidney disease but that discussion is beyond the scope of this article; a few important concepts are reviewed. The development of proteinuria, micro or macro, parallels the progression of CKD and typically progresses over 10 to 15 years [16,18,19]. Micro-albuminuria (MA) is defined as albuminuria that is detected in urine at levels of 30 mg/d to 299 mg/d [20]. If the excretion of albumin exceeds these parameters, macroalbuminuria, or overt proteinuria, is said to exist and heralds even greater CVD risk [16,18,19].

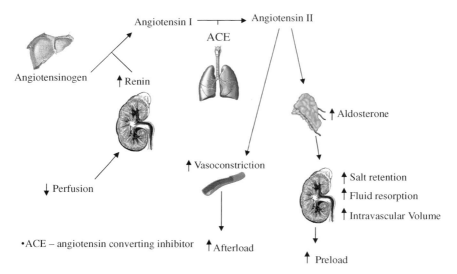

Fig. 1. Flowchart for the rennin–angiotensin–aldosterone system.

MA represents increased permeability of the glomerulus, often paralleling, and therefore a marker of, vascular endothelial dysfunction [21,22]. Furthermore, the presence of MA, alone or with decreased renal function, predicts increased morbidity and mortality [4,22–24]. Patients who develop MA are 20 times more likely to die of a CVD event [22–24].

Diabetic patients often develop microvascular (eg, retinopathy, nephropathy, neuropathy) and macrovascular complications (eg, coronary artery disease [CAD], peripheral vascular disease, cerebrovascular disease). Eighty percent of diabetic patients will succumb to the macrovascular complications [2–4,6]. Concomitant HTN and diabetes accelerate CVD end points, such as CAD, cerebrovascular disease, and stroke.

Evaluation

Often, HTN is not treated adequately in the United States, especially in the diabetic and elderly populations [2–4,6]. In evaluating patients for treatment of HTN, accurate BP measurement is necessary; the auscultatory method is preferred (Box 1). If HTN is detected during an office visit, especially in a patient who has diabetes, the clinician should check at least two measurements with a size appropriate cuff. It is paramount that initiation of medical therapy be prompt once HTN is documented in a diabetic patient.

The new JNC-VII guidelines have attempted to simplify the classification scheme for HTN (Table 1). In addition, the Committee identified a new population of patients, the prehypertensive. These patients have a systolic BP of 120 mm Hg to 139 mm Hg or a diastolic BP of 80 mm Hg to 89 mm Hg. The Committee combined what previously had been labeled as stages II and III HTN. Identification of the prehypertensive subgroup was based upon this

---

Box 1. Methods of blood pressure evaluation

- In-office: patient sitting in chair, two readings 5 minutes apart with a size appropriate cuff and using auscultatory method. Confirm in contralateral arm.
- Ambulatory BP monitoring: evaluation of "white-coat HTN." Absence of "nocturnal dipping" (10%–20% decrease in BP during sleep).
- Patient self-check: useful in determining response to therapy and improving adherence. Evaluation of "white-coat HTN."

Adapted from Chobanian AV, Bakris GL, Black HR, et al. Seventh Report of the Joint National Committee on Prevention, Detection, Evaluation, and Treatment of High Blood Pressure. Hypertension 2003;42:1206–52.

Table 1
Joint National Committee VII blood pressure classification scheme

| Category | Blood pressure (mm Hg) | |
	Systolic	Diastolic
Normal	<120	and <80
Pre-HTN	120–139	or 80–89
Stage 1 HTN	140–1549	or 90–99
Stage 2 HTN	≥160	or ≥100

Adapted from Chobanian AV, Bakris GL, Black HR, et al. Seventh report of the Joint National Committee on Prevention, Detection, Evaluation, and Treatment of High Blood Pressure. Hypertension 2003;42:1206–52.

population's predilection for developing more advanced HTN and the value of instituting lifestyle changes at this level of BP. One of the major contributions in the JNC-VII recommendations is the need for earlier and more aggressive combination therapy. If the BP is more than 20/10 mm Hg over goal on both checks, initiation with two-drug therapy is appropriate and should be instituted on that visit, in addition to education regarding lifestyle modifications [11]. Lifestyle modifications include smoking cessation, weight loss, the "Dietary Approaches to Stop Hypertension" (DASH) eating plan, increasing activity level, and reducing alcohol consumption [25–27].

Clinicians often delay making a diagnosis of HTN and opt to have patients check their BP at home or do ambulatory BP monitoring to evaluate for possible "white coat" HTN. Although these tools are not needed to make a diagnosis of HTN, they may be useful to determine the presence of drug resistance and evaluate hypotensive symptoms, episodic HTN, or autonomic dysfunction. In diabetic patients, autonomic dysfunction is common and manifests most often as orthostatic or postural hypotension.

Because of the increased propensity of diabetic patients to manifest orthostatic BP changes, measurements of BP should be performed in the supine and standing positions [2–4,6]. Postural hypotension is defined as a decrease in systolic BP of more than 20 mm Hg when associated with orthostatic signs and symptoms, such as lightheadedness/dizziness, dimming of vision, nausea, or diaphoresis [4]. In true autonomic neuropathy, a compensatory increase in pulse rate of more than 15 beats per minute should not be evident. Although the presence of postural hypotension in diabetic patients suggests autonomic dysfunction, other possible treatable causes should be considered, such as volume depletion, medications, and cardiac or metabolic etiologies. As discussed below, in diabetic patients who have autonomic dysfunction, one should be cautious in the use of diuretics and veno/vasodilators (eg, nitrates, α and central adrenergic blockers).

Other characteristics of HTN that are associated with diabetes include a "disproportionate elevation in systolic BP and a loss of nocturnal dipping of BP and heart rate" [4]. This "nondipping" seems to be due, in part, to dysautonomia that often is present in diabetic patients. This dysautonomia is characterized by reduced relative parasympathetic activity and may contribute to the fivefold to sevenfold increase in sudden death in diabetic patients [4].

Treatment

After HTN is confirmed, pharmacologic and nonpharmacologic interventions should be implemented right away [4]. For the prehypertensive, instituting lifestyle modification is paramount, along with some consideration of medication therapy (Fig. 2).

Weight reduction and increased aerobic activity are considered essential in treating the metabolic syndrome; both strategies were shown to improve HTN, insulin resistance, and dyslipidemia [25–27]. Adopting the DASH eating plan, which consists of a low sodium, high potassium, low calorie (800–1500/d), and high fiber should be a part of the treatment regimen [26]. Coupled with diet, increased physical activity, such as walking or reducing sedentary time is necessary [27]. Thirty to 45 minutes of walking three to five days a week was shown to improve lipid profiles, BP, and insulin resistance [25–27].

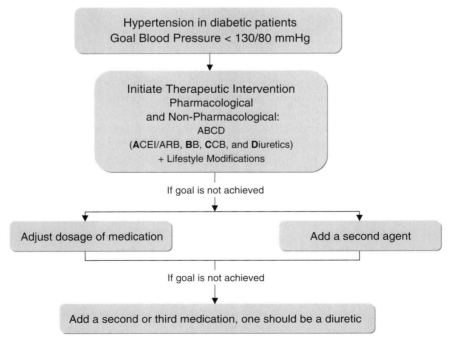

Fig. 2. Algorithm for antihypertensive therapy. Lifestyle modifications should emphasize weight reduction, increased activity, and smoking cessation. CCB, calcium channel blocker.

The United Kingdom Prospective Diabetes Study (UKPDS) demonstrated that tight BP control may be more of a benefit than tight glycemic control for CV outcomes in type 2 diabetics [13].

Diabetic patients who have HTN are a particularly high-risk group with regard to complications. In an analysis from a health maintenance organization in California, the cost of care for this group was six times higher than at baseline [28]. A 1% reduction in A1c, from 10% to 9%, produced a cost savings in diabetics; however, the cost savings that were noted in those who had diabetes that was complicated by HTN and CVD was more than $4000 for the same 1% reduction in glycosulated hemoglobin (HbA1c). Thus, it is possible that more intensive control of glycemia, HTN, and dyslipidemia will be most cost effective in the most high-risk population. In a recent report from the Centers for Disease Control Diabetes Cost-Effectiveness Group, similar findings were demonstrated with intensive glycemic and hypertensive control [29]. This group's model of analysis was similar to that of the UKPDS; their outcome measure in cost per quality-adjusted life-year gained in 1997 U.S. dollars resulted in similar cost savings of more than $4000.

Drug therapy

Angiotensin-converting enzyme inhibitors

There is significant evidence that interruption of the RAAS can provide cardioprotection. Data from trials, such as the Captopril Prevention Project; the Losartan Intervention For Endpoint reduction; and the Micro-HOPE, a substudy of the Heart Outcomes Prevention Evaluation (HOPE) trial, showed that ACEI may provide cardiovascular benefits as well as possible improvement in insulin resistance and prevention of diabetes [14,15,30–32]. Most notably, ACEIs also demonstrated the ability to slow progression of nephropathy in microalbuminuric, normotensive type 2 diabetics [33] as compared with other antihypertensives [33,34].

The mechanisms of ACEI to preserve kidney function seem to include antihypertensive effects and a reduction in membrane permeability to albumin, mesangial matrix expansion, and intraglomerular pressure [10,35]. Combined, these properties can lead to an ability to reduce proteinuria. In addition to the previously discussed benefits that RAAS blockade may have on adipocytes and obesity, this mechanism also can be implicated in the increasing data that these agents have a direct effect on improvement of insulin sensitivity [2,4,5].

After initiation of therapy, monitoring of renal function and potassium is imperative; however, a slight increase in serum creatinine (Cr) may be expected, usually secondary to intravascular depletion [36]. In the absence of heart failure, if there is an increase in serum Cr by more than 30% or a continual increase within the first 2 months of therapy, bilateral renal artery stenosis or chronic volume depletion should be excluded [10,36]. Most cases of inordinate increases in Cr are caused by volume depletion and are corrected by normalizing volume status [36].

Angiotensin receptor blockers

Other medications that have received considerable attention in recent years are the ARBs. Specifically, ARBs block the angiotensin-I receptor that is responsible for the effects of angiotensin-II [31,37–39]. ARB antihypertensive efficacy is roughly equivalent to ACEI; however, they have an improved side effect profile as compared with ACEIs—in particular, a much reduced incidence of cough [31,37–39]. RAAS blockade with an ACEI or an ARB may reduce the incidence of new-onset diabetes compared with other antihypertensive medication, such as BBs or thiazides [4,37]. ARBs also are effective in reducing renal disease progression and were shown to reduce albuminuria and time to Cr doubling in the studies, Reduction of Endpoint in NIDDM with Losartan (RENAAL) and the Irbesartan in Diabetic Nephropathy Trial [31,38]. This was shown again in Irbesartan in Microalbuminuria II, but only with reducing the progression of nephropathy, not in slowing progression of the decline of Cr clearance [40]. These studies have yet to elucidate whether the use of an ARB is comparable to an ACEI in diabetic patients who have early stage nephropathy. In patients who have nephrotic syndrome, there is evidence that combination therapy is beneficial in reducing the level of proteinuria [41]. ARBs were shown to be equal to ACEI in patients who had left ventricular hypertrophy, heart failure, and post-myocardial infarction [37]. Use of these agents might be expected to lead to reduced CVD risk and improved outcomes.

Thiazide diuretics

Other agents with significant data to support their use in hypertensive diabetics are low-dose thiazides. Thiazides were shown to reduce cardiovascular events and slow renal disease progression [11,42]. In the largest hypertensive study to date, the Antihypertensive and Lipid-Lowering treatment to prevent Heart Attack Trial (ALLHAT) looked at ACEI or calcium-channel blockers versus diuretics. It was confirmed that thiazide diuretics comparably reduce all-cause mortality, such as stroke, CAD, and heart failure [35]. ALLHAT also confirmed that thiazides should be considered as first-line therapy for many hypertensive patients [10,35]. The use of chlorthalidone has been controversial as a result of the increased incidence of new diabetes in the chlorthalidone group, compared with the amlodipine or lisinopril groups. In clinical practice, chlorothiazide and hydrochlorthiazide have replaced chlorthalidone.

It is important to understand the CVD risk that is associated with new onset diabetes in patients who have HTN who are on treatment. The report of Verdecchia et al [43] addressed this issue and discovered two important findings. First, the use of diuretics and the baseline plasma glucose were independent predictors of new onset diabetes after 6 years. Second, the occurrence of new onset diabetes in patients who had treated HTN conveyed a risk that was statistically similar to that of the patients who had HTN and diabetes at the beginning of the study. It is now believed that CVD disease risk starts well before the recognized clinical onset of diabetes.

Unlike at higher dosages, at lower dosages, electrolyte disturbances and adverse effects on lipid and carbohydrate metabolism are uncommon with thiazide therapy [4]; however, diuretics were shown to worsen insulin resistance and it is known that hyperinsulinemia promotes salt retention which potentiates a volume-expanded state for diabetics [4,35]. Nevertheless, using a thiazide diuretic in the antihypertensive repertoire consistently improved cardiovascular outcomes, even in those who had diabetes [23].

Calcium antagonists

It was shown that nondihydropyridine calcium antagonists (NDHPCA), such as verapamil and diltiazem, confer a significant degree of renal protection. Not to the degree of ACEI alone, but in combination therapy, NHDPCA and ACEI had additive effects of reducing albuminuria [44]. There is recent evidence from ALLHAT [37] and RENAAL [31] that dihydropyridine calcium antagonists also are nephroprotective, especially when used in conjunction with RAAS inhibitors. Thus, calcium antagonists often are useful as second- or third-line therapy, in addition to the above-mentioned agents [4,5].

β-Blockers

BBs are effective agents in the diabetic population that has HTN, especially in patients who have concomitant micro- and macrovascular complications. This was demonstrated in the UKPDS, wherein atenolol was comparable to captopril in reduction of cardiovascular outcomes [13,28]. Despite this evidence, BB use often is complicated by side effects, such as adverse effects on glucose and lipid profiles; they have been implicated in new-onset diabetes in obese patients [45,46]. This drug class is further complicated by peripheral vasoconstriction that can compromise the peripheral circulation; however, using vasodilating BBs, such as carvedilol, induced vasodilatation and improved insulin sensitivity [47–49].

Most BB use is in diabetics who have evidence of CAD, such as anginal symptoms, including anginal equivalents, or postmyocardial infarction [4,50,51]. BBs, such as carvedilol and atenolol, were demonstrated to reduce albuminuria, especially in combination with RAAS blockade [52]. Carvedilol even was shown to reduce progression of nephropathy [53]. Despite concerns, BBs are safe to use in diabetics who have HTN, especially in those who have ischemic heart disease or congestive heart failure [4,5].

α-Antagonists

α-Antagonists also may be used in diabetic HTN. Despite conflicting literature, these agents are noted to be at least neutral or to improve the glucose and lipid profiles relative to BBs or thiazide diuretics [54]. Their benefit in slowing progression of renal disease does not extend beyond what would be expected from their effect on BP alone.

Summary

HTN in patients who have diabetes should be managed aggressively; the goal BP of less than 130/80 mm Hg should be attained if clinicians seek to reduce cardiovascular morbidity and mortality for these patients. Along with instituting medical therapy after HTN is detected, lifestyle modifications need to be managed aggressively, together with strict glycemic and lipid control. Early management and optimization of treatment of HTN can delay and possibly prevent progression of cardiovascular complications, such as CAD, CKD, peripheral vascular disease, and cerebrovascular disease. Studied approaches to treat HTN in diabetics have included ACEIs and ARBs. Either class of medication, generally in combination with a thiazide diuretic, should be considered as initial therapy [4,10]. Calcium antagonists, BBs, and α-antagonists also have a role in this population of patients, usually as third- and fourth-line add-ons. The importance of using agents that block RAAS is becoming understood better. Typically, three or more antihypertensive medications plus lifestyle interventions are required to achieve a goal BP of less than 130/80 mm Hg.

Managing patients who have diabetes and HTN is a dynamic, ever-changing challenge. Early and aggressive antihypertensive therapy pays off; it is hoped that the insights in this article enable clinicians to meet the challenge more successfully.

References

[1] American Diabetes Association National Diabetes Fact Sheet. Available at: http://www.diabetes.org/diabetes-statistics/national-diabetes-fact-sheet.jsp. Accessed on May 24, 2004.

[2] McFarlane S, Gizycki HV, Winer N, et al. Control of cardiovascular risk factors in patients with diabetes and hypertension at urban academic medical centers. Diabetes Care 2002;25:718–23.

[3] McFarlane SI, Banerji M, Sowers JR. Insulin resistance and cardiovascular disease. J Clin Endocrinol Metab 2001;86(2):713–8.

[4] Sowers JR. Recommendations for special populations: diabetes mellitus and the metabolic syndrome. Am J Hypertens 2003;16(11):41S–5S.

[5] American Diabetes Association. Hypertension management in adults with diabetes: clinical practice recommendations 2004. Diabetes Care 2004;27(Suppl 1):S65–7.

[6] Bakris GL, Williams M, Dworkin L, et al. Preserving renal function in adults with hypertension and diabetes: a consensus approach. National Kidney Foundation Hypertension and Diabetes Executive Committees Working Group. Am J Kidney Dis 2000;36: 646–61.

[7] Gress TW, Nieto FJ, Shahar E, et al. Hypertension and antihypertensive therapy as risk factors for type 2 diabetes mellitus: Atherosclerosis Risk in Communities Study. N Engl J Med 2000;342:905–12.

[8] Sowers JR. Diabetic nephropathy and concomitant hypertension: a review of recent ADA recommendations. Am J Clin Proc 2002;3:27–33.

[9] American Diabetes Association. Treatment of hypertension in adults with diabetes: clinical practice recommendations 2002. Diabetes Care 2002;25(Suppl 1):S71–89.

[10] Chobanian AV, Bakris GL, Black HR, et al. Seventh Report of the Joint National Committee on Prevention, Detection, Evaluation, and Treatment of High Blood Pressure. Hypertension 2003;42:1206–52.

[11] Mann JF, Gerstein HC, Yi QL, et al. Development of renal disease in people at high cardiovascular risk: results of the HOPE randomized study. J Am Soc Nephrol 2003;14: 641–7.

[12] Lewington S, Clarke R, Qizilbash N, et al. Age-specific relevance of usual blood pressure to vascular mortality. A meta-analysis of individual data for one-million adults in 61 prospective studies. Lancet 2002;360:1903–13.

[13] UKPDS Group. UK Prospective Diabetes Study 38: tight blood pressure control and risk of macrovascular and microvascular complications in type 2 diabetes. BMJ 1998;317: 703–17.

[14] Hansson L, Lindholm LH, Niskanen L, et al. Effect of angiotensin-converting-enzyme inhibition compared with conventional therapy on cardiovascular morbidity and mortality in hypertension; the Captopril Prevention Project (CAPP) randomized trial. Lancet 1999; 353:611–6.

[15] Yusuf S, Sleight P, Pogue J, et al. Effects of an angiotensin-converting enzyme inhibitor, ramipril, on cardiovascular events in high-risk patients: the Heart Outcomes Prevention Evaluation. N Engl J Med 2000;342:145–53.

[16] Eknoyan G, Hostetter T, Bakris GL, et al. Proteinuria and other markers of chronic kidney disease: a position statement of the National Kidney Foundation (NKF) and The National Institute of Diabetes and Digestive and Kidney Diseases (NIDDK). Am J Kidney Dis 2003; 42:617–22.

[17] Janke J, Engeli S, Gorzelniak K, et al. Mature adipocytes inhibit in vitro differentiation of human preadipocytes via angiotensin type 1 receptors. Diabetes 2002;51:1699–707.

[18] Dineen SF, Gerstein HC. The association of microalbuminuria and mortality in non-insulin-dependent diabetes mellitus: a systematic overview of the literature. Arch Intern Med 1997; 157:1413–8.

[19] Bakris GL. Microalbuminuria: prognosticator implications. Curr Opin Nephrol Hypertens 1996;5:219–23.

[20] American Diabetes Asssociation. Nephropathy in diabetes: clinical practice recommendations 2004. Diabetes Care 2004;27(Suppl 1):S79–83.

[21] Bakris GL, Walsh MF, Sowers JR. Endothelium/mesangium interactions: role of insulin-like growth factors. In: Sowers JR, editor. Endocrinology of the vasculature. Totowa (NJ): Humana; 1996. p. 341–56.

[22] Garg JP, Bakris GL. Microalbuminuria: marker of vascular dysfunction, risk factor for cardiovascular disease. Vasc Med 2002;7:35–43.

[23] Ljungman S, Wikstrand J, Hartford M, et al. Urinary albumin excretion—a predictor of risk of cardiovascular disease. A prospective 10 year follow-up of middle-aged non-diabetic normal and hypertensive men. Am J Hypertens 1996;9:770–8.

[24] Kidney Disease Outcome Quality Initiative clinical practice guidelines for chronic kidney disease: evaluation, classification, and stratification. Am J Kidney Dis 2002;39:S1–246.

[25] Halbert JA, Silagy CA, Finucane P, et al. Exercise training and blood lipid levels in hyperlipidemic and normolipidemic adults: a meta-analysis of randomized, controlled trials. Eur J Clin Nutr 1999;53:514–22.

[26] Sacks FM, Svetky LP, Vollmer WM, et al. Effects on blood pressure of reduced dietary sodium and the Dietary Approaches to Stop Hypertension (DASH) diet. DASH-Sodium Collaborative Research Group. N Engl J Med 2001;344:3–10.

[27] Whelton SP, Chin A, Xin X, et al. Effect of aerobic exercise on blood pressure: a meta-analysis of randomized, controlled trials. Ann Intern Med 2002;136:493–503.

[28] UKPDS Group. Efficacy of atenolol and captopril in reducing risk of macrovascular and microvascular complications in type 2 diabetes. BMJ 1998;317:713–20.

[29] Cost-effectiveness of Intensive Glycemic Control. Intensified hypertension control, and serum cholesterol reduction for type 2 diabetes. CDC Diabetes Cost-effectiveness Group. JAMA 2002;287(19):2542–51.

[30] Effects of ramipril on cardiovascular and microvascular outcomes in peoples with diabetes mellitus: results of the HOPR study and MICRO-HOPE substudy. Lancet 2000; 355:253–9.

[31] Brenner BM, Cooper ME, de Zeeuw D, et al. Effects of losartan on renal and cardiovascular outcomes in patients with type 2 diabetes and nephropathy. New Engl J Med 2001;345: 861–9.

[32] Dahlof B, Devereux R, Kjeldsen S, et al. Cardiovascular morbidity and mortality in the Losartan Intervention For Endpoint Reduction in Hypertension Study, a randomised trial against atenolol. Lancet 2002;359:995–1003.

[33] Ravid M, Archmani R, Lishner M. Long-term renoprotective effect of angiotensin-converting enzyme inhibition in non-insulin dependent diabetes mellitus; A 7-year follow-up study. Arch Intern Med 1996;156:286–9.

[34] Bakris GL, Smith AC, Richardson DJ, et al. Impact of an ACE inhibitor and calcium antagonist on microalbuminuria and lipid subfractions in type 2 diabetes: a randomized, multi-center pilot study. J Hum Hypertens 2002;16:185–91.

[35] Major outcomes in high-risk hypertensive patients randomized to angiotensin-converting-enzyme inhibitor or calcium channel blocker vs diuretic: The Antihypertensive and Lipid-Lowering Treatment to Prevent Heart Attack Trial (ALLHAT). JAMA 2002;288:2981–97.

[36] Bakris GL, Weir MR. Angiotensin-converting enzyme inhibitor associated elevations in serum creatinine: is this a cause for concern? Arch Intern Med 2000;160:685–93.

[37] Pfeffer MA, McMurray JJ, Velazquez EJ, et al. Valsartan, captopril or both in myocardial infarction complicated by heart failure, left ventricular dysfunction, or both. N Engl J Med 2001;349:1893–906.

[38] Lewis EJ, Hunsicker LG, Clarke WR, et al. Renoprotective effect of the angiotensin-receptor antagonist irbesartan in patients with nephropathy due to type 2 diabetes. N Engl J Med 2001;345:851–60.

[39] Bakris GL, Weir MR, Shanifar S, et al. Effects of blood pressure level on progression of diabetic nephropathy: results form the RENAAL study. Arch Intern Med 2003;163: 1555–65.

[40] Parving HH, Lehnert H, Brochner-Mortensen J, et al. The effect of irbesartan on the development of diabetic nephropathy in patients with type 2 diabetes. N Engl J Med 2001; 345(12):870–8.

[41] Ferrari P, Marti HP, Pfister M, Frey FJ. Additive antiproteinuric effect of combined ACE inhibition and angiotensin II receptor blockade. J Hypertens 2002;20(1):125–30.

[42] Curb JD, Pressel SL, Cutler JA, et al for the Systolic Hypertension in the Elderly Program. (SHEP) Cooperative Research Group. Effect of diuretic-based antihypertensive treatment on cardiovascular disease risk in older diabetic patients with isolated systolic hypertension. JAMA 1996;276:1886–92.

[43] Verdecchia P, Borgioni C, Angeli F, et al. Adverse prognostic significance of new onset diabetes in treated hypertensive subjects. Hypertension 2004;43:963–9.

[44] Bakris GL, Weir MR, DeQuattro V, et al. Effects of an ACE inhibitor/calcium antagonist combination on proteinuria in diabetic nephropathy. Kidney Int 1998;54:1283–9.

[45] Mykkanen L, Kuusisto J, Pyorala K, et al. Increased risk of non-insulin-dependent diabetes mellitus in elderly hypertensive patients. J Hypertens 1994;12:1425–32.

[46] Gress TW, Nieto FJ, Shahar E, et al. Hypertension and antihypertensive therapy as risk factors for type 2 diabetes mellitus. Atherosclerosis Risk in Communities Study. N Engl J Med 2000;342:905–12.

[47] Jacob S, Rett K, Wickelmayr M, et al. Differential effect of chronic treatment with two beta-blocking agents on insulin sensitivity: the carvedilol-metoprolol study. J Hypertens 1996;14: 489–94.

[48] Jacob S, Balletshofer B, Henriksen EJ, et al. Beta-blocking agents in patients with insulin resistance: effects of vasodilating beta-blockers. Blood Press 1999;8:261–8.

[49] Giugliano D, Acampora R, Marfella R, et al. Metabolic and cardiovascular effects of carvedilol and atenolol in non-insulin-dependent diabetes mellitus and hypertension. A randomised, controlled trial. Ann Intern Med 1997;126:955–9.

[50] Dargie HJ. Effect of carvedilol on outcome after myocardial infarction in patients with left-ventricular dysfunction: the CAPRICORN randomized trial. Lancet 2001;357:1385–90.

[51] Poole-Wilson PA, Swedberg K, Cleland JG, et al. Comparison of carvedilol and metoprolol on clinical outcomes in patients with chronic heart failure in the Carvedilol Or Metoprolol European Trial (COMET): a randomized controlled trial. Lancet 2003;362:7–13.

[52] Giugliano D, Acampora R, Marfella R, et al. Metabolic and cardiovascular effects of carvedilol and atenolol in non-insulin-dependent diabetes mellitus and hypertension. A randomised, controlled trial. Ann Intern Med 1997;126:955–9.

[53] Fassbinder W, Quarder O, Waltz A. Treatment with carvedilol is associated with a significant reduction in microalbuminuria: a multi-center, randomized study. Int J Clin Pract 1999;53: 519–20.

[54] Bakris GL, Weir MR, Sowers JR. Therapeutic challenges in the obese diabetic patients with hypertension. Am J Med 1996;101:33S–46S.

ELSEVIER
SAUNDERS

Endocrinol Metab Clin N Am
34 (2005) 77–98

ENDOCRINOLOGY
AND METABOLISM
CLINICS
OF NORTH AMERICA

Glycemic Management of Type 2 Diabetes: An Emerging Strategy with Oral Agents, Insulins, and Combinations

Matthew C. Riddle, MD

Division of Endocrinology, Diabetes, and Clinical Nutrition,
Oregon Health and Science University, 3181 SW Sam Jackson Park Drive,
Portland, OR 97239-3098, USA

We have long known, but now understand more fully that type 2 diabetes is common, complex, and as treated presently, leads to severe medical consequences. In type 1 diabetes, hyperglycemia is the leading cause of harm. In type 2 diabetes, despite a well-documented contribution from other abnormalities that together have come to be known as the metabolic syndrome, hyperglycemia also contributes greatly to illness. Doubts as to whether treating hyperglycemia can improve medical outcomes in type 2 diabetes have been dispelled by the findings of the Kumamoto Study and the United Kingdom Prospective Diabetes Study (UKPDS) [1–3]. Moreover, in the last decade, the number of classes of antihyperglycemic agents that were approved in the United States for treating this disorder has increased from two (insulin secretagogues, insulin) to five (metformin, α-glucosidase inhibitors [AGIs], thiazolidinediones [TZDs]). Within each class, the individual choices have multiplied.

Despite these events, glycemic control in type 2 diabetes in the United States has not improved. The most recent analysis from the National Health and Nutrition Evaluation Survey shows a trend toward worsening of the mean glycohemoglobin (A1c) of patients who are known to have diabetes, from 7.6% (1988–1994) to 7.8% (1999–2000) [4]. Moreover, studies of groups of patients in well-organized health systems confirm that pharmacotherapy generally is started late and not titrated aggressively. For example, a recent report found that patients typically were started on

The author has received honoraria for consulting services or lecture presentations, or research grant support from the following manufacturers of products that are used for treating diabetes: Amylin, Sanofi-Aventis, GlaxoSmithKline, Lilly, and NovoNordisk.

E-mail address: riddlem@ohsu.edu

0889-8529/05/$ - see front matter © 2005 Elsevier Inc. All rights reserved.
doi:10.1016/j.ecl.2004.12.002

a single oral agent only when A1c averaged 8.7% and had been greater than 8% for an average of 9 months [5]. A second oral agent was added to metformin when A1c averaged 8.8% (after 15 months of exposure to A1c that was greater than 8%) or to a sulfonylurea when A1c averaged 9.1% (21 months greater than 8%). Insulin was started when, on metformin plus sulfonylurea, A1c averaged 9.6% (23 months greater than 8%). In another health system, insulin was started when A1c averaged 9.3% and the resulting improvement after a year was only to 8.4%; this was close to the mean value for their insulin-using patients overall [6].

Presumably, multiple factors underlie this nationwide failure of therapy, which is likely to be similar in most countries. These include financial constraints; reluctance of patients to use some therapies, notably insulin; and lack of conviction by medical providers (and perhaps more important, by reimbursers) that treating diabetes is effective and worthwhile. Lack of agreement on a simple and evidence-based strategy for pharmacotherapy has been another barrier. This article reviews available pharmacotherapeutic options, discusses some principles of treatment, and proposes a unified strategy.

Antihyperglycemic agents

Table 1 shows the classes of antihyperglycemic agents that are available in the United States, including different formulations and dosages. It is a long list, and most formulary managers and physicians will select only a subset for routine use. Table 2 lists formulations in which two individual agents are combined. Table 3 displays several important properties of each class of agents. Excellent reviews provide more detailed information on these agents and their use [7–16].

Mechanisms of action

Each class has a distinctive mechanism of action. The insulin secreta-gogues—sulfonylureas and two nonsulfonylurea agents (repaglinide and nateglinide)—bind to elements of the ATP-dependent potassium channel complex in membranes of pancreatic β cells [17]. By doing so they potentiate glucose-dependent insulin secretion (especially when used chronically), or provoke insulin secretion independent of current glucose levels with the potential to cause hypoglycemia (especially when used initially or in-termittently). They are less effective or ineffective when the mass of β cells is reduced or their function is impaired. Metformin acts mainly at the liver to reduce hepatic glucose production by a mechanism that is not understood completely [18]. In effect, it potentiates the suppressive effects of insulin on hepatic glucose production. Metformin also can prevent weight gain or lead

Table 1
Antihyperglycemic agents widely available in the United States

Agent	Trade name/generic brand	Dosage(s)
Secretagogues		
Sulfonylureas		
Chlorpropamide	Diabinese (Pfizer, New York, NY)	100 mg, 250 mg
	Generic	100 mg, 250 mg
Glimepiride	Amaryl (Sanofi-Aventis, Bridgewater, NJ)	1 mg, 2 mg, 4 mg
Glipizide	Glucotrol (Pfizer)	5 mg, 10 mg
	Glucotrol XL (Pfizer)	2.5 mg, 5 mg, 10 mg
	Generic glipizide	5 mg, 10 mg
	Generic glipizide XL	2.5 mg, 5 mg, 10 mg
Glyburide	DiaBeta (Sanofi-Aventis)	1.25 mg, 2.5 mg, 5 mg
	Glynase (Pharmacia-Upjohn [Pfizer])	1.5 mg, 3 mg, 6 mg
	Micronase (Pharmacia-Upjohn [Pfizer])	1.25 mg, 2.5 mg, 5 mg
	Generic	1.25 mg, 2.5 mg, 5 mg
	Generic micronized	1.5 mg, 3 mg, 6 mg
Tolazamide	Tolinase (Pharmacia-Upjohn [Pfizer])	100 mg, 250 mg, 500 mg
	Generic	100 mg, 250 mg, 500 mg
Tolbutamide	Orinase (Pharmacia-Upjohn [Pfizer])	500 mg
	Generic	500 mg
Non-sulfonylurea secretagogues		
	Nateglinide Starlix (Novartis, East Hanover, NJ)	60 mg, 120 mg
	Repaglinide Prandin (NovoNordisk, Princeton, NJ)	0.5 mg, 1 mg, 2 mg
Biguanide		
Metformin	Glucophage (Bristol-Myers Squibb, Lawrenceville, NJ)	500 mg, 850 mg, 1000 mg
	Glucophage XR (Bristol-Myers Squibb, Lawrenceville, NJ)	500 mg, 750 mg, 1000 mg
	Generic	500 mg, 850 mg, 1000 mg
α-Glucosidase inhibitors		
Acarbose	Precose (Bayer)	25 mg, 50 mg, 100 mg
Miglitol	Glyset (Pharmacia-Upjohn [Pfizer])	25 mg, 50 mg, 100 mg
Thiazolidinediones		
Pioglitazone	Actos (Takeda, Linconshire, IL)	15 mg, 30 mg, 45 mg
Rosiglitazone	Avandia (GlaxoSmithKline, Philadelphia, PA)	2 mg, 4 mg, 8 mg
Long-acting insulins		
NPH	Humulin N (Lilly, Indianapolis, IN)	10-mL vial, 3-mL pen
	Novolin N (NovoNordisk)	10-mL vial, 3-mL pen
Lente	Humulin L (Lilly)	10-mL vial
Ultralente	Humulin U (Lilly)	10-mL vial
Glargine	Lantus (Sanofi-Aventis)	10-mL vial
Short- or rapid-acting insulins		
Regular	Humulin R (Lilly)	100 U/mL: 10-mL vial; 500 U/mL: 20-mL vial
	Novolin R (NovoNordisk)	10-mL vial, 3-mL cartridge
Aspart	Novolog (NovoNordisk)	10-mL vial, 3-mL cartridge, 3-mL pen
Lispro	Humalog (Lilly)	10-mL vial, 3-mL pen

Abbreviation: NPH, neutral protamine Hagedorn.

Table 2
Combined formulations of antihyperglycemic agents available in the United States

Agent	Trade name	Dosage(s)
Secretagogue + metformin		
Glipzide + metformin	Metaglip (Bristol-Myers Squibb)	2.5 mg/250 mg
		2.5 mg/500 mg
		5 mg/500 mg
Glyburide + metformin	Glucovance (Bristol-Myers Squibb)	1.25 mg/250 mg
		2.5 mg/500 mg
		5 mg/500 mg
Thiazolidinedione + metformin		
Rosiglitazone + metformin	Avandamet (GlaxoSmithKline)	1 mg/500 mg
		2 mg/500 mg
		4 mg/500 mg
		2 mg/1000 mg
		4 mg/1000 mg
Long-acting with short or rapid-acting insulins		
NPH + regular	Humulin 70/30 (Lilly)	3-mL pen
	Humulin 50/50 (Lilly)	10-mL vial
	Novolin 70/30 (NovoNordisk)	10-mL vial,
		3-mL cartridge
Analogue mixtures		
Protamine aspart + aspart	Novolog 70/30 (NovoNordisk)	10-mL vial, 3-mL pen
Protamine lispro + lispro	Humalog mix 75/25 (Lilly)	10-mL vial, 3-mL pen

to weight loss, in some cases as a result of unpleasant gastrointestinal side effects, but also in many patients who do not have such symptoms [19,20]. AGIs act within the intestinal lumen to impair the action of enzymes that digest complex carbohydrates and some disaccharides, thereby delaying their absorption until food has passed further down the small intestine [21]. When the balance of AGI dosage and carbohydrate load is correct, this action blunts postprandial increments of glucose without unwanted effects. Beyond their effect on glycemic patterns, AGIs may have favorable effects on the secretion of gut peptides, such as glucagon-like peptide (GLP)-1 [22]. TZDs bind to the peroxisome-proliferator–activated receptor-γ and the resulting complex alters expression of many genes. The best understood effects of this process are cellular replication and an increase of sensitivity to insulin in adipose tissue [23]. Treatment with TZDs suppresses release of free fatty acids and increases secretion of the hormone, adiponectin [24,25], with resulting favorable effects on insulin sensitivity in the liver and in muscle. Injected insulin has multiple effects on fuel metabolism. At low blood levels it suppresses endogenous glucose production (mainly in the liver, but also in the kidney) by direct effects on these tissues and by reducing mobilization of free fatty acids and glycerol from adipose tissue and amino acids from muscle; all of these favor endogenous glucose production [26,27]. At increased levels, such as are normally seen after meals, insulin promotes glucose uptake by muscle [27].

Table 3
Some properties of classes of antihyperglycemic agents

Parameter	Secretagogues	Metformin	AGIs	TZDs	Insulins
Mechanism of action	Potentiate insulin secretion	Suppresses liver glucose production	Delay intestinal CHO absorbtion	Improve insulin sensitivity (fat, liver, and muscle)	Suppress glucose production; enhance glucose uptake
A1c reduction (%)	1.5–2.0	1.5–2.0	0.5–1.0	0.75–2.0	Limited by hypoglycemia only
Adverse effects	Hypoglycemia, weight gain	Nausea, diarrhea, lactic acidosis	Flatulence, diarrhea	Edema, congestive heart failure, weight gain, anemia	Hypoglycemia, weight gain
Nonglycemic effects	None	Reduces CV risk markers; limits weight gain	Reduce CV risk markers	Reduce CV risk markers	Reduce CV risk markers
Evidence for benefit					
Microvascular	Strong	Strong	None	None	Strong
Macrovascular	None	Moderate	Weak	Weak	Moderate

Abbreviation: CHO, carbohydrate.

Effect on A1c

Most oral antihyperglycemic agents can reduce A1c by 1.5% to 2.0% from a typical baseline of 8.5% to 9.5% [7–9]. Specifically, the sulfonylureas; the nonsulfonylurea secretagogue, repaglinide; metformin; and the TZDs, pioglitazone and rosiglitazone, all have this ability, depending on the baseline A1c (see later discussion). By comparison, the AGIs, acarbose and miglitol, and the nonsulfonylurea secretagogue, nateglinide, typically reduce A1c by 0.5% to 1.0%. Insulin has unlimited ability to reduce glucose levels, but its clinical efficacy is limited in practice by the risk of hypoglycemia, especially when it is delivered in nonphysiologic patterns. Reductions of A1c by 2.0% or more may occur when insulin is started for type 2 diabetes, however [28].

Complicating the general statements above is the observation that the reduction of A1c is affected by the starting value—the greater the baseline, the greater the therapeutic effect. This is due, in part, to regression to the mean—the statistical observation that high outliers tend to return toward a population mean upon retesting. In the case of extremely high A1c values, this might be related to a stressful event that occurred before the original test. The phenomenon also is due to reversal of the adverse effects of poor metabolic control (glucotoxicity and lipotoxicity) on insulin secretion and insulin action [29–31]. Also, not much reduction of A1c is possible when starting values are close to normal. Fig. 1 shows experimental data that illustrate this phenomenon in a group of patients who had short duration of diabetes (~3 years), and therefore, substantial β-cell reserve [32]. Patients in this study received no antihyperglycemic therapy for at least 8 weeks and were treated with the sulfonylurea, glyburide, or with metformin, with titration to what was considered an optimal dosage. (A third arm that used

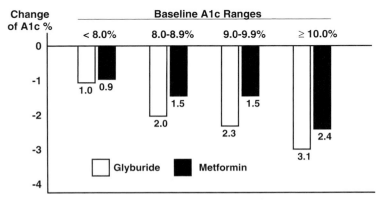

Fig. 1. Change of A1c from baseline after 4 months of monotherapy with glyburide (n = 151, mean final dosage 7.6 mg/d) or metformin (n = 164, mean dosage 1796 mg/d), with values shown separately for four ranges of baseline A1c values. (*Data from* Garber AJ, Donovan DS, Dandona P, et al. Efficacy of glyburide/metformin tablets compared with initial monotherapy in type 2 diabetes. J Clin Endocrinol Metab 2003;88:3598–604.)

a combination glyburide/metformin tablets is not pertinent to the present discussion.) Mean baseline A1c was 8.6%; the value after 4 months averaged 6.8% with glyburide and 6.9% with metformin and 68% and 62% of the patients, respectively, reached the 7% target. The greatest reductions from baseline were seen in those patients whose baseline A1c was greater than 10% (−3.1% with glyburide and −2.4% with metformin), whereas the smallest reductions were in patients whose starting A1c was less than 8% (−0.9% and −1.0%). Most patients whose starting A1c was less than 9% reached the 7% target. Despite excellent reductions of A1c, many of the patients whose starting values were greater than 9% did not reach 7% with oral monotherapy, even in the group of patients who had a short duration of diabetes. In summary, although starting A1c values of greater than 9% suggest greater than average therapeutic response may be seen with any class of agents, the likelihood of reaching the treatment target from a baseline of more than 9% with a single agent is much less than when treatment is started when glycemic control is better. Also, the effect of baseline A1c on therapeutic responses should be kept in mind when assessing the results of clinical trials, especially when comparisons with other agents not used in the trial are implied.

The change of glycemic patterns that lead to a reduction of A1c is not the same for all agents. Secretagogues (other than nateglinide), metformin, and TZDs mainly improve overnight and preprandial (basal) glucose control, whereas the AGIs and nateglinide mainly reduce the increments of glucose after meals. The longer-acting (basal) insulins mainly control overnight and between-meal glycemia. Regular insulin and the rapid-acting insulin analogs have effects that are focused more on prandial glucose control.

Adverse effects

Each class of agents has characteristic unwanted effects. For secretagogues these are modest weight gain and potential hypoglycemia [11]. Metformin causes nausea or diarrhea in about 5% of patients at low dosages and up to 20% or 30% at 2000 mg to 2500 mg daily [33,34]. Because of its exclusively renal clearance and the risk of lactic acidosis with high blood levels, Metformin cannot be used by patients who have renal impairment. AGIs frequently cause flatulence or diarrhea, and like metformin, should be titrated from small to larger dosages over weeks of treatment to minimize these symptoms [13]. TZDs often cause weight gain or fluid retention—both of which can be significant—and also may cause mild anemia [35,36]. The rare, but severe, liver toxicity that led to withdrawal of troglitazone from use apparently does not occur with the other TZDs [37]. Because of the potential to precipitate congestive heart failure, which is rare but well-documented [38,39], TZDs should not be used in patients who have impaired myocardial function. In addition to hypoglycemia, insulin often causes moderate weight gain.

Evidence for medical benefit

Compared with treatments for hypertension and dyslipidemia, antihyperglycemic agents have been studied in few trials with medical end points. Proof of benefit for microvascular complications in type 2 diabetes is strong for sulfonylureas, metformin, and insulin [1–3]. Corresponding evidence for AGIs and TZDs is not available, because, in part, of the shorter time that these have been used; however; it generally is assumed that similar benefits will occur when glycemic control is improved by them. Proof that any of these agents can reduce the frequency of (or mortality from) cardiovascular (CV) events is not as strong, and this possibility is explored in depth elsewhere in this issue. Insulin is the agent with the strongest evidence for an effect on mortality and CV outcomes [40,41]. Findings from a substudy of the UKPDS that suggested that metformin can reduce CV events and CV mortality compared with diet therapy also are encouraging [3]; however, few patients were studied and the results showed no statistical difference from the effects of insulin or a sulfonylurea, so this important observation needs confirmation. A recent study suggests that the AGI, acarbose, may have a favorable effect on CV outcomes [42], but concerns have been raised about the methods that were used in this secondary analysis [43].

Time-course of action

The duration of action after a single dose differs significantly between individual agents and specific formulations of agents within each class. These differences are well-known and always must be considered by the prescriber. In addition, the timing of onset of glycemic effects when each class of agents is started deserves comment. Insulin has the most rapid effects and suppresses plasma glucose concentrations within minutes of administration of short- or rapid-acting forms. Orally-administered secretagogues act within hours; the full effect of a given dosing schedule usually is achieved within a week or two. Partly because of the need to titrate dosage gradually to minimize gastrointestinal side effects, metformin and AGIs typically require a month or more to reach full efficacy [34,44]. For reasons that are not well-understood, TZDs have a gradual onset of action and often do not reach full effect for several months after initiation [45].

Differences between secretagogues

Within each class, the various agents and formulations are, except for their time-course of action, generally more similar than different; however, certain secretagogues have differences that may be clinically important. Because chlorpropamide is cleared mainly by the kidney and can cause serious hypoglycemia when used in the presence of renal insufficiency, and also can cause a syndrome of water intoxication, it is no longer used widely.

Also, the available formulations of glipizide have markedly different pharmacokinetics that dramatically alter their potency (relative effectiveness at a given dosage). Five mg of extended-release glipizide (glipizide XL), once daily, is enough to provide full efficacy [46] compared with 10 mg, twice daily, for conventional glipizide. But the most important and controversial issue regarding individual secretagogues concerns glyburide. This sulfonyl-urea was shown to interfere with myocardial ischemic preconditioning—a process that is believed to be protective in ischemic heart disease [47]. This provides a rationale for the apparent CV risk that was associated with treatment with tolbutamide (which probably also impairs ischemic pre-conditioning) in the University Group Diabetes Program (UGDP) study [48]. Because of the UGDP, the package inserts of sulfonylureas still include a "black box" warning of possible CV risk. Not all secretagogues seem to share glyburide's adverse effect on preconditioning; especially good evidence shows that glimepiride is free of it [49]. In addition, glyburide has been associated with greater rates of hypoglycemia than other sulfonylureas [2,50,51]. For these two reasons, glyburide's status as the most widely used secretagogue no longer seems appropriate [52].

Principles of antihyperglycemic pharmacotherapy

Define a specific target

Some general principles for treating hyperglycemia in type 2 diabetes have emerged from experience and clinical studies. The most basic of these is the need for a specific target for therapy. Intervention trials that attempted to confirm that treatment of hyperglycemia will reduce morbidity and mortality mainly addressed microvascular complications. Mean glycemic control achieved in these trials has been to A1c values in the range of 7.0% to 7.3%, with at least 25% reduction of microvascular events with each 1% (absolute) reduction of A1c [1–3]. Thus, objective evidence supports striving for glycemic control at least to 7% A1c to minimize eye, nerve, and kidney complications. Certain patients, especially the extremely old or otherwise frail, may have less ambitious targets assigned, such as 7.5% or 8% A1c; however, most patients should seek 7% A1c. Having a consensus target (7% A1c or less) is a major advance [53]. The target should serve as a trigger for initiating therapy and a goal for ongoing treatment. Should trials that are underway confirm that seeking even better glycemic control can reduce CV events, this target may have to be revised.

Treat to target

In the past, most studies of treatments for hyperglycemia have enrolled patients who had poor glycemic control, and have ended with A1c levels far greater than 7%. There are several reasons. One is that most patients begin pharmacotherapy when A1c is more than 9%. Another is that regulatory agencies (and others) have judged therapies by their ability to reduce A1c from baseline. Because these responses are greater when the baseline is increased, patients who have poor glycemic control have been chosen for many early studies of new agents. Yet another reason is that until recently, most studies examined the effects of a single agent, and the therapeutic power of each is limited, except for insulin. Definition of the 7% target led to a new concept, best exemplified by the Treat-to-Target Trial [54]. In this study, 756 subjects who had a mean A1c of 8.6% were randomized to begin neutral protamine Hagedorn (NPH) insulin or insulin glargine at bedtime to supplement basal insulin, while their previous (one or two) oral therapies were continued. Insulin dosage was increased systematically to seek a fasting plasma glucose of 100 mg/dL as a titration target. Nearly 60% of the subjects achieved A1c of 7% or less. In the future, most clinical trials are likely to include the proportion of patients that reaches a defined glycemic target as an important measure of success. This emphasis should favor earlier escalation of treatment and greater use of combinations of agents in trials and in the clinical management of patients.

Know the efficacy of treatments

Under favorable conditions, the most commonly used agents can reduce A1c by an average of 1.5% to 2.0% from baseline (see Table 3). When baseline A1c is less than 9%, monotherapy with a sulfonylurea, repaglinide, metformin, or a TZD has an excellent chance of reducing A1c to 7% or less. Treatment with an AGI or nateglinide is much less likely to succeed because of the lesser therapeutic power of these agents, unless A1c is less than 8% initially. When A1c is more than 9% at baseline, treatment with any single agent, except insulin, probably will not succeed fully.

Advance therapy using combinations

The progressive nature of type 2 diabetes is well-established; decline of β-cell function over time contributes more to this process than worsening of insulin resistance [55,56]. When the underlying physiologic defects are severe, more than one agent may be needed. Even when initial therapy is successful, further therapy will be needed over time. The rate of this progression, on a population basis, was demonstrated in the UKPDS [56]. Monotherapy with a sulfonylurea, metformin, or basal insulin leads to initial success followed by a steady increase of A1c by 0.2% to 0.3% yearly. Thus, a typical patient whose A1c is 6.5% after initial therapy would be expected to have A1c of 7.5% in 3 to 5 years. Addition of a second agent would re-establish control, but if the agent that was used initially was stopped, no improvement would be likely. For example, discontinuation of glyburide upon initiation of metformin usually leads to no important change of A1c, whereas addition of the second agent improves control almost as much as when metformin is used as initial monotherapy (Fig. 2) [34]. The

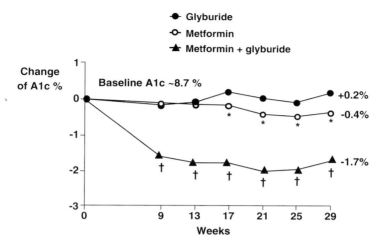

Fig. 2. Change of A1c from baseline during 29 weeks of treatment of patients who previously were taking glyburide 20 mg/d, with randomization to continued glyburide (n = 209), switch to metformin (n = 210), or addition of metformin to glyburide (n = 213). At Week 29, 90% of patients in the metformin-only group and 70% of the group that was assigned to metformin plus glyburide were taking 2500 mg of metformin daily. The daggers indicate $P < .001$ for differences between combination therapy and glyburide alone, and the asterisks indicate $P < .01$ for differences between metformin and glyburide monotherapy. (*Adapted from* DeFronzo RA, Goodman AM, and the Multicenter Metformin Study Group. Efficacy of metformin in patients with noninsulin-dependent diabetes mellitus. N Engl J Med 1995;333:541–9; with permission.)

principle demonstrated here is that progression of therapy is expected and that treatments should be added rather than substituted. Although the therapeutic effects of agents in different classes are additive, owing to their differing mechanisms of action, their side effects are not; this permits combination therapy to be well-tolerated. Combination therapy is essential to success in treating type 2 diabetes.

Start with standard methods

The large number of available treatments poses a challenge for busy physicians. There are more than 90 individual antihyperglycemic prescription options (see Tables 1 and 2), and remembering the idiosyncrasies, dosages, and typical schedule for administration of each agent is no simple task. Many physicians and most health systems are eager to have a simple "algorithm" to guide therapy for type 2 diabetes. Ideally, such a standardized scheme would require few choices for the typical patient, so that no flow chart or printed guidebook need be consulted. Only recently have sufficient evidence and experience become available to provide such guidance. The rest of this article is devoted to this task.

Individualize options when necessary

Despite the need for a simple way to treat typical patients, especially early in the course of type 2 diabetes, individualized management is necessary for many patients from the outset, and nearly all patients later in the course of diabetes. Therefore, individualized treatment options must be used when standard treatments are not appropriate or fail to maintain glycemic targets without undue side effects. Beyond implementing standard therapies, physicians must recognize triggers for deviating from the standard scheme, and choose alternative methods. These "nonstandard" treatments should not be regarded as second-rate, but more appropriate in specific situations.

Standard methods

When A1c is more than 7% but no greater than 8%, and no significant effort at improving lifestyle has been made, nonpharmacologic therapy may be tried; however, sustained success with this alone has proven difficult [55–57]. Moreover, many patients already have made some effort to improve eating and exercise behaviors. Therefore, the typical patient who has type 2 diabetes with A1c that is more than 7% should be considered for oral pharmacotherapy immediately, in addition to continued lifestyle efforts.

Sulfonylureas, metformin, and insulin have the best evidence for medical benefit and, from long experience with their use, the best understood therapeutic effects and side effects. For these reasons, they should be considered the standard therapies. Each of them is best suited to certain situations.

Starting therapy: monotherapy with a sulfonylurea or metformin

Most often, pharmacotherapy for type 2 diabetes is started for patients who do not have an acute illness and who have minimal symptoms. In this setting, a sulfonylurea or metformin is appropriate initial therapy. Because most patients will need these two agents together soon, which of them is used first usually is not important; however, a few factors should be considered. First, patients who have a greater A1c will benefit from the more rapid onset of action of a sulfonylurea, and this choice is less likely to cause unpleasant side effects for patients who already do not feel entirely well. Second, patients who have lower A1c levels may benefit from metformin's lack of risk of hypoglycemia, even with excellent glycemic control. Also, obese patients who have major concerns about further gain may prefer metformin. The tendency to assign obese patients to metformin and the less obese to sulfonylurea has little evidence to support it, however, because adiposity does not predict the glycemic effects of either class significantly. In general, patients whose A1c is more than 8% may be considered good candidates for a sulfonylurea and those whose A1c is between 7% and 8% are better suited to metformin.

Despite the potential pitfalls in recommending individual therapies in a class, it seems necessary to suggest the most logical choice of sulfonylureas. The most convenient are those that are fully effective when taken once daily. Three are available in the United States: chlorpropamide, glimepiride, and glipizide XL. Chlorpropamide has specific disadvantages that were mentioned previously, but the other two are used widely, and each has advantages. Glipizide XL is available as generic; has maximal effect at 5 mg. once daily [46]; and also is available as a 2.5-mg capsule with at least half maximal effectiveness. Glimepiride has maximal effect at 4 mg, once daily, and comes in 1-mg, 2-mg, and 4-mg tablets that are scored and easily broken in two. The 1-mg dosage has at least half maximal effectiveness [58]. Both agents have less tendency to cause hypoglycemia than glyburide. In the case of metformin, the main choice is between the conventional formulation and an extended-release form. Either form should be started at 500 mg, once or twice daily, with increase of dosage no more often than weekly to minimize side effects. The first 500 mg of metformin is not a trivial dose, having perhaps 30% of metformin's maximal effectiveness [33]. Because there is not much difference in the dosage, effectiveness, or side effects of the conventional and extended release forms of metformin, there seems little reason to prefer one over the other. Both are available as generic.

Oral combination therapy

Patients whose baseline A1c is more than 9% often need to add a second oral agent within a few months of therapy. Others will have gradual worsening of control and need combination therapy later. The combination of a sulfonylurea plus metformin is well-tested and should be the standard approach for typical patients [59,60]. This raises the question of whether to use these two agents as separate formulations, or as the combination tablet that is now available [32]. The main argument in favor of combined formulations is that fewer tablets will be needed, with possible improved medication adherence; however, four tablets are needed for full efficacy of the metformin/glipizide or metformin/glyburide formulations. In contrast, one glipizide XL capsule or glimepiride tablet plus two metformin tablets daily will yield full efficacy. Thus, the combination formulations are not always more convenient. Moreover, they do not allow separate adjustment of dosage when a side effect specific to one agent occurs. There seems to be no strong reason why separately formulated metformin and long-acting sulfonylurea preparations should not remain the standard options for early combination therapy.

Adding insulin to oral agents

When two oral agents fail to maintain target-level control, a third oral agent must be added or insulin must be started. Addition of a TZD to establish a three oral agent regimen is discussed widely [61–63] and can be

effective for many patients, especially those whose baseline A1c values are
no more than 8% (see later discussion). Based on its greater evidence-base
and greater reliability when initial A1c values are higher, starting insulin
probably still deserves to be the usual approach. Insulin can be started
several ways: (1) oral agents can be discontinued and two or more daily
injections of insulin can be substituted; (2) the sulfonylurea may be stopped
and two or more insulin injections added while metformin is continued; (3)
one or both oral agents can be continued and multiple dosages of mealtime
insulin can be started; or (4) a single injection of basal insulin added may be
added while oral therapy continues. The last option, is simple, effective, and
well-tolerated and causes the least weight gain [64]. Especially because of its
simplicity, adding basal insulin to oral therapies is best suited to being the
standard way to start insulin.

Fig. 3 shows data from the Treat-to-Target Trial that illustrate this
method [52]. Patients entered this trial taking one or two oral agents and had
A1c of 8.6% at baseline. More than 70% were taking a sulfonylurea and
metformin. Human NPH or glargine insulin was added at bedtime and
the dosage was increased systematically based on once-daily self-testing
of glucose, with (plasma-referenced) fasting glucose of 100 mg/dL as
the titration target. Almost 60% of patients in this trial reached the 7% A1c
target with each insulin, but there was considerably less nocturnal
hypoglycemia with glargine than with NPH insulin. The mean insulin
dosage used was between 0.45 units/kg body weight and 0.50 units/kg body

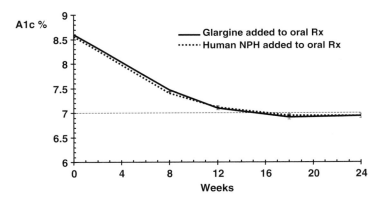

Fig. 3. A1c during 24 weeks of treatment with a single dose of insulin glargine (N = 367) or
human NPH insulin (N = 389) taken at bedtime added to previous oral therapies, starting with
10 units daily and with systematic weekly titration of dosage. Final A1c values for the 91% of
patients who completed the protocol were 6.9% in each group; 58% and 57% of those
randomized had A1c up to 7% (*horizontal dashed line*) with glargine and NPH, respectively.
(*Adapted from* Riddle MC, Rosenstock J, Gerich J, the Insulin Glargine 4002 Study
Investigators. The Treat-to-Target Trial. Randomized addition of glargine or human NPH
insulin to oral therapy of type 2 diabetic patients. Diabetes Care 2003;26:3080–6; with
permission.)

weight. Other studies showed that systematically titrating a basal insulin while continuing oral agents can improve glycemic control reliably [65–68]. Several features of this method suggest that it could be applied widely. Only one routine glucose test and one daily insulin injection are required. The process of increasing the insulin at regular intervals (eg, weekly) can be based on a simple algorithm that is understood easily and performed by the patient.

Individualized options

The simplified approach that was outlined above is suitable for most patients who have type 2 diabetes; in most cases, it should maintain control for up to 10 years after diagnosis. Like all algorithms, it will not always apply or be effective. For these situations, a regimen that is suited to the patient and the situation is needed. Ideally, individualized decisions should be made by a physician who has extra experience and training in diabetes. At least five circumstances call for such individualization (Fig. 4).

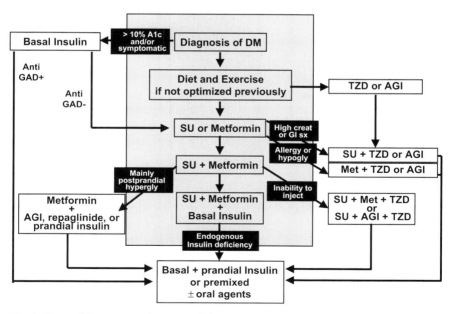

Fig. 4. Sequential treatments for type 2 diabetes. The treatments within the shaded rectangle are proposed, on the basis of evidence for medical benefits and well-known patterns of adverse effects, as standard therapies. Clinical situations that may trigger individualized use of other regimens are shown, with these alternative methods appearing outside of the shaded rectangle. Most patients who have type 2 diabetes may eventually require basal plus prandial insulin, with or without oral therapy as well, as shown at the bottom of the diagram. creat, creatinine; DM, diabetes mellitus; GI sx, gastrointestinal symptoms; Met, metformin; SU, sulfonylurea.

Symptomatic hyperglycemia or other acute illness

Insulin may be the best initial therapy when the patient has overt symptoms that are due to hyperglycemia. In this situation, A1c generally is more than 10% and the patient may have excessive urine output, weight loss, fatigue, blurred vision, or prominent neuropathic symptoms. Also, insulin is by far the best option when treatment must be started during a severe illness, such as a vascular event, major trauma, or systemic infection. All patients should have a rapid therapeutic response to insulin, and with improved glycemic control many patients may become more responsive to oral therapies and may be able to switch to oral agents alone after using insulin initially. Others, especially those who prove to have late-onset type 1 diabetes (also called latent autoimmune diabetes of adulthood) will need ongoing treatment with insulin. Late type 1 diabetes is common and occurs in at least 1 of 10 persons who have adult-onset diabetes; it is especially common among those who have a sudden onset before age 40 and with near-normal body weight [69,70]. Finding a positive blood test for anti–glutamic acid decarboxylase antibodies goes far toward confirming this diagnosis. When initial therapy with insulin can be discontinued because of recovery from an acute illness or marked improvement of metabolic control, a standard oral therapy approach may be instituted.

When a patient who is taking treatment for diabetes is hospitalized for a major illness, individualized insulin treatment may become necessary for a time [71], and oral therapies may have to be stopped temporarily. Oral agents are much less effective in the hospital setting because of the tendency of acute illnesses to suppress the endogenous insulin secretion that is needed for an effective response to oral agents. In addition, oral agents have the potential for serious adverse effects in the setting of major illness (eg, interference with ischemic preconditioning by some sulfonylureas, lactic acidosis with metformin, marked fluid retention with TZDs).

Contraindications to, or side effects from, sulfonylureas or metformin

Metformin is contraindicated when serum creatinine values are greater than 1.4 mg/dL for women or 1.5 mg/dL for men, and causes intolerable gastrointestinal symptoms even at low dosages in a few patients. Sulfonylureas usually are well-tolerated, but occasionally cause allergic or gastrointestinal symptoms. More often, even glipizide XL or glimepiride may cause more hypoglycemia than is acceptable, especially if used when A1c is elevated only slightly or when postprandial hyperglycemia is the main concern. In these settings, the problematic agent may be replaced by a TZD or an AGI, either as monotherapy or in combination with another agent. A TZD with metformin, TZD with sulfonylurea, AGI with metformin, and AGI with sulfonylurea are effective regimens [72–75]. Also, the nonsulfonylurea secretagogues may be used effectively in combination with metformin or a TZD [76–78].

Difficulty with starting insulin

When two oral agents no longer maintain target A1c values, for some patients, a third oral agent, usually a TZD, is more appropriate than insulin. Several factors that favor this individualized choice are limitation of dexterity, vision, or mental capacity; allergy to insulin; aversion to injections; and unusual risk of hypoglycemia, as in the elderly or those who have marked variability of food intake. Therapy with three oral agents can be effective [61–63]. For example, a recent study compared adding pioglitazone or bedtime NPH insulin to previous treatment with metformin plus a secretagogue [62]. Adding pioglitazone reduced mean A1c from 9.7% to 7.8%, whereas adding insulin reduced A1c from 10.1% to 7.8% in this trial. Weight gain was similar; insulin caused more hypoglycemia, whereas the TZD caused more edema. Adding a TZD as the third agent seems most attractive when A1c at baseline is 8% or less and the 7% target is more likely to be reached with additional oral therapy. While we wait for the results of trials that compare medical outcomes of treatment with TZDs versus other agents, in some cases, physicians and patients may have strong individual preferences in deciding which agent to add as the third agent. Finally, it is likely that using three oral agents will delay, rather than avoid, the need for insulin.

Another alternative to starting basal insulin is the introduction of twice-daily premixed insulin with the aim of providing basal and prandial support with a simple regimen. Little evidence is available to show that this method can restore excellent glycemic control without prominent hypoglycemia, but for patients for whom limited glycemic goals are appropriate this may be a reasonable approach.

Mainly postprandial hyperglycemia

Some patients have much more pronounced postprandial hyperglycemia than fasting hyperglycemia, either with or without oral antihyperglycemic treatment. For them, initial treatment with regular or rapid-acting insulin at mealtimes, rather than with basal insulin, may be considered despite its greater complexity [79–82]. Situations in which this pattern is common include gestational diabetes (when insulin alone rather than with oral therapy is the standard method); diabetes that is due to pancreatitis; during treatment with glucocorticoids; and among Asian populations who eat extremely high carbohydrate meals. In any of these settings, basal insulin may have to be added subsequently to result in a full basal bolus insulin regimen. Patients who have mainly postprandial hyperglycemia (and are not pregnant) may have good results with nateglinide or repaglinide with each meal, either as initial therapy or as a second intervention after initial treatment with metformin or a TZD. Similarly, nonpregnant patients who have mainly postprandial hyperglycemia may respond well to mealtime doses of an AGI.

Failure to maintain glycemic control with oral agents plus basal insulin

Continued decline of β-cell function often leads to the need for multiple injections of insulin. At this point, individualization of all aspects of antihyperglycemic therapy (eg, which oral agents to continue, when to add further insulin injections, what kinds of insulin to use, how to match dosage to glucose tests) becomes mandatory. Intensive insulin therapy, which demands more training and experience from patients and providers, poses a challenge which has not been met well by most health systems. Under the best conditions, patients who are successful with simple regimens for 10 or more years are able to make the transition to complex, individualized regimens smoothly and maintain good metabolic control. Tactics for effective management of type 2 diabetes using multiple injections of insulin have not been studied as carefully as for type 1 diabetes. This is an important concern, but is beyond the scope of this article.

Summary

The many antihyperglycemic preparations are best used for type 2 diabetes in a logical sequence, using combinations of agents, with clear targets for glycemic control. On the basis of long familiarity, proven benefit and known side effects, and low cost, the sulfonylureas, metformin, and insulin still deserve to be the standard treatments. As shown in the central shaded area of Fig. 4, standard treatment begins with monotherapy and progresses to oral combination therapy and then to two oral agents plus basal insulin. Several triggers for deviation from the standard methods are identified (see Fig. 4). The incidence of each of the conditions that require early individualized treatment has not been studied, but it seems reasonable to estimate no more than 10% each for a strongly symptomatic presentation, inability to use a sulfonylurea or metformin, inability to use insulin, or an early need for prandial therapy. If this estimate is correct, approximately two thirds of patients who are diagnosed with type 2 diabetes should do well with standard therapy for up to 10 years using the standard methods shown. Eventually, many more will need individualized treatment to maintain glycemic control. This scheme is certain to evolve as further information on the nonglycemic benefits (or hazards) of the various therapies appears and as new treatments are released. Notably, agents that mimic or potentiate the effects of gastrointestinal peptides, such as amylin and GLP-1 analogues and dipeptidyl peptidase IV inhibitors, are likely to alter the current algorithm. For now, systematic application of the scheme (see Fig. 4) should improve the success of treatment greatly from its currently disappointing level.

Acknowledgments

The author wishes to thank Dr. Diane Karl for advice on preparation of the manuscript.

References

[1] Ohkubo Y, Kishikawa H, Araki E, et al. Intensive insulin therapy prevents the progression of diabetic microvascular complications in Japanese patients with non-insulin-dependent diabetes mellitus: a randomized prospective 6-year study. Diabetes Res Clin Pract 1995;28: 103–17.

[2] Prospective Diabetes Study UK. (UKPDS) Group. Intensive blood-glucose control with sulphonylureas or insulin compared with conventional treatment and risk of complications in patients with type 2 diabetes (UKPDS 33). Lancet 1998;352:837–53.

[3] Prospective Diabetes Study UK. (UKPDS) Group. Effect of intensive blood-glucose control with metformin on complications in overweight patients with type 2 diabetes (UKPDS 34). Lancet 1998;352:854–65.

[4] Saydah SH, Fradkin J, Cowie CC. Poor control of risk factors for vascular disease among adults with previously diagnosed diabetes. JAMA 2004;291:335–42.

[5] Brown JB, Nichols GA, Perry A. The burden of treatment failure in type 2 diabetes. Diabetes Care 2004;27:1535–40.

[6] Hayward RA, Manning WG, Kaplan SJ, et al. Starting insulin therapy in patients with type 2 diabetes. Effectiveness, complications, and resource utilization. JAMA 1997;278:1663–9.

[7] Inzucchi SE. Oral antihyperglycemic therapy for type 2 diabetes. JAMA 2002;287:360–72.

[8] Lebovitz HE. Oral therapies for diabetic hyperglycemia. Endo Metab Clin North Am 2001; 30:909–33.

[9] DeFronzo RA. Pharmacologic therapy for type 2 diabetes mellitus. Ann Intern Med 1999; 131:281–303.

[10] Mudaliar S, Edelman SV. Insulin therapy in type 2 diabetes. Endo Metab Clin North Am 2001;30:935–82.

[11] Lebovitz HE. Insulin secretagogues. Sulfonylureas and meglitinides. In: Leroith D, Taylor SI, Olefsky JM, editors. Diabetes mellitus: a fundamental and clinical text. Philadelphia: Lippincott Williams & Wilkins; 2000. p. 769–78.

[12] Garber AJ. Metformin. In: Leroith D, Taylor SI, Olefsky JM, editors. Diabetes mellitus: a fundamental and clinical text. Philadelphia: Lippincott Williams & Wilkins; 2000. p. 778–87.

[13] Lebovitz HE. Alpha-glucosidase inhibitors. Endo Metab Clin North Am 1997;26:539–51.

[14] Foyt HL, Ghazzi MN, Hanley RM, et al. Thiazolidinediones. In: Leroith D, Taylor SI, Olefsky JM, editors. Diabetes mellitus: a fundamental and clinical text. Philadelphia: Lippincott Williams & Wilkins; 2000. p. 788–97.

[15] Burge MR, Schade DS. Insulins. Endo Metab Clin North Am 1997;26:575–98.

[16] Bolli GB, DiMarchi RD, Park GD, et al. Insulin analogues and their potential in the management of diabetes mellitus. Diabetologia 1999;42:1151–67.

[17] Ashcroft FM. Mechanisms of the glycaemic effects of sulfonylureas. Horm Metab Res 1996; 28:456–63.

[18] Cusi K, DeFronzo RA. Metformin: a review of its metabolic effects. Diabetes Rev 1998;6: 89–131.

[19] United Kingdom Prospective Diabetes Study Group. United Kingdom Prospective Diabetes Study (UKPDS) 13. Relative efficacy of randomly allocated diet, sulphonylurea, insulin, or metformin in patients with newly diagnosed non-insulin dependent diabetes followed for three years. BMJ 1995;310:83–8.

[20] Stuvoll M, Numjhan N, Perriello G, et al. Metabolic effects of metformin in non-insulin-dependent diabetes mellitus. N Engl J Med 1995;333:550–4.

[21] Bischoff H. Pharmacology of α-glucosidase inhibition. Eur J Clin Invest 1994;24(Suppl 3): 3–10.

[22] Qualmann C, Nauck MA, Holst JJ, et al. Glucagon-like peptide 1 (7–36 amide) secretion to luminal sucrose from the upper and lower gut: a study using glucosidase inhibition (acarbose). Scand J Gastroenterol 1995;30:872–96.

[23] Furnsinn C, Waldhausl W. Thiazolidinediones: metabolic actions in vitro. Diabetologia 2002;45:1211–23.

[24] Yang WS, Jeng CY, We TJ, et al. Synthetic peroxisome proliferator-activated receptor-gamma agonist, rosiglitazone, increases plasma levels of adiponectin in type 2 diabetic patients. Diabetes Care 2002;25:376–80.

[25] Hirose H, Kawai T, Yamamoto Y, et al. Effects of pioglitazone on metabolic parameters, body fat distribution and serum adiponectin levels in Japanese male patients with type 2 diabetes. Metabolism 2002;51:314–7.

[26] Rizza RA, Mandarino LJ, Gerich JE. Dose-response characteristics for effects of insulin on production and utilization of glucose in man. Am J Physiol 1981;240:E630–9.

[27] Lewis GF, Zinman B, Groenewoud Y, et al. Hepatic glucose production is regulated both by direct hepatic and extrahepatic effects of insulin in humans. Diabetes 1996;45:454–62.

[28] Yki-Jarivinen H. Combination therapies with insulin in type 2 diabetes. Diabetes Care 2001; 24:758–67.

[29] Rossetti L, Giaccari A, DeFronzo RA. Glucose toxicity. Diabetes Care 1990;13:610–30.

[30] Yki-Jarivinen H. Glucose toxicity. Endocr Rev 1992;13:415–29.

[31] Leahy JL. β-cell dysfunction with chronic hyperglycemia: the overworked β-cell hypothesis. Diab Rev 1996;4:298–319.

[32] Garber AJ, Donovan DS, Dandona P, et al. Efficacy of glyburide-metformin tablets compared with initial monotherapy in type 2 diabetes. J Clin Endocrinol Metab 2003;88: 3598–604.

[33] Garber AJ, Duncan TG, Goodman AM, et al. Efficacy of metformin in type II diabetes: results of a double-blind, placebo-controlled, dose-response trial. Am J Med 1997;103: 491–7.

[34] DeFronzo RA, Goodman AM, and the Multicenter Metformin Study Group. Efficacy of metformin in patients with non-insulin-dependent diabetes mellitus. N Engl J Med 1995;333: 541–9.

[35] Aronoff S, Rosenblatt S, Braithwaite S, et al. The Pioglitazone 001 Study Group. Pioglitazone hydrochloride monotherapy improves glycemic control in the treatment of patients with type 2 diabetes. Diabetes Care 2000;23:1605–11.

[36] Phillips LS, Grunberger G, Miller E, et al for the Rosiglitazone Clinical Trials Study Group. Once and twice-daily dosing with rosiglitazone improves glycemic control in patients with type 2 diabetes. Diabetes Care 2001;24:308–15.

[37] Lebovitz HE, Kreider M, Freed MI. Evaluation of liver function in type 2 diabetic patients during clinical trials. Diabetes Care 2002;25:815–21.

[38] Nesto RW, Bell D, Bonow RO, et al. Thiazolidinedione use, fluid retention, and congestive heart failure. A consensus statement from the American Heart Association and the American Diabetes Association. Diabetes Care 2004;27:256–63.

[39] Tang WH, Francis GS, Hoofwerf BJ, et al. Fluid retention after initiation of thiazolidinedione therapy in diabetic patients with established chronic heart failure. J Am Coll Cardiol 2003;41:1394–8.

[40] Malmberg K for the DIGAMI (Diabetes Mellitus, Insulin Glucose Infusion in Acute Myocardial Infarction) Study Group Prospective randomized study of intensive insulin treatment on long-term survival after acute myocardial infarction in patients with diabetes mellitus. BMJ 1997;314:1512–5.

[41] Furnary AP, Wu YX, Bookin SO. Effect of hyperglycemia and continuous intravenous insulin infusions on outcomes of cardiac surgical procedures: The Portland Diabetic Project. Endocr Pract 2004;10(Suppl 2):21–33.

[42] Chiasson J-L, Josse RG, Gomis R, et al for The STOP-NIDDM Trial Research Group. Acarbose treatment and the risk of cardiovascular disease and hypertension in patients with impaired glucose tolerance. The STOP-NIDDM Trial. JAMA 2003;290:486–94.

[43] Kaiser T, Sawicki PT. Acarbose for patients with hypertension and impaired glucose tolerance [letter]. JAMA 2003;290:3066.

[44] Chiasson J-L, Josse RG, Hunt JA, et al. The efficacy of acarbose in the treatment of patients with non-insulin-dependent diabetes mellitus. Ann Intern Med 1994;121:928–35.

[45] Lebovitz HE, Dole JF, Patwardhan R, et al for the Rosiglitazone Clinical Trials Study Group. Rosiglitazone monotherapy is effective in patients with type 2 diabetes. J Clin Endocrinol Metab 2001;86:280–8.

[46] Simonson DC, Kourides IA, Fineglos M, et al. The Glipizide Gastrointestinal Therapeutic System Study Group. Efficacy, safety, and dose-response characteristics of glipizide gastrointestinal therapeutic system on glycemic control and insulin secretion in NIDDM. Diabetes Care 1997;20:597–606.

[47] Kloner RA, Yellon D. Does ischemic preconditioning occur in patients? J Am Coll Cardiol 1994;24:1133–42.

[48] Meinert CL, Knatterud GL, Prout TE, et al. A study of the effects of hypoglycemic agents on vascular complications in patients with adult-onset diabetes. II. Mortality results. Diabetes 1970;19(Suppl 2):789–830.

[49] Lee T-M, Chou T-F. Impairment of myocardial protection in type 2 diabetic patients. J Clin Endocrinol Metab 2003;88:531–7.

[50] Holstein A, Plashke A, Egberts E-H. Lower incidence of severe hypoglycemia in patients with type 2 diabetes treated with glipempiride versus glibenclamide. Diabetes Metab Res Rev 2001;17:467–73.

[51] Schorr RI, Ray WA, Daugherty JR, et al. Incidence and risk factors for serious hypoglycemia in older persons using insulin or sulfonylureas. J Am Geriatr Soc 1996;44:751–5.

[52] Riddle MC. Sulfonylureas differ in effects on ischemic preconditioning—is it time to retire glyburide? J Clin Endocrinol Metab 2003;88:528–30.

[53] American Diabetes Association. Standards of medical care in diabetes. Diabetes Care 2004; 27(Suppl 1):S15–35.

[54] Riddle MC, Rosenstock J, Gerich J, for the Insulin Glargine 4002 Study Investigators. The Treat-to-Target Trial. Randomized addition of glargine or human NPH insulin to oral therapy of type 2 diabetic patients. Diabetes Care 2003;26:3080–6.

[55] Hadden DR, Blair ALT, Wilson EA, et al. Natural history of diabetes presenting age 40–69 years: a prospective study of the influence of intensive dietary therapy. Quart J Med 1986;59: 579–98.

[56] Prospective Diabetes Study UK 16. Overview of 6 years' therapy of type II diabetes: a progressive disease. Diabetes 1995;44:1249–58.

[57] UK Prospective Study Group. UK Prospective Diabetes Study 7. Response of fasting plasma glucose to diet therapy in newly presenting type II diabetic patients. Metabolism 1990;39:905–12.

[58] Goldberg RB, Holvey SM, Schneider J, the Glimepiride Protocol No. 201 Study Group. A dose-response study of glimepiride in patients with NIDDM who have previously received sulfonylurea agents. Diabetes Care 1996;19:849–56.

[59] Riddle M. Combining sulfonylureas and other oral agents. Am J Med 2000;108(Suppl 6A): 15S–22S.

[60] Hermann LS, Shersten B, Bitzen P-O, et al. Therapeutic comparison of metformin and sulfonylurea, alone and in various combinations: a double-blind controlled study. Diabetes Care 1994;17:1100–9.

[61] Dailey GI, Noor MA, Park J, et al. Glyburide/metformin tablets in combination with rosiglitazone improve glycemic control in patients with type 2 diabetes: a randomized, double-blind trial. Am J Med 2003;116:223–9.

[62] Aljabri H, Kozak S, Thompson D. A comparison of adding pioglitazone or insulin to patients with type 2 diabetes in poor control on maximal doses of sulphonylurea and metformin: a prospective, randomized, 16 week trial. Am J Med 2003;116:230–5.

[63] Schwartz SS, Sievers R, Strange P, et al for the INS-2061 Study Team. Insulin 70/30 mix plus metformin versus triple oral therapy in the treatment of type 2 diabetes after failure of two oral drugs: efficacy, safety, and cost analysis. Diabetes Care 2003;26:2238–43.

[64] Yki-Jarvinen H, Kauppila M, Kujansuu I, et al. Comparison of insulin regimens in patients with non-insulin-dependent diabetes mellitus. N Engl J Med 1992;327:1426–33.

[65] Shank ML, DelPrato S, DeFronzo RA. Bedtime insulin/daytime glipizide. Effective therapy for sulfonylurea failures in NIDDM. Diabetes 1995;44:165–72.

[66] Riddle MC, Schneider J, and the Glimepiride Combination Group. Beginning insulin treatment of obese patients with evening 70/30 insulin plus glimepiride versus insulin alone. Diabetes Care 1998;21:1052–7.

[67] Yki-Jarvinen H, Dressler A, Ziemen M, The HOE 901/3002 Study Group. Less nocturnal hypoglycemia and better post-dinner glucose control with bedtime insulin glargine compared with bedtime NPH insulin during insulin combination therapy in type 2 diabetes. Diabetes Care 2000;23:1130–6.

[68] Fritsche A, Schweitzer MA, Haring H-U, The 4001 Study Group. Glimepiride combined with morning insulin glargine, bedtime neutral protamine hagedorn, or bedtime insulin glargine in patients with type 2 diabetes. Ann Intern Med 2003;138:952–9.

[69] Tuomi T, Carlsson A-L, Haiyan L, et al. Clinical and genetic characteristics of type 2 with and without GAD antibodies. Diabetes 1999;48:150–7.

[70] Tuomi T, Groop LC, Zimmet PZ, et al. Antibodies to glutamic acid decarboxylase reveal latent autoimmune diabetes mellitus in adults with a non-insulin-dependent onset of disease. Diabetes 1993;42:359–62.

[71] Clement S, Braithwaite SS, Magee MF, et al. Management of diabetes and hyperglycemia in hospitals. Diabetes Care 2004;27:553–91.

[72] Fonseca V, Rosenstock J, Patwardhan R, et al. Effect of metformin and rosiglitazone combination therapy in patients with type 2 diabetes mellitus. JAMA 2000;283:1695–702.

[73] Hanefeld M, Brunetti P, Schernthaner GH, et al on behalf of the QUARTED Study Group. One-year glycemic control with a sulfonylurea plus pioglitazone versus a sulfonylurea plus metformin in patients with type 2 diabetes. Diabetes Care 2004;27:141–7.

[74] Phillips P, Karrasch J, Scott R, et al. Acarbose improves glycemic control in overweight type 2 diabetic patients insufficiently treated with metformin. Diabetes Care 2003;26:269–73.

[75] Costa B, Pinol C. Acarbose in ambulatory treatment of non-insulin-dependent diabetes mellitus associated to imminent sulfonylurea failure: a randomized multicentric trial in primary health-care. Diabetes Res Clin Pract 1997;38:33–40.

[76] Raskin P, Klaff L, McGill J, et al. Efficacy and safety of combination therapy. Repaglinide plus metformin versus nateglinide plus metformin. Diabetes Care 2003;26:2063–8.

[77] Rosenstock J, Shen SG, Gatlin MR, et al. Combination therapy with nateglinide and a thiazolidinedione improves glycemic control in type 2 diabetes. Diabetes Care 2002;25:1529–33.

[78] Fonseca V, Grunberger G, Gupta S, et al. Addition of nateglinide to rosiglitazone monotherapy suppresses mealtime hyperglycemia and improves overall glycemic control. Diabetes Care 2003;26:1685–90.

[79] Landstedt-Hallin L, Adamson U, Arner P, et al. Comparison of bedtime NPH or preprandial regular insulin combined with glibenclamide in secondary sulfonylurea failure. Diabetes Care 1995;18:1183–6.

[80] Feinglos MN, Thacker CH, English J, et al. Modification of postprandial hyperglycemia with insulin lispro improves glucose control in patients with type 2 diabetes. Diabetes Care 1997;20:1539–42.

[81] Bastyr EJ, Stuart CA, Brodows RG, et al for the IOEZ Study Group. Therapy focused on lowering postprandial glucose, not fasting glucose, may be superior for lowering HbA1c. Diabetes Care 2000;23:1236–41.

[82] Poulsen MK, Henricksen JE, Hother-Nielsen O, et al. The combined effect of triple therapy with rosiglitazone, metformin, and insulin aspart in type 2 diabetic patients. Diabetes Care 2003;26:3273–9.

ELSEVIER
SAUNDERS

Endocrinol Metab Clin N Am
34 (2005) 99–116

ENDOCRINOLOGY
AND METABOLISM
CLINICS
OF NORTH AMERICA

Hospital Management of Diabetes

Etie S. Moghissi, MD, FACP, FACE[a],*, Irl B. Hirsch, MD[b,c],*

[a]Inpatient Diabetes and Metabolic Control Task Force,
American Association of Clinical Endocrinologists, 501 East Hardy Street,
Suite 110, Inglewood, CA 90301, USA
[b]Division of Metabolism, Endocrinology, and Nutrition, Department of Medicine,
University of Washington Medical Center, 1959 NE Pacific Street,
Box 356176, Seattle, WA 98195, USA
[c]Diabetes Care Center, University of Washington Medical Center,
Seattle, WA, USA

Diabetes remains a major cause of death and disability and is a growing global concern. The age-adjusted prevalence of type 2 diabetes in the United States increased by more than 55% from 1990 to 2000 [1]. It is estimated that one out of three individuals born in 2000 will develop diabetes in their lifetime [2].

Chronic complications of diabetes, especially cardiovascular disease, result in hospitalization in many patients with diabetes. In 2001, more than 4.6 million hospitalizations were associated with diabetes, accounting for nearly 17 million hospital days at a cost of over $40 billion [3].

Mounting observational and interventional evidence consistently indicates that hyperglycemia in the hospital setting is associated with increased mortality and morbidity and that meticulous glycemic control can improve clinical outcomes [4–7]. The purpose of this article is to review the evidence, discuss the importance of striving for good glycemic control in the hospital setting, and emphasize the need for additional outcome research studies to further examine the currently recommended in-hospital glycemic guidelines.

Dr. Morghissi is the former Vice-Chair of the Statement on Inpatient Diabetes and Metabolic Control writing panel of the American Association of Clinical Endocrinologists.

* Corresponding authors. Division of Metabolism, Endocrinology, and Nutrition, Department of Medicine, University of Washington Medical Center, 1959 NE Pacific Street, Box 356176, Seattle, WA 98195 (I.B. Hirsch).

E-mail addresses: emoghissi@pol.net (E.S. Moghissi); ihirsch@u.washington.edu (I.B. Hirsch).

0889-8529/05/$ - see front matter © 2005 Elsevier Inc. All rights reserved.
doi:10.1016/j.ecl.2004.11.001

The article concludes with a discussion of strategies for achieving tight glycemic targets.

Hyperglycemia in the hospital setting

Hyperglycemia is a frequent finding in hospitalized patients. With the escalating incidence of diabetes in the United States, the number of patients with diabetes who require hospitalization has also increased. Between 1980 and 2001, the age-adjusted hospital discharge rate for diabetes as any-listed diagnosis in the general population increased over 49% from 109.0 to 162.4 per 10,000 in the general population [8]. A rapidly growing body of evidence clearly suggests that meticulous glycemic control improves clinical outcomes, including reduced mortality and infection rates [4–7]; however, until recently there were no established guidelines or standards for management of diabetes in the hospital setting.

In a recent consensus conference cosponsored by the American Association of Clinical Endocrinologists, American College of Endocrinology, American Diabetes Association, Endocrine Society, American Association of Diabetes Educators, American Heart Association, American Society of Anesthesiologists, Society of Critical Care Medicine, Society of Hospital Medicine, and Society of Thoracic Surgeons, a position statement was developed by the American College of Endocrinology with recommendations for glycemic targets in the hospital setting [9]. During the 2-day conference, experts reviewed extensive data and deliberated regarding the most appropriate targets for glycemic control in the hospital setting [9]. The upper limits of normal for glycemic targets are shown in Box 1.

Role of intravenous insulin therapy in critically ill patients

Hyperglycemia is very common in critically ill patients in the intensive care unit (ICU), even among patients with no prior history of diabetes. This

---

Box 1. Upper limits for glycemic targets

Intensive care unit
    110 mg/dL (6.1 mmol/L)

Noncritical care units
    Preprandial
    110 mg/dL (6.1 mmol/L)
    Maximal glucose
    180 mg/dL (10.0 mmol/L)

Data from American College of Endocrinology. Position statement on inpatient diabetes and metabolic control. Endocr Pract 2004;10:77–82.

"stress hyperglycemia" is believed to be due to insulin resistance in the liver and the skeletal muscle. Until recently, it was felt that mild to moderate degrees of hyperglycemia was inconsequential or perhaps even adaptive to ensure there was enough substrate to provide enough energy.

Van den Berghe and colleagues [5] challenged this notion in a prospective, randomized control study. They studied 1548 mechanically ventilated adults who were admitted to a surgical ICU. These patients were randomized to receive either intensive insulin therapy with target blood glucose of 80 to 110 mg/dL or conventional therapy to maintain blood glucose between 180 and 200 mg/dL; insulin infusion was initiated in the conventional group if blood glucose exceeded 215 mg/dL. The primary outcome measure was all-cause mortality in the ICU. Secondary outcome measures included in-hospital mortality, duration of ICU stay, and need for ICU ventilator support for more than 14 days.

The intensive insulin therapy group showed a significant reduction in ICU mortality compared with the conventional therapy group, 4.6% and 8% respectively ($P < 0.04$). The mortality reduction was only evident in patients who stayed in the ICU more than 5 days, 10.6% versus 20.2% ($P = 0.005$). In addition, the intensive therapy group had significant reductions in in-hospital mortality (-34%), sepsis (-46%), acute renal failure requiring dialysis or hemofiltration (-41%), rate of transfusion (-50%), and polyneuropathy (-44%).

Impact of hyperglycemia and intravenous insulin infusion on the outcome of myocardial infarction

More than 80% of deaths associated with diabetes are from cardiovascular disease, of which 75% are a result of coronary artery disease [10]. Although the mortality from coronary artery disease has declined in the general population, this decline has not been as significant in individuals with diabetes. Insulin resistance and abnormal glucose tolerance is even more common in patients with acute coronary syndrome as evidenced by a recent study showing that only one third of all patients had a normal glucose tolerance test 3 months after the acute event [11]. These results are consistent with a 2002 prospective study by Norhammar and colleagues [12], who looked at outcomes in 181 consecutive patients admitted to the coronary care units of two hospitals in Sweden with acute myocardial infarction but no diagnosis of diabetes and a blood glucose concentration of less than 200 mg/dL (11.1 mmol/L). Subjects underwent standardized oral glucose tolerance tests (75-g glucose load) at discharge and again 3 months later. Fifty-eight of 164 (35%) and 58 of 144 (40%) individuals had impaired glucose tolerance at discharge and after 3 months, respectively, whereas 51 of 164 (31%) and 36 of 144 (25%) had previously undiagnosed diabetes mellitus.

It is well established that the short- and long-term prognosis of diabetic patients sustaining acute myocardial infarction is poor and is associated with increased mortality and morbidity [13]. A meta-analysis of 15 studies reported that hyperglycemia (glucose > 110 mg/dL), with or without a prior history of diabetes, is associated with increases in in-hospital mortality and congestive heart failure in patients admitted for acute myocardial infarction [14].

The DIGAMI study demonstrated that the unfavorable long-term prognosis could be improved by insulin treatment [4], extending findings from previous reports [15–17]. In the DIGAMI study, 620 patients with acute myocardial infarction and hyperglycemia (with and without prior history of diabetes) were randomized to either intravenous (IV) insulin-glucose infusion for at least 24 hours, followed by multidose subcutaneous insulin treatment for at least 3 months or to a control group, which received conventional treatment that generally included sulfonylurea therapy. The conventional treatment group was used as the control arm; therapy was left to the discretion of the treating physicians. Standard therapy for acute myocardial infarction was applied to all subjects. The baseline character-istics were similar between the two groups. The primary end point of the study was 3-month mortality; the secondary end point was 1-year mortality.

Results showed that the mortality at 1 year was significantly reduced in the infusion group (19%) compared with the control group (26%). The long-term results (3.4 years of follow-up) showed a persistent relative mortality reduction of 25% ($P = 0.011$) in the insulin-treated group, which corresponds to an absolute mortality reduction of 11%. Risk reduction was even more significant in patients who were considered "low risk": a group of 272 patients with no prior history of insulin therapy. In this group, there was a 58% reduction in mortality at discharge ($P < 0.05$), a 50% reduction at 12 months, and a 45% reduction at 3.4 years ($P = 0.004$).

Impact of insulin therapy on nonglycemic parameters of metabolic control

Insulin promotes glucose oxidation, which is beneficial in ischemic situations [18]. Increased levels of circulating free fatty acids (FFAs) are a common finding in a setting of myocardial ischemia [19]. FFA oxidation is detrimental to the myocardium because of an increased oxygen demand and to a direct inhibition of glucose oxidation [20]. In addition, increased FFA use during ischemia causes accumulation of FFA metabolites. These in turn are toxic to the myocardium and can provoke arrhythmia and exacerbate mechanical dysfunction [19]. Furthermore, the Paris Prospective Study reported FFAs as a predictor of sudden death [21], and the infusion of FFAs can induce ventricular fibrillation [19,22].

Proinflammatory cytokines are also likely involved in the morbidity and mortality of severe illness [23,24]. These cytokines appear to promote acute thrombosis, sepsis, heart failure, the cachexia of malignancy, and are involved in the pathogenesis of atherosclerosis. The regulation of these cytokines (and the acute phase proteins they modulate) is complex and not fully understood. However, one fact remains clear: exogenous insulin, when infused to normal or near-normal blood glucose levels, can inhibit some of these macrophage and monocyte products [25–27].

There are two other possible mechanisms through which insulin may independently improve outcomes in critically ill patients. First, it suppresses the growth factors involved in acute thrombosis, which may be important during acute myocardial infarction [28]. Second, it stimulates endothelial nitric oxide synthase, which results in the synthesis of nitric oxide and potentially results in vascular vasodilation [29].

Impact of hyperglycemia and intravenous insulin infusion on cardiac surgery outcome

The prevalence of diabetes among patients undergoing coronary artery bypass graft (CABG) is as high as 28%, and diabetes is an independent risk factor for CABG-related death [30]. In addition, postoperative hyperglycemia ($\geq$200 mg/dL) is a predictor of infectious complications in patients undergoing coronary artery surgery [31] and is associated with surgical-site infection [32]. In a study of 1000 patients undergoing cardiothoracic surgery at a large university hospital setting, hyperglycemia in the first 48 postoperative hours was associated with a twofold higher rate of surgical-site infection compared with the normoglycemic group [32].

It has been shown that IV insulin during the postoperative period improves outcome. Zerr and colleagues [33] were able to demonstrate that use of IV insulin in the first 3 postoperative days significantly reduces morbidity in cardiac surgery patients, specifically in reducing deep sternal wound infection. This retrospective study involved 1585 patients with diabetes who underwent cardiac surgery between 1987 and 1993. The study looked at the rate of deep wound infection in patients treated before and after September 1991, when a protocol of postoperative continuous IV insulin to maintain a blood glucose level of less than 200 mg/dL was initiated. Patients treated with IV insulin infusion to maintain glucose levels below 200 mg/dL had a significantly lower incidence ($P < 0.02$) of deep wound infection, from 2.8% before the implementation of IV insulin therapy to 0.74% the third year after the implementation. In a subsequent publication, Furnary and colleagues [34] reported that continuous insulin infusion added an independently protective effect against death (odds ratio 0.50, $P = .005$) to the constellation of risk factors described in the Society of Thoracic Surgeons risk model [30]. They concluded that diabetes per se is not a true risk factor for death after CABG; rather, it is the underlying glycometabolic state of the myocardium that independently affects postoperative mortality.

Relationship between glycemic control and stroke outcome

Observational studies suggest a correlation between blood glucose level, mortality and morbidity, and functional recovery in patients who have suffered a stroke. Capes and colleagues [35] performed a meta-analysis of 26 studies published between 1996 and 2000 and reported that in patients with no history of diabetes who had an ischemic stroke, even a moderately elevated glucose level (>110 mg/dL) is associated with a threefold higher risk of in-hospital or 30-day mortality and an increased risk of poor functional recovery compared with those with lower glucose levels. This meta-analysis was limited by several factors, including the use of pooled studies with different inclusion and exclusion criteria, definitions of hyperglycemia, and concomitant treatment; nevertheless, the strong association between admission hyperglycemia and poor prognosis suggests that glucose level is an important prognostic factor for morbidity and mortality after stroke.

Other studies suggest similar correlation between blood glucose level and mortality and morbidity in stroke patients [36,37]. These observational studies highlight the need for interventional controlled trials to investigate the impact of targeted glycemic control on the outcome of acute stroke both in patients with and without a known history of diabetes.

Hyperglycemia and infection

The association between hyperglycemia and infection has long been recognized [38,39]. Pomposelli and coworkers [38] found that early postoperative glucose control predicts nosocomial infection in diabetic patients. In this study, 97 patients with diabetes undergoing surgery were studied. On postoperative day 1, a single glucose level of more than 220 mg/dL was shown to be a sensitive predictor of nosocomial infection at a rate 2.7 times higher than in patients who had blood glucose levels below 220 mg/dL. In a separate evaluation that excluded patients with minor urinary tract infection from the analysis, the rate of severe infection such as sepsis, pneumonia, and wound infection was increased to 5.7%.

In 1499 patients studied between 1987 and 1994, Furnary and colleagues [6] found that hyperglycemia in the first 48 hours following surgery was an independent risk factor for deep sternal wound infection; patients with glucose levels above 200 mg/dL had a risk 2.2 times higher than those patients with glucose levels of less than 200 mg/dL. Control of hyperglycemia with IV insulin in these patients resulted in a 66% reduction of this serious complication to a rate similar to that of nondiabetic subjects.

The association between hyperglycemia and increased infection may be attributed to impaired immune function. Phagocyte dysfunction appears to be the primary problem, including impaired adherence, chemotaxis, phagocytosis, bacterial killing, and respiratory burst [40–50]. Other abnormalities of impaired immune function associated with hyperglycemia include nonenzymatic glycation of immunoglobulins and reduced T-lymphocyte populations [51]. The effect on peripheral lymphocytes associated with hyperglycemia is reversed when glucose levels are lowered [52].

Good glycemic control reduces cost and length of hospital stay

Although the association between hyperglycemia and adverse outcomes is well supported [53–56], prospective studies for using glucose reduction as a means of reducing length of hospitalization are few, and cost-effectiveness analyses are even fewer in number.

Several studies have shown a relationship between improved inpatient glucose control and decreased hospital length of stay [34,57–62]. Furnary and colleagues [62] showed that length of stay was increased by 1 day for each 50-mg/dL increase above 150 mg/dL in the mean glucose during the first 3 postoperative days ($P < 0.001$). An intensive IV insulin regimen was associated with 23% reduction in length of hospital stay. This resulted in a net savings of more than $680 per patient.

In a nonrandomized, retrospective review, Levetan and associates [58] reported that diabetes team consultation resulted in a 56% shorter hospitalization than those patients with no consultation and proposed a cost saving of $2353 per patients who were managed by the diabetes team. From the studies available, the cost benefit of improved glycemic control appears to be apparent; however, more rigorous analyses of cost effectiveness are warranted.

The use of intravenous insulin in the hospital

In the ICU, the data support the use of IV insulin both for critically ill patients (especially those who have had recent surgery) and for those with hyperglycemia during an acute myocardial infarction [9,63]. There is also general consensus that IV insulin should be used for metabolically unstable patients with widely fluctuating blood glucose levels, regardless of their location in the hospital [9,63]. However, IV insulin infusions are infrequently used on general medical and surgical wards. Typical "sliding scale" insulin is not effective in the manner that it is typically used [64], and yet it is part of our medical culture [65].

IV insulin infusions have been used to manage diabetes for more than 20 years and have a proven record of safety and efficacy [66]. An insulin drip has more predictable bioavailability, is easier and quicker to titrate, and is safer than subcutaneous insulin in patients who are not eating or who may be suddenly switched to no-eating status.

There are a wide variety of insulin infusion protocols, but there are no studies in which algorithms are compared with one another. It is apparent that protocols have to be adapted to each specific hospital environment and that no one protocol would be likely to be effective at all hospitals. As an example, Appendix 1 presents the protocol used by the author at the University of Washington Medical Center in Seattle, Washington [67].

Several aspects of the IV insulin protocol need to be emphasized. First, there must be enough bedside glucose testing to ensure optimum patient safety. The ideal frequency of glucose testing has not been systematically studied. At the University of Washington, we generally initiate the protocol with hourly glucose measurements, at least until the blood glucose is stable [67]. Next, the protocol should include some mechanism for changing infusion rate if there have been significant alterations in blood glucose. Some of the most widely used protocols have this feature [68,69].

Next, enough glucose needs to be provided to prevent both hypoglycemia and starvation ketosis. Again, the ideal amount has not been systematically studied, but most authors suggest 5 to 10 g each hour. If ketonuria occurs despite well-controlled blood glucose levels, the amount of glucose needs to be increased.

The University of Washington Medical Center is a 400-bed teaching hospital where numerous IV insulin infusion protocols have been used since 1991. Each service had their own protocol, but in July of 2002 the insulin infusion algorithms were all standardized to a protocol adapted from the Markovitz report (see Appendix 1) [68]. Instead of introducing the protocol throughout the entire hospital at the same time, each nursing unit was transitioned sequentially until they were comfortable with the new protocol. This took over a year to accomplish, but we found satisfaction from nurses and physicians to be high, and the protocol was found to be quite safe [70]. Compared with the old protocol, which resulted in over 40% of blood glucose values above 180 mg/dL, we found only 16.7% of blood glucose levels greater than this value. Likewise, hypoglycemia was rare with the new protocol. Only 3% had one blood glucose measurement below 40 mg/dL, and 16% had one reading below 60 mg/dL. On the old protocol, this compares to 14% and 30% below 40 mg/dL and 60 mg/dL, respectively.

It is clear that for these types of protocols to work effectively, there must be an understanding of the general philosophies of insulin therapy among endocrinologists, cardiologists, surgeons, anesthesiologists, primary care physicians, nurses, and hospital pharmacists. Often a significant amount of education will be required for those not very familiar with insulin therapy.

According to the American College of Endocrinology position statement on inpatient diabetes and metabolic control [9], implementation of these protocols requires assessment of hospital systems for safety and quality of care; adjustments may be required for appropriate provision of diabetes care, including timely delivery of meal trays, point-of-care blood glucose testing, and the administration of diabetes medications. It is also recommended that nursing staff receive adequate and ongoing in-service training on the specialized needs of the inpatient with diabetes, especially with regard to insulin therapy. A team approach to implementation is also recommended. In addition to the physician, the team may include specialty staff such as a certified diabetes educator. Diabetes educators and nursing staff should collaborate in providing basic "survival skills" when needed to allow for a safe discharge. Finally, discharge planning should be initiated well in advance, exploring community resources and arranging for follow-up of diabetic issues.

The use of subcutaneous insulin therapy in the hospital

When addressing subcutaneous (SC) insulin therapy, it is important that the definitions of insulin therapy are appreciated. Differences between physiologic and nonphysiologic insulin replacement, basal and prandial insulin replacement, and the difference between a supplement and an adjustment need to be clear [66]. The insulin supplement (or "correction dose") needs to be differentiated from sliding scale insulin [34,66].

Neutral protamine Hagedorn and regular insulin have been traditionally used for basal and prandial glucose coverage, respectively. We believe that the use of current insulin analogs minimizes hypoglycemia and increases flexibility [71]. It is important to appreciate that even though studies have not been performed, rapid-acting analogs (lispro or aspart) should theoretically be more effective and safer as correction dose insulin than regular insulin. This is because their more rapid onset and shorter duration of action makes them more predictable. By the same token, it is our opinion that, although using a pure basal insulin (eg, insulin glargine) to treat acute hyperglycemia will result in failure, glargine does provide a much more predictable basal delivery of insulin compared with neutral protamine Hagedorn or ultralente insulin.

Appendix 1 presents a sample SC order form that was developed and implemented at the University of Washington Medical Center to improve safety and efficacy of SC insulin [67]. Compared with the IV insulin infusion protocols, there is much less experience with these SC protocols. However, our protocol has resulted in several advantages, including some that were unexpected (Appendix 2). First, like all hospital protocols, having a uniform SC insulin algorithm results in standardization of therapy. Any problems can be rectified and there can be immediate quality improvements in the entire hospital system. Second, the protocol is designed to improve glucose control to better match the new guidelines [9]. Third, and perhaps most importantly, an SC insulin protocol that differentiates basal insulin replacement, prandial insulin replacement, and correction dose insulin can educate both younger and older physicians in current strategies for insulin use [71]. This last benefit was unexpected. Over the years there have been numerous attempts to better educate physicians about both the basics and the subtleties of insulin therapy, but surveys have reported that physicians do not have a good understanding of how to best use insulin, especially in the United States [72,73]. By using an SC protocol for hospitalized patients on a daily basis, physicians learn how to adjust insulin appropriately, including the best use of correction dose insulin. We believe that in relatively short amounts of time, medical and surgical residents of all specialties could become quite knowledgeable about the use of SC insulin by simply working with the protocol for their hospitalized patients. Only prospective trials will be able to confirm these beliefs.

Summary

The evidence continues to strengthen our understanding that improved glycemic control with the use of insulin therapy may significantly improve morbidity and mortality in hospitalized patients with hyperglycemia, with or without a previous diagnosis of diabetes. However, many questions remain concerning the impact and relative contributions of blood glucose and insulin per se. Nevertheless, the publication of numerous and consistent studies have made it clear that the topic of glycemic management in the hospital requires a larger priority among clinicians caring for these patients.

The recently published guidelines by the American Association of Clinical Endocrinologists are the first formal recommendations on this topic [9], but national guidelines for blood glucose levels cannot take into account all of the different challenges facing different hospitals. This suggests that each institution will require individualization of protocols even though the ultimate metabolic goals are identical. Furthermore, it is not realistic to expect those unfamiliar with diabetes therapy to appreciate all of the nuances and vagaries of insulin treatment. Like any medical treatment, a significant amount of time will need to be invested by the providers involved with the care of these patients before a mastery of the therapy can be achieved. Nevertheless, because the rewards to our patients can be significant, we need to strive to improve the systems where we work. Individual clinicians with vast experience in diabetes care cannot be successful for the inpatient with diabetes unless the hospital has systems in place to effectively and efficiently facilitate the management of the metabolic needs of this population.

The main challenge now is the safe and effective implementation of these guidelines in both small and large hospitals given the limited level of resources available in today's medical environment. Therefore, our single most important recommendation is to ensure that all clinicians involved in the management of these patients are in agreement about general philosophies of diabetes management. We would recommend that there are "champions" for each discipline: endocrinology, cardiology, anesthesiology, surgery, nursing, and pharmacy, all of which have developed hospital-specific guidelines for glycemic management. These recommendations can be slowly adapted, one unit at a time, until the entire hospital has transitioned to a more "diabetes-friendly" environment. The ultimate goal of well-controlled glycemia with minimal hypoglycemia should be possible for most hospitals, and we hope this review will assist clinicians in achieving this objective.

We await additional outcome research with carefully controlled studies to confirm the value of these recommendations at different levels of glycemic control. We believe that we can already state with confidence that the preliminary evidence shows that, like outpatient diabetes management, metabolic control matters during acute illness.

Appendix 1. Example of a standardized intravenous insulin infusion

General guidelines

- Goal blood glucose level: usually 80 to 180 mg/dL (80 to 110 mg/dL for the ICU)
- Standard drip: 100 U/100 mL 0.9% NaCl by way of an infusion device (1 U/1 cc)
- Surgical patients who have received an oral diabetes medication within 24 hours should start when blood glucose level is above 120 mg/dL. All other patients can start when blood glucose level is 70 mg/dL or more
- Insulin infusions should be discontinued when a patient is eating and has received first dose of subcutaneous insulin

Intravenous fluids

- Most patients will need 5 to 10 g of glucose per hour
- D_5W or $D_5W1/2NS$ at 100 to 200 mL per hour or equivalent (total parenteral nutrition, enteral feeds, and so forth)

Initiating the infusion

- Algorithm 1: start here for most patients.
- Algorithm 2: for patients not controlled with algorithm 1, or start here if status post (s/p) CABG, s/p solid organ transplant or islet cell transplant, receiving glucocorticoids, or patient with diabetes receiving more than 80 U/d of insulin as an outpatient
- Algorithm 3: for patients not controlled with algorithm 2; no patients start here without authorization from the endocrine service
- Algorithm 4: for patients not controlled with algorithm 3; no patients start here

Patients not controlled with the above algorithms require an endocrine consult.

Algorithm 1		Algorithm 2		Algorithm 3		Algorithm 4	
BG	Units/hour	BG	Units/hour	BG	Units/hour	BG	Units/hour
< 70	Off	< 70	Off	< 70	Off	< 70	Off
70–109	0.2	70–109	0.5	70–109	1	70–109	1.5
110–119	0.5	110–119	1	110–119	2	110–119	3
120–149	1	120–149	1.5	120–149	3	120–149	5
150–179	1.5	150–179	2	150–179	4	150–179	7
180–209	2	180–209	3	180–209	5	180–209	9
210–239	2	210–239	4	210–239	6	210–239	12
240–269	3	240–269	5	240–269	8	240–269	16
270–299	3	270–299	6	270–299	10	270–299	20
300–329	4	300–329	7	300–329	12	300–329	24
330–359	4	330–359	8	330–359	14	> 330	28
> 360	6	> 360	12	> 360	16	—	—

< 60 = hypoglycemia (see below for treatment).
Abbreviation: BG, blood glucose.

Moving from algorithm to algorithm

- Moving up: an algorithm failure is defined as a blood glucose level outside the goal range (see above goal), and the blood glucose does not change by at least 60 mg/dL within 1 hour
- Moving down: when blood glucose level is less than 70 mg/dL × 2

Patient monitoring

- Goal blood glucose level: 80 to 180 mg/dL
- Check capillary blood glucose level every hour until it is within goal range for 4 hours, then decrease to every 2 hours for 4 hours; if it remains stable, decrease to every 4 hours
- Hourly monitoring may be indicated for critically ill patients even if they have stable blood glucose

Treatment of hypoglycemia (blood glucose level < 60 mg/dL)

- Discontinue insulin drip AND
- Give $D_{50}W$ IV (patient awake, 25 mL [1/2 amp]; patient not awake, 50 mL [1 amp])
- Recheck blood glucose level every 20 minutes and repeat 25 mL of $D_{50}W$ IV if it is below 60 mg/dL; restart drip once blood glucose is above 70 mg/dL × 2 checks; restart drip with lower algorithm (see *Moving Down*)

When to notify the physician

- If there is any blood glucose change greater than 100 mg/dL in 1 hour
- If blood glucose level is above 360 mg/dL
- For hypoglycemia that has not resolved within 20 minutes of administering 50 mL of $D_{50}W$ IV and discontinuing the insulin drip

Adapted from Trence DL, Kelly JL, Hirsch IB. The rationale and management of hyperglycemia for in-patients with cardiovascular disease: time for change. J Clin Endocrinol Metab 2003;88:2430–7; with permission.

Appendix 2. Example of standardized subcutaneous insulin orders

Blood glucose monitoring

- Before meals and at bedtime
- _____ hours after meals
- 2:00 to 3:00 AM

Insulin orders	Breakfast	Lunch	Dinner	Bedtime
Prandial	Give____units of: Lispro Aspart Regular	Give____units of: Lispro Aspart Regular	Give____units of: Lispro Aspart Regular	—
Basal	Give____units of: NPH Lente Ultralente Glargine	—	Give____units of: NPH Lente Ultralente Glargine	Give____units of: NPH Lente Ultralente Glargine

Goal premeal blood glucose: 80–150 mg/dL.

Suggested lag times for prandial insulin:

- Aspart/Lispro: 0 to 15 minutes before eating
- Regular: 30 minutes before eating

If blood glucose is < 60 mg/dL:

A. If patient can take orally, give 15 g of fast-acting carbohydrate (4-oz fruit juice/nondiet soda, 8-oz nonfat milk, or 3 to 4 glucose tablets)
B. If patient cannot take orally, give 25 mL of D50 as IV push
C. Check finger capillary glucose every 15 minutes and repeat above if blood glucose is < 80 mg/dL

Premeal "correction dose" algorithm for hyperglycemia to be administered in addition to scheduled insulin dose to correct premeal hyperglycemia.

- Lispro
- Aspart

Algorithm	Premeal BG	Additional insulin (units)
Low-dose[a]	150–199	1
	200–249	2
	250–299	3
	300–349	4
	> 349	5
Medium-dose[b]	150–199	1
	200–249	3
	250–299	5
	300–349	7
	> 349	8
High-dose[c]	150–199	2
	200–249	4
	250–299	7
	300–349	10
	> 349	12
Individualized	150–199	
	200–249	
	250–299	
	300–349	
	> 349	

Abbreviation: BG, blood glucose.
[a] For patients requiring ≤ 40 U of insulin per day.
[b] For patients requiring 40–80 U of insulin per day.
[c] For patients requiring > 80 U of insulin per day.

General insulin dosing recommendations

Patients with type 1 diabetes

This patient must have insulin to prevent ketosis. Even if the patient is not eating, he/she will need at least basal insulin (NPH/lente/ultralente/glargine) to prevent ketosis.

1. When admitting a patient with type 1 diabetes, continue the basal insulin that the patient was taking at home at the same dose. If the patient will not be eating, use an insulin drip rather than subcutaneous insulin. The prandial insulin (regular/lispro/aspart) may require adjustment depending on the patient's situation. If the patient is eating much less, the prandial insulin will need to be reduced. Many hospitalized patients are under significant metabolic stress (infection, glucocorticoids, and so forth) and may require larger doses of prandial insulin despite eating less.
2. If a patient is newly diagnosed, the usual daily insulin requirement is 0.5 to 0.7 U/kg/d. Half should be given as basal insulin and the remainder as prandial insulin.

Patients with type 2 diabetes

1. If patient is using insulin at home, continue the outpatient regimen and adjust as needed.
2. If patient has not been using insulin previously, the usual total daily insulin requirement is 0.4 to 1.0 U/kg/d.
3. Individual insulin doses vary widely and adjustments should be made based on the bedside and laboratory glucose levels.

Note: Individual insulin doses vary widely, and adjustments should be based on bedside and laboratory glucose levels.

Adapted from Trence DL, Kelly JL, Hirsch IB. The rationale and management of hyperglycemia for in-patients with cardiovascular disease: time for change. J Clin Endocrinol Metab 2003;88:2430–87; with permission.

References

[1] Centers for Disease Control and Prevention (CDC). Diabetes fact sheet. Available at: http://diabetes.org/diabetes-statistics/national-diabetes-fact-sheet.jsp. Accessed February 20, 2004.
[2] Narayan KMV, Boyle JP, Thompson TJ, et al. Lifetime risk for diabetes mellitus in the United States. JAMA 2003;290:1884–90.
[3] Hogan P, Dall T, Nikolov P. American Diabetes Association. Economic costs of diabetes in the US in 2002. Diabetes Care 2003;26:917–32.
[4] Malmberg K, Norhammar A, Wedel H, et al. Glycometabolic state at admission: important risk marker of mortality in conventionally treated patients with diabetes mellitus and acute myocardial infarction: long-term results from the Diabetes and Insulin-Glucose Infusion in Acute Myocardial Infarction (DIGAMI) study. Circulation 1999;99:2626–32.
[5] Van den Berghe G, Wouters P, Weekers F, et al. Intensive insulin therapy in the critically ill patients. N Engl J Med 2001;345:1359–67.
[6] Furnary AP, Zerr KJ, Grunkemeier GL, et al. Continuous intravenous insulin infusion reduces the incidence of deep sternal wound infection in diabetic patients after cardiac surgical procedures. Ann Thorac Surg 1999;67:352–60 [discussion: 360–2].
[7] Lazar HL, Chipkin SR, Fitzgerald CA, et al. Tight glycemic control in diabetic coronary artery bypass graft patients improves perioperative outcomes and decreases recurrent ischemic events. Circulation 2004;109:1497–502.
[8] Centers for Disease Control and Prevention. Diabetes Public Health Resource. Available at: http://www.cdc.gov/diabetes/statistics. Accessed February 20, 2004.
[9] American College of Endocrinology. Position statement on inpatient diabetes and metabolic control. Endocr Pract 2004;10:77–82.
[10] Webster MW, Scott RS. What cardiologists need to know about diabetes. Lancet 1997;350(Suppl):123–8.
[11] Tenerz A, Norhammar A, Silveira A, et al. Diabetes, insulin resistance, and the metabolic syndrome in patients with acute myocardial infarction without previously known diabetes. Diabetes Care 2003;26:2770–6.
[12] Norhammar A, Tenerz A, Nilsson G, et al. Glucose metabolism in patients with acute myocardial infarction and no previous diagnosis of diabetes mellitus: a prospective study. Lancet 2002;359:2140–4.
[13] Abbott R, Kannel W, Wilson P. The impact of diabetes on survival following myocardial infarction in men and women. JAMA 1988;260:3456–60.

[14] Capes SE, Hunt D, Malmberg K, et al. Stress hyperglycemia and increased risk of death after myocardial infarction in patients with and without diabetes: a systematic overview. Lancet 2000;355:773–8.

[15] Malmberg K, Ryden L, Efendic S, et al. A randomized trial of insulin-glucose infusion followed by subcutaneous insulin treatment in diabetic patients with acute myocardial infarction: effects on one year mortality. J Am Coll Cardiol 1995;26:57–65.

[16] Malmberg K, Ryden L, Hamsten A, et al. Effects of insulin treatment on cause-specific one-year mortality and morbidity in diabetic patients with acute myocardial infarction. Eur Heart J 1996;17:1337–44.

[17] Malmberg K. Prospective randomized study of intensive insulin treatment on long-term survival after acute myocardial infarction in patients with diabetes mellitus. BMJ 1997;314: 1512–5.

[18] Perdomo G, Commerford SR, Richard A-MT, et al. Increased beta-oxidation in muscle cells enhances insulin-stimulated glucose metabolism and protects against fatty acid induced insulin resistance despite intramyocellular lipid accumulation. J Biol Chem 2004;279(26): 27177–86.

[19] Oliver MF, Opie LH. Effects of glucose and fatty acids on myocardial ischaemia and arrhythmias. Lancet 1994;343:155–8.

[20] Lopaschuk GD, Wambolt RB, Barr RL. An imbalance between glycolysis and glucose oxidation is a possible explanation for the detrimental effects of high levels of fatty acids during aerobic reperfusion of ischemic hearts. J Pharmacol Exp Ther 1993;264:135–44.

[21] Jouven X, Charles MA, Desnos M, et al. Circulating nonesterified fatty acid level as a predictive risk factor for sudden death in the population. Circulation 2001;104:756–61.

[22] Hirsch IB. Impact of insulin therapy on non-glycemic effects during acute illness. Endo Pract 2004;10(Suppl 2):63–70.

[23] Gabay C, Kushner I. Acute phase proteins and other systemic responses to inflammation. N Engl J Med 1999;340:448–54.

[24] Zeidler C, Kanz L, Hurkuck KL. In vivo effects of interleukin-6 on thrombopoiesis in healthy and irradiated primates. Blood 1992;80:2740–5.

[25] Dandona P, Aljada A, Bandyopadhyay A. The potential therapeutic role of insulin in acute myocardial infarction in patients admitted to intensive care and in those with unspecified hyperglycemia. Diabetes Care 2003;26:516–9.

[26] Dandona P, Aljzcz Z, Mohanty P, et al. Insulin inhibits intranuclear factor κβ and stimulates κβ in mononuclear cells in obese subjects: evidence for an anti-inflammatory effect. J Clin Endocrinol Metab 2001;86:3257–65.

[27] Aljada A, Ghanim H, Saadeh R, et al. Insulin inhibits NF-κβ and MCP-1 expression in human aortic endothelial cells. J Clin Endocrinol Metab 2001;86:450–3.

[28] Ghanim H, Mohanty P, Aljada A, et al. Insulin reduces the pro-inflammatory transcription factor, activation protein-1 (AP-1), in mononuclear cells (MNC) and plasma matrix metalloproteinase-9 (MMP-9) concentration. Diabetes 2001;50(Suppl 1):A408.

[29] Steinberg HO, Brechtel G, Johnson N, et al. Insulin-mediated skeletal muscle vasodilation is nitric-oxide dependent. A novel action of insulin to increase nitric oxide release. J Clin Invest 1994;94:1172–9.

[30] Edwards FH, Grover FL, Shroyer AL, et al. The Society of Thoracic Surgeons, National Cardiac Surgery Database: current risk assessment. Ann Thorac Surg 1997;63:903–8.

[31] Golden SH, Pear-Vigilance C, Kao WH, et al. Preoperative glycemic control and the risk of infectious complications in a cohort of adult with diabetes. Diabetes Care 1999;22:1408–14.

[32] Latham R, Lancaster AD, Covington JF, et al. The association of diabetes and glucose control with surgical site infection among cardiothoracic surgery patients. Infect Control Hosp Epidemil 2001;22:607–12.

[33] Zerr KJ, Furnary AP, Grunkemeier GL, et al. Glucose control lowers the risk of wound infection in diabetics after open heart operations. Ann Thorac Surg 1997;63:356–61.

[34] Furnary AP, Gao G, Grunkemeier GL, et al. Continuous insulin infusion reduces mortality in patients with diabetes undergoing coronary artery bypass grafting. J Thorac Cardiovasc Surg 2003;125:1007–21.

[35] Capes SE, Hunt D, Malmberg K, et al. Stress hyperglycemia and prognosis of stroke in non diabetic and diabetic patients: a systematic overview. Stroke 2001;32:2426–32.

[36] Williams LS, Rotich J, Qi R, et al. Effects of admission hyperglycemia on mortality and costs in acute ischemic stroke. Neurology 2002;59:67–71.

[37] Pulsinelli WA, Levy DE, Sigsbee B, et al. Increased damage after ischemic stroke in patients with hyperglycemia with or without established diabetes mellitus. Am J Med 1983; 74:540–4.

[38] Pomposelli JJ, Baxter JK III, Babineau TJ, et al. Early postoperative glucose control predicts nosocomial infection rate in diabetic patients. J Parenter Enteral Nutr 1998;22:77–81.

[39] Golden SH, Peart-Vigilance C, Kao WH, et al. Perioperative glycemic control and the risk of infectious complications in a cohort of adults with diabetes. Diabetes Care 1999;22: 1408–14.

[40] Joshi N, Caputo G, Weitekamp M, et al. Infections in patients with diabetes mellitus. N Engl J Med 1999;341:1906–12.

[41] Wheat L. Infection and diabetes mellitus. Diabetes Care 1980;3:187–97.

[42] Mowat A, Baum J. Chemotaxis of polymorphonuclear leukocytes from patients with diabetes mellitus. N Engl J Med 1971;284:621–7.

[43] Bagdade J, Root R, Bulger R. Impaired leukocyte function in patients with poorly controlled diabetes. Diabetes 1974;23:9–15.

[44] Bagdade JD, Stewart M, Walters E. Impaired granulocyte adherence. A reversible defect in host defense in patients with poorly controlled diabetes. Diabetes 1978;27:677–81.

[45] van Oss CJ, Border JR. Influence of intermittent hyperglycemic glucose levels on the phagocytosis of microorganisms by human granulocytes in vitro. Immunol Commun 1978;7: 669–76.

[46] Davidson N, Sowden J, Fletcher J. Defective phagocytosis in insulin-controlled diabetics: evidence for a reaction between glucose and opsonizing proteins. J Clin Pathol 1984;37: 783–6.

[47] Alexiewicz J, Kumar D, Smogorzewski M, et al. Polymorphonuclear leukocytes in non-insulin-dependent diabetes mellitus: abnormalities in metabolism and function. Ann Intern Med 1995;123:919–24.

[48] Leibovici L, Yehezkelli Y, Porter A, et al. Influence of diabetes mellitus and glycemic control on the characteristics and outcome of common infections. Diabet Med 1996;13:457–63.

[49] Kwoun M, Ling P, Lydon E, et al. Immunologic effects of acute hyperglycemia in nondiabetic rats. J Parenter Enteral Nutr 1997;21:91–5.

[50] McManus L, Bloodworth R, Prihoda T, et al. Agonist-dependent failure of neutrophil function in diabetes correlates with extent of hyperglycemia. J Leukoc Biol 2001;70: 395–404.

[51] Black CT, Hennessey PJ, Andrassy RJ. Short-term hyperglycemia depresses immunity through nonenzymatic glycosylation of circulating immunoglobulin. J Trauma 1990;30: 830–2 [discussion: 832–3].

[52] Bouter KP, Meyling FH, Hoekstra JB, et al. Influence of blood glucose levels on peripheral lymphocytes in patients with diabetes mellitus. Diabetes Res 1992;19:77–80.

[53] Selby JV, Ray GT, Zhang D, et al. Excess costs of medical care for patients with diabetes in a managed care population. Diabetes Care 1997;20:1396–402.

[54] Weir CJ, Murray GD, Dyker AG, et al. Is hyperglycaemia an independent predictor of poor outcome after acute stroke? Results of a long term follow up study. BMJ 1997;314:1303–6.

[55] Wahab NN, Cowden EA, Pearce NJ, et al. ICONS Investigators. Is blood glucose an independent predictor of mortality in acute myocardial infarction in the thrombolytic era? J Am Coll Cardiol 2002;40:1748–54.

[56] Umpierrez GE, Isaacs SD, Bazargan N, et al. Hyperglycemia: an independent marker of in-hospital mortality in patients with undiagnosed diabetes. J Clin Endocrinol Metab 2002; 87:978–82.

[57] Koproski J, Pretto Z, Poretsky L. Effects of an intervention by a diabetes team in hospitalized patients with diabetes. Diabetes Care 1997;20:1553–5.

[58] Levetan CS, Salas JR, Wilets IF, et al. Impact of endocrine and diabetes team consultation on hospital length of stay for patients with diabetes. Am J Med 1995;99:22–8.

[59] Levetan CS, Passaro MD, Jablonski KA, et al. Effect of physician specialty on outcomes in diabetic ketoacidosis. Diabetes Care 1999;22:1790–5.

[60] Almbrand B, Johannesson M, Sjostrand B, et al. Cost-effectiveness of intense insulin treatment after acute myocardial infarction in patients with diabetes mellitus; results from the DIGAMI study. Eur Heart J 2000;21:733–9.

[61] Zhan C, Miller MR. Excess length of stay, charges, and mortality attributable to medical injuries during hospitalization. JAMA 2003;290:1868–74.

[62] Furnary AP, Chaugle H, Zerr KJ, et al. Postoperative hyperglycemia prolongs length of stay in diabetic CABG patients. Circulation 2000;102:II–556.

[63] Clement S, Braithwait SS, Magee MF, et al. Management of diabetes and hyperglycemia in hospitals. Diabetes Care 2004;27:553–91.

[64] Queale WS, Seidler AJ, Brancati FL. Glycemic control and sliding scale insulin use in medical inpatients with diabetes mellitus. Arch Intern Med 1997;157:545–52.

[65] Hirsch IB, Farkas-Hirsch R. Sliding scale or sliding scare: it's all sliding nonsense. Diabetes Spectrum 2001;14:79–81.

[66] Hirsch IB, Paauw DS, Brunzell J. Inpatient management of adults with diabetes. Diabetes Care 1995;18:870–8.

[67] Trence DL, Kelly JL, Hirsch IB. The rationale and management of hyperglycemia for in-patients with cardiovascular disease: time for change. J Clin Endocrinol Metab 2003;88: 2430–87.

[68] Markovitz L, Wiechmann R, Harris N, et al. Description and evaluation of a glycemic management protocol for diabetic patients undergoing heart surgery. Endocr Pract 2002;8: 10–8.

[69] Albert Starr Academic Center for Cardiac Surgery. Star Wood Research. Available at: http://www.starrwood.com/research/insulin.html. Accessed March 14, 2004.

[70] Ku SY, Sayre CA, Hirsch IB, et al. New insulin infusion protocol improves blood control in hospitalized patients without increasing hypoglycemia. Jt Comm J Qual Improv, in press.

[71] Dewitt DE, Hirsch IB. Outpatient therapy for type 1 and type 2 diabetes: scientific review. JAMA 2003;289:2254–64.

[72] Tabak AG, Tamas G, Zgibor J, et al. Targets and reality: a comparison of healthcare indicators in the US (Pittsburgh Epidemiology of Diabetes Complications Study) and Hungary (DiabCare Hungary). Diabetes Care 2000;23:1284–9.

[73] Haywood RA, Manning WG, Kaplan SH, et al. Starting insulin therapy in patients with type 2 diabetes: effectiveness, complications, and resource utilization. JAMA 1997;278:1663–9.

Endocrinol Metab Clin N Am
34 (2005) 117–135

ENDOCRINOLOGY
AND METABOLISM
CLINICS
OF NORTH AMERICA

Potential Cardiovascular Benefits of Insulin Sensitizers

Biju P. Kunhiraman, MD[a], Ali Jawa, MD[a],
Vivian A. Fonseca, MD[b,c,*]

[a]Section of Endocrinology, Diabetes, and Metabolism, Tulane University and Hospital,
1430 Tulane Avenue, New Orleans, LA 70112, USA
[b]Department of Medicine and Pharmacology, Tulane University Medical Center,
1430 Tulane Avenue, New Orleans, LA 70112, USA
[c]Veterans Affairs Hospital, New Orleans, LA, USA

Type 2 diabetes mellitus is a progressive disorder that is caused by a combination of insulin resistance (IR) in the skeletal muscle, adipose tissue, and liver and is burdened further by increasingly impaired pancreatic secretion. It is characterized by metabolic abnormalities that begin several years before the onset of overt hyperglycemia and end with substantial vascular disability [1]. Several epidemiologic studies have shown that hyperinsulinemia that reflects IR is an independent risk factor for cardiovascular disease [2]. Correction of IR, therefore, may be important in the management of type 2 diabetes and may decrease the risk for cardiovascular disease.

Many of the features of IR that are present before the onset of hyperglycemia continue to operate after the onset of hyperglycemia and may be exacerbated by the glucose-mediated tissue effect [3,4]. Insulin resistance contributes to the development of atherosclerosis through multiple recognizable risk factors, such as hypertension, dyslipidemia, and hypercoagulability (Fig. 1) [5].

Patients who have diabetes have a greatly increased relative risk of cardiovascular disease when compared with patients who do not have diabetes [6]. Much of the morbidity and mortality in type 2 diabetes is

Diabetes research at Tulane University Health Sciences Center is supported in part by Susan Harling Robinson Fellowship in Diabetes Research and the Tullis-Tulane Alumni Chair in Diabetes.

* Corresponding author. Department of Medicine and Pharmacology, 1430 Tulane Avenue (SI 53), Tulane University Medical Center, New Orleans, LA 70112.
E-mail address: vfonseca@tulane.edu (V.A. Fonseca).

0889-8529/05/$ - see front matter © 2005 Elsevier Inc. All rights reserved.
doi:10.1016/j.ecl.2004.11.005

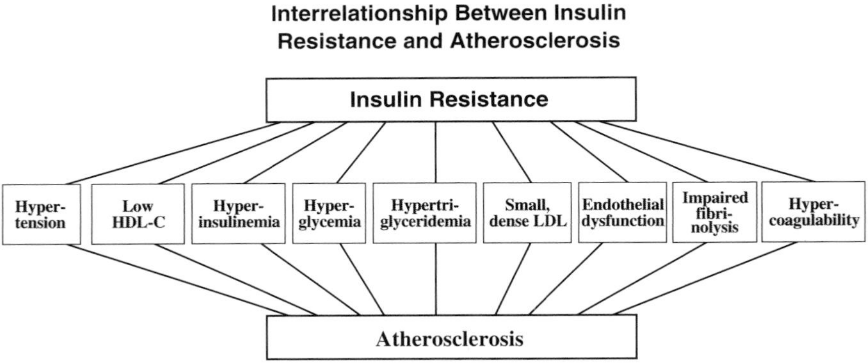

**Interrelationship Between Insulin
Resistance and Atherosclerosis**

Fig. 1. Insulin resistance contributes to the development of atherosclerosis through multiple recognizable risk factors [95,96]. HDL-C, high-density lipoprotein cholesterol; LDL-C, low-density lipoprotein cholesterol.

associated with coronary artery disease, congestive heart failure, and sudden cardiac death. In patients who have established cardiovascular disease, the rate of subsequent cardiovascular events is significantly greater than in individuals who do not have diabetes [7] and is associated with greatly increased morbidity and mortality. Recent advances in invasive cardiology and medical therapy have led to a significant reduction in cardiovascular mortality in nondiabetic men and women. The U.S. reduction in cardiovascular mortality in men who have diabetes, however, has been modest and not statistically significant [8]; mortality rates increased during a 10-year period in women who had diabetes.

Insulin resistance contributes to hyperglycemia in type 2 diabetes and plays a pathophysiologic role in a variety of other metabolic abnormalities, including high levels of plasma triglycerides, low levels of high-density lipoprotein (HDL) cholesterol, hypertension, abnormal fibrinolysis, and coronary heart disease [9,10]. This cluster of abnormalities has been recognized as the IR syndrome or the metabolic syndrome (Table 1) [5,11].

Although controversial because of the small number of patients that was studied, the obesity substudy in the U.K. Prospective Diabetes Study demonstrated that patients who had type 2 diabetes who were treated with metformin had a 30% reduction in cardiovascular disease events and mortality compared with those who were given conventional treatment [12].

Metformin is the only drug that has been suggested to decrease cardiovascular events in patients who have type 2 diabetes, independent of glycemic control [12]. Although metformin inhibits hepatic gluconeogenesis, it also improves peripheral insulin sensitivity, possibly by reducing body weight.

Thiazolidinediones (TZDs) are a new class of compounds for the treatment of type 2 diabetes mellitus. The glucose lowering effects of these drugs are mediated primarily by decreasing IR at the level of the muscle, thereby increasing glucose uptake [13,14]. To a lesser extent, they decrease glucose production by the liver [15]. They act through the proliferator-activated receptor gamma (PPAR-γ) receptors, which are expressed in a variety of tissues, including adipose and vascular tissue.

PPAR-γ is a nuclear receptor that has a regulatory role in differentiation of cells, particularly adipocytes [16]. In addition, TZDs decrease plasma free fatty acid concentrations and may improve insulin sensitivity indirectly by this decrease in free fatty acids [17]. Because free fatty acids are involved in glucose and lipid metabolism [18] and have deleterious effects on the vasculature [19], this reduction in plasma free fatty acids may have a beneficial effect on cardiovascular disease.

Because IR may play a pathophysiologic role in cardiovascular disease, it was proposed that drugs that directly improve insulin sensitivity, such as TZDs, may correct other abnormalities of the IR syndrome in addition to improving hyperglycemia. Thus, treatment of patients with type 2 diabetes with these agents may confer benefits beyond the lowering of glucose [20]. Because of their beneficial effects on IR, the vascular effect of TZDs is a subject of considerable research interest (Table 2).

The purpose of this article is to assess the potential cardioprotective effects of insulin sensitizers, mainly the TZDs, in patients who have type 2 diabetes (Table 3). We focus on the potential to improve the various components of the metabolic syndrome (eg, dyslipidemia, hypertension, impaired fibrinolysis). The current recommended approach to each of the risk factors is addressed and an attempt is made to develop a strategy for reducing cardiovascular risk in patients who have diabetes, in general, and for those who have established cardiovascular disease, in particular. Some of these principles also may apply to individuals who have impaired glucose tolerance, many of whom have features of the IR syndrome.

Table 1

Risk determinants for the diagnosis of the metabolic syndrome as defined by the Adult Treatment Panel III

Risk factor	Defining level
Abdominal obesity (waist circumference)	
Men	> 40 in (> 102 cm)
Women	> 35 in (> 88 cm)
TGs	$\geq$ 150 mg/dL
HDL-C	
Men	< 40 mg/dL
Women	< 50 mg/dL
Blood pressure	$\geq$ 130/$\geq$ 85 mm Hg
Fasting glucose	$\geq$ 110 mg/dL

Data from Haffner SM. Management of dyslipidemia in adults with diabetes. Diabetes Care 1998;21(1):160–78.

Table 2
Ongoing studies involving thiazolidinediones

Study [Ref.]	Main objective	Medications	Endpoint	
			Primary	Secondary
ADOPT [97]	Look at long-term outcome of TZD monotherapy	Rosiglitazone, metformin, or glyburide	Time to monotherapy failure	IS, β-cell preservation, microalbuminuria, PAI-1, CRP, fibrinogen levels
BARI 2D [98]	Compare CV benefits of insulin sensitizers vs insulin-providing therapy (SU or insulin)	Rosiglitazone ± metformin vs SU ± insulin	5-y mortality	Rates of MI, ischemic events, PAI-1 activity, LV function, angina, QOL, subsequent revascularization procedures (CABG and PCI)
DREAM [99]	Look at the use of TZD and ACEI in preventing progression of IGT to T2DM	Rosiglitazone + placebo, or rosiglitazone + ramipril, or ramipril + placebo, or placebo alone	Development of diabetes	Microvascular complications
PIPOD	Evaluate TZD monotherapy to prevent progression of GDM-associated IR to T2DM	Pioglitazone	Development of T2DM	
PROACTIVE [100]	Evaluate TZD therapy in insulin resistant patients	Pioglitazone	Mortality or cardiovascular events	
RECORD	Evaluate glycemic control and CV events in T2DM	Combination therapy: metformin, rosiglitazone, + SU	Time to combined CV end point	Multiple CV and glycemic end points

Abbreviations: ACEI, angiotensin-converting enzyme inhibitor; ADOPT, Avandia Diabetes Outcomes and Progression Trial; BARI-2D, Bypass Angioplasty Revascularization Intervention T2DM; CABG, Coronary artery bypass graft; CV, cardiovascular; DREAM, Diabetes Reduction Assessment with Ramipril and Rosiglitazone Medication; GDM, gestational diabetes mellitus; IGT, impaired glucose tolerance; IS, insulin sensitivity; LV, left ventricular; PAI-1, plasminogen activator inhibitor type 1; PCI, percutaneous coronary intervention; PIPOD, Pioglitazone for the Prevention of Diabetes; PROACTIVE, Prospective Pioglitazone Clinical Trial in Macrovascular Events; QOL, Quality of Life; RECORD, Rosiglitazone Evaluated for Cardiac Outcomes and Regulation of Glycemia in Diabetes; SU, sulphonylureas; T2DM, type 2 diabetes mellitus.

Adapted from Zarich SM. Treating the diabetic patient: appropriate care for glycemic control and cardiovascular disease risk factors; Rev Cardiovasc Med 2003;4(Suppl 5):S19–28.

Table 3
Effects of the thiazolidinediones on cardiovascular risk factors

Risk factor	Effect
Inflammation lipids	Decreases the effects of TNF-α Inhibits NF-κB Decreases ICAM/VCAM expression Decreases Sd-LDL Increases HDL Decreases triglycerides
Coagulation/fibrinolysis	Decreases PAI-1 Decreases fibrinogen levels
Microalbuminuria	Decreases microalbuminuria
Direct vascular effects	Decreases carotid Intima-media thickness and inflammation Decreases blood pressure Induces coronary artery relaxation by decreasing cytosolic calcium Regulates monocyte/macrophage function in atherosclerotic lesions Decreases vascular smooth muscle cell migration Decreases calcium influx and attenuates vascular contraction Decreases renal artery/mesangial cell proliferation
Obesity	Decreases visceral obesity Increases adiponectin Decreases CRP

Abbreviations: CRP, C-reactive protein; ICAM, intercellular adhesion molecule; VCAM, vascular cell adhesion molecule; HDL, high-density lipoprotein; NF-κB, nuclear factor kappa-B; PAI-1, plasminogen activator inhibitor type-1; Sd-LDL, small dense low-density lipoprotein; TNF-α, tumor necrosis factor-alpha.

Recent studies have demonstrated the importance of nontraditional risk factors for cardiovascular disease in diabetes [21]. Traditional and non-traditional risk factors for cardiovascular disease that have been described in patients who have diabetes are outlined in Box 1. Many of the nontraditional risk factors have been found to be associated with IR [22]. Clearly, in patients with diabetes, reduction of blood pressure and improvement in dyslipidemia can impact adverse cardiovascular outcomes.

Insulin sensitizers and lipid metabolism

Lipid abnormalities are present in 30% to 50% of patients who have type 2 diabetes [7]. The characteristic pattern of dyslipidemia in patients who have diabetes and IR includes decreased HDL cholesterol (HDL-C); elevated triglyceride (TG) levels; and an increase in small, dense low-density lipoprotein (LDL) particles, which are more atherogenic. Metformin modestly decreases LDL and increases HDL and has variable effects on TGs [23]. In combination with a sulfonylurea or as monotherapy, it recently

> **Box 1. Traditional and nontraditional risk factors for cardiovascular disease in patients who have diabetes**
>
> *Traditional (established) risk factors*
> Hypertension
> Lipids
> Obesity
> Smoking
>
> *Nontraditional risk factors*
> Abnormal fibrinolysis (fibrinogen, plasminogen activator
>   inhibitor type-1)
> Microalbuminuria
> Endothelial dysfunction
> Markers of inflammation (C-reactive protein, tumor necrosis
>   factor-α, interleukin-6)
> Homocysteine
> Hypercoagulation
>
> ---
>
> *Data from* Saito I, Folsom AR, Brancati FL, et al. Nontraditional risk factors for coronary heart disease incidence among persons with diabetes: the Atherosclerosis Risk in Communities (ARIC) Study. Ann Intern Med 2000;133(2):81–91.

was shown to decrease some nontraditional cardiac risk factors, including remnant lipoprotein cholesterol [24].

The effects of TZDs on lipid metabolism are more complex [25,26]. TZD monotherapy has been associated with a modest (8%–10%) increase in LDL levels, but there is little change in apolipoprotein B levels and a marked shift from small, dense to large, fluffy LDL phenotype. They also were shown to increase HDL significantly, especially in patients who had diabetes and HDL levels that were less than 35 mg/dL. The effects of TZDs on TGs are variable and correlate with the baseline TG level. All of the TZDs increase HDL-C, although only troglitazone and pioglitazone have been shown to decrease TGs consistently [27,28]. The LDL particles in patients who have type 2 diabetes mellitus tend to be smaller and dense which makes them more atherogenic. There is evidence that PPAR-γ may be an important regulator of foam cell gene expression and that oxidized LDL cholesterol regulates macrophage gene expression through these receptors [29]. Furthermore, PPAR-γ promotes the uptake of oxidized LDL cholesterol by macrophages [30]. Therefore, an interaction between PPAR-γ and oxidized LDL cholesterol may be important in the development of atherosclerosis in diabetic patients. Type 2 diabetes is associated with increased TG-rich particles, which trigger inflammation by activating the nuclear factor κB (NFκB) [31]. Type 2 diabetes mellitus also is associated with a low plasma HDL-C, and thus, a reduction in the activity of the protective effect of reverse cholesterol transport pathway [32].

Visceral adiposity causes enhanced lipolysis [33] and augmented free fatty acid (FFA) flux into the portal system. Increased FFA flow into the liver may induce hepatic IR, retard insulin clearance, and enhance lipid synthesis.

Hypertension

Evidence exists that IR contributes to hypertension [34–36]. If true, then improving insulin sensitivity should have the potential to lower blood pressure. The effects of TZDs on blood pressure were examined in several different experimental and clinical settings. Rosiglitazone treatment added onto the patient's usual antihypertensive regimen resulted in better blood pressure control and improved IR [37]. Raji et al [37] examined the effect of rosiglitazone on IR and blood pressure in patients who had essential hypertension. There were significant, albeit small, decreases in mean 24-hour systolic blood pressure; the decline in systolic blood pressure correlated with the improvement in insulin sensitivity. Rosiglitazone treatment of non-diabetic, hypertensive patients improved insulin sensitivity, reduced systolic and diastolic blood pressure, and induced favorable changes in markers of cardiovascular risk [37,38]. Scherbaum and colleagues also reported decreases in systolic blood pressure by pioglitazone in normotensive and hypertensive patients with type 2 diabetes [39].

A potential mechanism for TZD-mediated decreases in blood pressure may be improved insulin sensitivity, which promotes insulin-mediated vasodilatation. Alternative hypotheses for the decrease in blood pressure include inhibition of intracellular calcium and myocyte contractility [40,41] and endothelin-1 expression and secretion. In contrast with TZDs, metformin's effect on blood pressure is controversial, and, at best, minimal.

Endothelial function and vascular reactivity

Vascular endothelium is involved in the regulation of vascular tone, vessel permeability, and angiogenesis. Various paracrine vasodilatory and vasoconstrictor factors, most notably nitric oxide and endothelin-1, determine vascular tone [42,43].The endothelium plays a vital role in the maintenance of blood fluidity, vascular wall tone, and permeability. Endothelial dysfunction is central to many vascular diseases, including atherosclerosis and diabetic microangiopathy. Endothelial function is disturbed by many of the individual features of the IR syndrome, including hypertension, dyslipidemia, and hyperglycemia [44].

Insulin has several direct vascular actions that may contribute to vascular protection or injury. Vascular-protective effects of insulin include stimulation of endothelial cell production of the vasodilator, nitric oxide [45]. This, in turn, inhibits formation of lesions that are dependent on the migration and proliferation of vascular smooth muscle cells (VSMCs) [41], attenuates binding of inflammatory cells to the vascular wall, and inhibit thrombosis by reducing platelet adhesion and aggregation [46].

The ability of the blood vessels to dilate in response to stimuli, including ischemia, is called vascular reactivity or flow-mediated dilatation. Brachial artery vasoactivity is a noninvasive method of assessing endothelial function in vivo [47]. Impaired flow-mediated dilatation is seen with tobacco use, hypercholesterolemia, and diabetes mellitus. It was suggested that endothelial injury and abnormal flow-mediated dilatation may precede the structural changes that are related to atherosclerosis in these subjects.

A recent study showed that IR is a major contributor toward endothelial dysfunction in type 2 diabetes mellitus. Pistrosch et al [48] showed that IR is related to endothelial dysfunction, independent of glycemic control; endothelial IR may be an aspect of IR, in general. Most importantly, they showed that the IR and endothelial dysfunction are amenable to treatment by rosiglitazone, with up to a 60% reduction in IR. Results from their study also suggest that rosiglitazone may improve non-nitric oxide/prostacyclin–related endothelium-dependent vasodilatation. Improvement of vascular reactivity in obese, nondiabetic patients after treatment with rosiglitazone also was reported [49]. This improvement was associated with beneficial changes in several markers of inflammation and endothelial activation.

The TZDs act on the endothelium by way of various mechanisms, including increased nitric oxide synthesis and modulation of various cytokines, including adhesion molecules, that are involved in the atherosclerotic process [50–52]. Recently, metformin also was shown to improve endothelial function [53]; however, the effect is modest compared with the TZDs.

Vascular wall abnormalities

B-mode ultrasound is a noninvasive method for evaluating carotid intimal-medial complex thickness, which is an indicator for early atherosclerosis and is associated with IR [54,55]. This measurement may serve as a surrogate marker for atherosclerotic events because patients who have increased intimal-medial complex thickness have a greater rate of cardiovascular events over time [55]. Treatment with troglitazone significantly decreased intima-media thickness in patients who had type 2 diabetes [54]. Koshiyama and associates [56] recently reported a significant decrease in the intima-media thickness in patients who had type 2 diabetes who were treated with pioglitazone. It is possible that the TZD effects are directly cellular on the atherosclerotic process and not linked to the effects on IR.

In acute coronary events, plaque rupture is a core event. Exposure of the highly thrombogenic lipid core to circulating coagulation factors can lead to a progressive cascade that results in occlusion of the vessel. Matrix metalloproteinases (MMPs) that are produced by monocyte-derived macrophages and VSMCs contribute to this process [32]. TZDs inhibited the expression and functional activity of MMP-9 in human monocyte–derived macrophages and human VSMCs [57–59].

Fibrinolysis and coagulation

Decreased fibrinolytic activity, in association with elevated plasma plasminogen activator inhibitor type 1 (PAI-1), is associated with an increased risk for atherosclerosis and cardiovascular disease [60,61]. PAI-1 is the primary inhibitor of endogenous tissue plasminogen activator and is elevated in patients who have diabetes and in insulin-resistant nondiabetic individuals. Increased PAI-1 levels are recognized now as an integral part of the IR syndrome and correlate significantly with plasma insulin. Impaired fibrinolysis also is noted in other insulin-resistant states, such as the polycystic ovary syndrome [57]. Fonseca and colleagues [62] demonstrated a decrease in plasma PAI-1 levels in patients who had diabetes who were treated with a TZD. This observation was confirmed in several studies [63–65]. The postulated mechanism for the effect of the TZDs is by way of the activation of PPAR-γ and subsequent suppression of PAI-1.

In vitro studies with troglitazone demonstrated direct effect on the vessel wall that led to a decreased synthesis of PAI-1 and indirect effects on hepatic synthesis as a result of the attenuation of hyperinsulinemia [66]. Pioglitazone and rosiglitazone were found to have a similar effect [63,67]. Therefore, PAI-1 reduction may be a class effect of the insulin sensitizers. Metformin also reduces PAI-1, which supports the notion that these changes are mediated by a decrease in IR [61].

Inflammation

PPAR-γ ligands counter the effects of various inflammatory cytokines that are released after the endothelial injury. These agents also inhibit VSMC proliferation; down-regulate endothelial cell growth factor receptors; and suppress the movement of various other cells through inhibition of vascular cell adhesion molecule–1, intercellular adhesion molecule–1, and monocyte chemoattractant protein (MCP)-1. Animal studies demonstrated that pioglitazone has vasculoprotective effects in acute and chronic vascular injury [52,68]. Similarly, in a rat model, rosiglitazone reduced myocardial infarction size [69] and postischemic injury and improved aortic flow following reperfusion [70].

Like elevated PAI-1, increases in plasma concentrations of markers of inflammation, such as C-reactive protein (CRP), are associated with the IR syndrome and cardiovascular disease [71]. Fuell and colleagues [72] reported reductions in the proinflammatory markers, interleukin-6, CRP, and white blood cells, in patients who had type 2 diabetes and were treated with rosiglitazone, whereas Haffner and colleagues [73] reported a reduction in levels of MMP-9 and CRP in patients who had type 2 diabetes who were treated with rosiglitazone. These effects may be related to the decrease in IR and may have beneficial consequences for long-term cardiovascular risk. Satoh et al [74] showed that the potential antiatherogenic effects of pioglitazone (ie, decrease of CRP and pulse wave velocity) were independent of changes in parameters that were related to glucose metabolism.

Insulin and TZDs inhibit the expression of proinflammatory genes (NFκB-regulated genes) and suppress factors that are responsible for plaque rupture and thrombosis (eg, early growth response transcription factor–1, tissue factor), which could contribute to an antiatherogenic effect [75]. One study that evaluated troglitazone showed a profound reduction in the levels of NFκB—a molecule that induces inflammatory cytokines, such as tumor necrosis factor–α, MCP-1, adhesion molecules (soluble intercellular adhesion molecule–1), and reactive oxygen species. Thus, TZDs exert anti-inflammatory actions that may contribute to their putative antiatherosclerotic effects.

In a recent study, metformin decreased some cardiac risk factors (eg, soluble vascular cell adhesion molecule-1) when used as monotherapy or in combination with sulfonylureas, after a 12-week treatment period [24].

Adiponectin

Adipose tissue is not just an inert storage organ, but is an important endocrine organ that plays a key role in the integration of endocrine, metabolic, and inflammatory signals for the control of energy homeostasis [76]. It was shown to secrete a host of proteins called adipokines; adiponectin is one of the key players. Although adiponectin is secreted only by adipose tissue, its levels are decreased in obese humans, as opposed to other adipocytokines, whose levels are increased in obese people [77]. Levels are decreased in persons who have essential hypertension [78], diabetes, or coronary artery disease [79]. Adiponectin seems to play an important role in glucose and lipid metabolism in insulin sensitive tissues in human and animal models. It has significant insulin sensitizing and anti-inflammatory properties. The mechanism through which adiponectin exerts its actions are largely unknown. Infusion of adiponectin increased whole body insulin sensitivity in rodents [80]. TZDs [81] and weight loss [82] seem to increase the levels of adiponectin.

It has been shown that CRP mRNA is expressed in human adipose tissue. A significant inverse correlation has been observed between CRP and adiponectin mRNA [83].

Albuminuria

Urinary microalbuminuria is monitored routinely in clinical practice and is recognized as a marker of cardiovascular disease and diabetic nephropathy [84]. Current methods of reducing microalbuminuria include strict glycemic control and use of angiotensin-converting enzyme (ACE) or angiotensin receptor blocker (ARB) inhibitors. TZDs were shown to reduce microalbuminuria [85]. In a 52-week open trial of patients who had type 2 diabetes who were given rosiglitazone or glyburide, rosiglitazone significantly reduced urinary albumin:creatinine ratio compared with baseline (Fig. 2) [86]. PPAR-γ receptors are expressed in mesangial cells of animal models and inhibit mesangial cell proliferation and angiotensin II–induced PAI-1 expression [87]. Consequently, the TZD effect on microalbuminuria may represent an additional element to consider in the decision-making process for selecting antihyperglycemic agents that may have an additive benefit to ACE or ARB inhibitors in reducing microalbuminuria. The subsequent impact on the course and progression of diabetic nephropathy remains unknown, however.

Left ventricular mass, congestive heart failure, and type 2 diabetes

Ghazzi et al [27] investigated whether patients who had type 2 diabetes who were treated with troglitazone, 800 mg daily (a dosage larger than that used in clinical practice) or glyburide developed any cardiac mass increase or functional impairment. Two-dimensional echocardiography and pulsed Doppler demonstrated that troglitazone and glyburide did not change left ventricular mass index significantly over 48 weeks. Similar studies that were performed with rosiglitazone and pioglitazone also demonstrated no adverse effect on cardiac mass or function [39,88]. Nonetheless, the use of TZDs is contraindicated in patients who have advanced heart failure (New York Heart Association class III and IV) because of the expansion of plasma volume [89]. Certain aspects of the patient's disease profile need to be kept in mind when prescribing TZDs. Box 2 and Fig. 2 show these risk factors and the current guidelines for the use of TZDs in heart failure.

Congestive heart failure (CHF) was not seen frequently in trials using TZDs. The prevalence of CHF was less than 1% for rosiglitazone monotherapy or when rosiglitazone was added to sulfonylurea or metformin, and was similar to that observed during treatment with a placebo [90]. The incidence of CHF increased to 2% and 3% when rosiglitazone, 4 mg/d or 8 mg/d, respectively, was added to insulin therapy of the study population, compared with 1% in the group that was treated with insulin alone [90]. Pre-existing microvascular and cardiovascular comorbidity was more prevalent in those clinical trials in which rosiglitazone was added to insulin therapy than in those trials in which rosiglitazone was used alone and compared with placebo or combined with metformin or sulfonylureas. The patients who developed CHF on rosiglitazone plus insulin were older and had diabetes of longer duration.

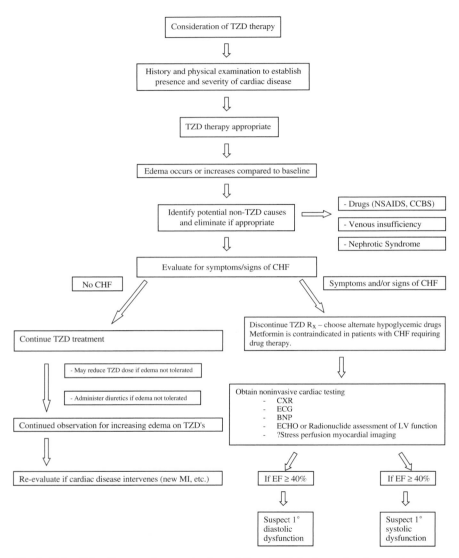

Fig. 2. Thiazolidinediones and congestive heart failure. BNP, brain natriuretic peptide; CCBs, calcium channel blockers; CHF, chronic heart failure; CXR, chest radiograph; ECG, electrocardiogram; ECHO, echocardiogram; EF, ejection failure; LV, left ventricular; MI, myocardial infarction; NSAIDs, nonsteroidal anti-inflammatory drugs. Copyright © 2004 American Diabetes Association ADA. (*From* Nesto RW, Bell D, Bonow RO, et al. Thiazolidinedione use, fluid retention, and congestive heart failure: a consensus statement from the American Heart Association and American Diabetes Association. Diabetes Care 2004;27(1):256–63; with permission.)

> **Box 2. Risk factors for heart failure in patients who are treated with thiazolidinediones**
>
> History of heart failure (either systolic or diastolic)
> History of myocardial infarction or symptomatic coronary
>   artery disease
> Hypertension
> Left ventricular hypertrophy
> Significant aortic or mitral valve heart disease
> Advanced age (> 70 y)
> Long-standing diabetes (> 10 y)
> Pre-existing edema or current treatment with loop diuretics
> Development of edema or weight gain on TZD therapy
> Insulin coadministration
> Chronic renal failure (creatinine > 2.0 mg/dL)
>
> ---
>
> *Data from* Nesto RW, Bell D, Bonow RO, et al. Thiazolidinedione use, fluid retention, and congestive heart failure: a consensus statement from the American Heart Association and American Diabetes Association. Diabetes Care 2004;27(1): 261.

The data on pioglitazone are similar [91]. In a placebo-controlled trial [91], 2 of 191 patients (1.1%) who received 15 mg of pioglitazone plus insulin and 2 of 188 (1.1%) patients who received 30 mg of pioglitazone plus insulin developed CHF, compared with none of the 187 patients who received insulin alone. All four of these patients had underlying coronary artery disease.

It is unlikely, however, that the drugs differ with regard to the risk of CHF because they incur similar degrees of volume expansion. In summary, the prevalence of CHF in TZD-treated patients is low but is definitely greater in patients who already are treated with insulin and receive larger dosages of the TZD and have other risk factors for CHF. Guidelines and recommendations have now been published and have to be followed while using TZDs in patients who have diabetes and heart failure [90].

Nichols and colleagues [89] reported that CHF was present in 11.8% of subjects who had type 2 diabetes and in 4.5% of the controls. Furthermore, in subjects who had diabetes who were free of CHF at baseline, they observed incident cases of CHF in 7.7% of subjects compared with only 3.4% of the control subjects. Thus, patients who have diabetes are at high risk for CHF; this should be considered when evaluating data relating to the use of medications for treating diabetes.

Metformin also is contraindicated in patients who have CHF. Diabetes management in patients who have CHF can be particularly difficult, probably related to the IR that is caused by sympathetic overactivity and the use of diuretics that can worsen hyperglycemia and often requires insulin therapy.

A study by Masoudi et al [91] showed that the use of metformin and TZDs has increased rapidly in Medicare beneficiaries who have diabetes and heart failure, despite explicit warnings against this practice from the US Food and Drug Administration.

The complexity of drug regimens that are used with multiple side effects and the perceived poor prognosis make diabetes management difficult. Insulin therapy may be the best option in patients who have CHF; however, it is not known whether improved control of diabetes and other risk factors will improve life expectancy. Any such approach will need to be proven safe and cost effective.

Combination therapy

Several studies showed that the combination of metformin or sulfonyl-ureas with a TZD improved glycemic control, insulin sensitivity, and β-cell function compared with metformin alone [92–94]. The RESULT study that was conducted by Rosenstock et al is the longest double-blind, placebo-controlled study that supports the notion of sustained effects with TZDs and possible β-cell preservation. A combination of metformin and a TZD is appealing theoretically because they have differing mechanisms of action with little or no risk of hypoglycemia. Both have shown cardiovascular risk reduction; however, sulfonylureas often are used to potentiate glycemic effects. Long-term studies are needed to determine whether such combinations will decrease cardiovascular events.

Summary

A multiple risk factor approach is needed in patients who have type 2 diabetes. Because many risk factors are linked with IR, treatment with insulin sensitizers has the potential to modulate these risk factors favorably. TZDs have many important effects beyond lowering blood glucose. By targeting IR, they improve many cardiovascular risk factors that are associated with the IR syndrome. In particular, they increase HDL-C, have anti-inflammatory effects, improve endothelial function and fibrinolysis, and decrease carotid intimal thickness; however, no evidence-based studies on cardiovascular outcomes are available to substantiate the potential cardioprotective effects of TZDs. Several clinical trials that were designed to investigate the effect that these agents have on reducing cardiovascular events are well under way.

References

[1] DeFronzo RA. Pathogenesis of type 2 (non-insulin dependent) diabetes mellitus: a balanced overview. Diabetologia 1992;35(4):389–97.
[2] Despres JP, Lamarche B, Mauriege P, et al. Hyperinsulinemia as an independent risk factor for ischemic heart disease. N Engl J Med 1996;334(15):952–7.

[3] Brunzell JD, Hokanson JE. Dyslipidemia of central obesity and insulin resistance. Diabetes Care 1999;22(Suppl 3):C10–3.

[4] Ginsberg HN. Insulin resistance and cardiovascular disease. J Clin Invest 2000;106(4): 453–8.

[5] Executive Summary of The Third Report of The National Cholesterol Education Program (NCEP) Expert Panel on Detection, Evaluation, and Treatment of High Blood Cholesterol in Adults (Adult Treatment Panel III). JAMA 2001;285(19):2486–97.

[6] Kannel WB, McGee DL. Diabetes and cardiovascular disease. The Framingham study. JAMA 1979;241(19):2035–8.

[7] Haffner SM. Management of dyslipidemia in adults with diabetes. Diabetes Care 1998; 21(1):160–78.

[8] Gu K, Cowie CC, Harris MI. Diabetes and decline in heart disease mortality in US adults. JAMA 1999;281(14):1291–7.

[9] Davidson MB. Is treatment of insulin resistance beneficial independent of glycemia? Diabetes Care 2003;26(11):3184–6.

[10] Reaven GM. Banting lecture 1988. Role of insulin resistance in human disease. Diabetes 1988;37(12):1595–607.

[11] Reaven GM, Lithell H, Landsberg L. Hypertension and associated metabolic abnormal-ities–the role of insulin resistance and the sympathoadrenal system. N Engl J Med 1996; 334(6):374–81.

[12] Effect of intensive blood-glucose control with metformin on complications in overweight patients with type 2 diabetes (UKPDS 34). UK Prospective Diabetes Study (UKPDS) Group. Lancet 1998;352(9131):854–65.

[13] Martens FM, Visseren FL, Lemay J, et al. Metabolic and additional vascular effects of thiazolidinediones. Drugs 2002;62(10):1463–80.

[14] Wagstaff AJ, Goa KL. Rosiglitazone: a review of its use in the management of type 2 diabetes mellitus. Drugs 2002;62(12):1805–37.

[15] Inzucchi SE, Maggs DG, Spollett GR, et al. Efficacy and metabolic effects of metformin and troglitazone in type II diabetes mellitus. N Engl J Med 1998;338(13):867–72.

[16] Kersten S, Desvergne B, Wahli W. Roles of PPARs in health and disease. Nature 2000; 405(6785):421–4.

[17] Olefsky JM. Treatment of insulin resistance with peroxisome proliferator-activated receptor gamma agonists. J Clin Invest 2000;106(4):467–72.

[18] Boden G, Chen X, Capulong E, et al. Effects of free fatty acids on gluconeogenesis and autoregulation of glucose production in type 2 diabetes. Diabetes 2001;50(4): 810–6.

[19] Steinberg HO, Paradisi G, Hook G, et al. Free fatty acid elevation impairs insulin-mediated vasodilation and nitric oxide production. Diabetes 2000;49(7):1231–8.

[20] Parulkar AA, Pendergrass ML, Granda-Ayala R, et al. Nonhypoglycemic effects of thiazolidinediones. Ann Intern Med 2001;134(1):61–71.

[21] Fonseca VA. Risk factors for coronary heart disease in diabetes. Ann Intern Med 2000; 133(2):154–6.

[22] Saito I, Folsom AR, Brancati FL, et al. Nontraditional risk factors for coronary heart disease incidence among persons with diabetes: the Atherosclerosis Risk in Communities (ARIC) Study. Ann Intern Med 2000;133(2):81–91.

[23] Kirpichnikov D, McFarlane SI, Sowers JR. Metformin: an update. Ann Intern Med 2002; 137(1):25–33.

[24] Abbasi F, Chu JW, McLaughlin T, et al. Effect of metformin treatment on multiple cardiovascular disease risk factors in patients with type 2 diabetes mellitus. Metabolism 2004;53(2):159–64.

[25] Freed MI, Ratner R, Marcovina SM, et al. Effects of rosiglitazone alone and in combination with atorvastatin on the metabolic abnormalities in type 2 diabetes mellitus. Am J Cardiol 2002;90(9):947–52.

[26] Rosenblatt S, Miskin B, Glazer NB, et al. The impact of pioglitazone on glycemic control and atherogenic dyslipidemia in patients with type 2 diabetes mellitus. Coron Artery Dis 2001;12(5):413–23.

[27] Ghazzi MN, Perez JE, Antonucci TK, et al. Cardiac and glycemic benefits of troglitazone treatment in NIDDM. The Troglitazone Study Group. Diabetes 1997;46(3):433–9.

[28] Suter SL, Nolan JJ, Wallace P, et al. Metabolic effects of new oral hypoglycemic agent CS-045 in NIDDM subjects. Diabetes Care 1992;15(2):193–203.

[29] Nagy L, Tontonoz P, Alvarez JG, et al. Oxidized LDL regulates macrophage gene expression through ligand activation of PPARgamma. Cell 1998;93(2):229–40.

[30] Tontonoz P, Nagy L, Alvarez JG, et al. PPARgamma promotes monocyte/macrophage differentiation and uptake of oxidized LDL. Cell 1998;93(2):241–52.

[31] Dichtl W, Nilsson L, Goncalves I, et al. Very low-density lipoprotein activates nuclear factor-kappaB in endothelial cells. Circ Res 1999;84(9):1085–94.

[32] Gotto AM Jr, Brinton EA. Assessing low levels of high-density lipoprotein cholesterol as a risk factor in coronary heart disease: a working group report and update. J Am Coll Cardiol 2004;43(5):717–24.

[33] Matsuzawa Y, Funahashi T, Nakamura T. Molecular mechanism of metabolic syndrome X: contribution of adipocytokines adipocyte-derived bioactive substances. Ann N Y Acad Sci 1999;892:146–54.

[34] DeFronzo RA. Insulin resistance: a multifaceted syndrome responsible for NIDDM, obesity, hypertension, dyslipidaemia and atherosclerosis. Neth J Med 1997;50(5):191–7.

[35] Ferrannini E, Natali A. Essential hypertension, metabolic disorders, and insulin resistance. Am Heart J 1991;121(4 Pt 2):1274–82.

[36] Natali A, Ferrannini E. Hypertension, insulin resistance, and the metabolic syndrome. Endocrinol Metab Clin North Am 2004;33(2):417–29.

[37] Raji A, Seely EW, Bekins SA, et al. Rosiglitazone improves insulin sensitivity and lowers blood pressure in hypertensive patients. Diabetes Care 2003;26(1):172–8.

[38] Bennett SM, Agrawal A, Elasha H, et al. Rosiglitazone improves insulin sensitivity, glucose tolerance and ambulatory blood pressure in subjects with impaired glucose tolerance. Diabet Med 2004;21:415–22.

[39] Scherbaum W, Goke B, for the German Pioglitazone Study Group. Pioglitazone reduces blood pressure in patients with type-2 diabetes mellitus. Diabetes 2001;50(Suppl):A462.

[40] Morikang E, Benson SC, Kurtz TW, et al. Effects of thiazolidinediones on growth and differentiation of human aorta and coronary myocytes. Am J Hypertens 1997;10(4 Pt 1): 440–6.

[41] Song J, Walsh MF, Igwe R, et al. Troglitazone reduces contraction by inhibition of vascular smooth muscle cell Ca2+ currents and not endothelial nitric oxide production. Diabetes 1997;46(4):659–64.

[42] Blackman DJ, Morris-Thurgood JA, Atherton JJ, et al. Endothelium-derived nitric oxide contributes to the regulation of venous tone in humans. Circulation 2000;101(2):165–70.

[43] Sobel BE. Coronary artery disease and fibrinolysis: from the blood to the vessel wall. Thromb Haemost 1999;82(Suppl 1):8–13.

[44] Tooke J. The association between insulin resistance and endotheliopathy. Diabetes Obes Metab 1999;1(Suppl 1):S17–22.

[45] Steinberg HO, Brechtel G, Johnson A, et al. Insulin-mediated skeletal muscle vasodilation is nitric oxide dependent. A novel action of insulin to increase nitric oxide release. J Clin Invest 1994;94(3):1172–9.

[46] Kahn NN, Bauman WA, Hatcher VB, et al. Inhibition of platelet aggregation and the stimulation of prostacyclin synthesis by insulin in humans. Am J Physiol 1993;265(6 Pt 2): H2160–7.

[47] Lehmann ED, Riley WA, Clarkson P, et al. Non-invasive assessment of cardiovascular disease in diabetes mellitus. Lancet 1997;350(Suppl 1):SI14–9.

[48] Pistrosch F, Passauer J, Fischer S, et al. In type 2 diabetes, rosiglitazone therapy for insulin resistance ameliorates endothelial dysfunction independent of glucose control. Diabetes Care 2004;27(2):484–90.

[49] Mohanty P, Aljada A, Ghanim H, et al. Rosiglitazone improves vascular reactivity, inhibits reactive oxygen species (ROS) generation, reduces p47phox subunit expression in mononuclear cells (MNC) and reduces C reactive protein (CRP) and monocyte chemotactic protein-1 (MCP-1): evidence of a potent anti-inflammatory effect. Diabetes 2001;50(Suppl 2):A68.

[50] Cominacini L, Garbin U, Pasini AF, et al. The expression of adhesion molecules on endothelial cells is inhibited by troglitazone through its antioxidant activity. Cell Adhes Commun 1999;7(3):223–31.

[51] Ohta MY, Nagai Y, Takamura T, et al. Inhibitory effect of troglitazone on TNF-alpha-induced expression of monocyte chemoattractant protein-1 (MCP-1) in human endothelial cells. Diabetes Res Clin Pract 2000;48(3):171–6.

[52] Yoshimoto T, Naruse M, Shizume H, et al. Vasculo-protective effects of insulin sensitizing agent pioglitazone in neointimal thickening and hypertensive vascular hypertrophy. Atherosclerosis 1999;145(2):333–40.

[53] Mather KJ, Verma S, Anderson TJ. Improved endothelial function with metformin in type 2 diabetes mellitus. J Am Coll Cardiol 2001;37(5):1344–50.

[54] Minamikawa J, Tanaka S, Yamauchi M, et al. Potent inhibitory effect of troglitazone on carotid arterial wall thickness in type 2 diabetes. J Clin Endocrinol Metab 1998;83(5):1818–20.

[55] O'Leary DH, Polak JF, Kronmal RA, et al. Carotid-artery intima and media thickness as a risk factor for myocardial infarction and stroke in older adults. Cardiovascular Health Study Collaborative Research Group. N Engl J Med 1999;340(1):14–22.

[56] Koshiyama H, Shimono D, Kuwamura N, et al. Rapid communication: inhibitory effect of pioglitazone on carotid arterial wall thickness in type 2 diabetes. J Clin Endocrinol Metab 2001;86(7):3452–6.

[57] Ehrmann DA, Schneider DJ, Sobel BE, et al. Troglitazone improves defects in insulin action, insulin secretion, ovarian steroidogenesis, and fibrinolysis in women with polycystic ovary syndrome. J Clin Endocrinol Metab 1997;82(7):2108–16.

[58] Jiang C, Ting AT, Seed B. PPAR-gamma agonists inhibit production of monocyte inflammatory cytokines. Nature 1998;391(6662):82–6.

[59] Marx N, Sukhova G, Murphy C, et al. Macrophages in human atheroma contain PPARgamma: differentiation-dependent peroxisomal proliferator-activated receptor gamma (PPARgamma) expression and reduction of MMP-9 activity through PPAR-gamma activation in mononuclear phagocytes in vitro. Am J Pathol 1998;153(1):17–23.

[60] Davidson MB. Clinical implications of insulin resistance syndromes. Am J Med 1995;99(4):420–6.

[61] Nagi DK, Yudkin JS. Effects of metformin on insulin resistance, risk factors for cardiovascular disease, and plasminogen activator inhibitor in NIDDM subjects. A study of two ethnic groups. Diabetes Care 1993;16(4):621–9.

[62] Fonseca VA, Reynolds T, Hemphill D, et al. Effect of troglitazone on fibrinolysis and activated coagulation in patients with non-insulin-dependent diabetes mellitus. J Diabetes Complications 1998;12(4):181–6.

[63] Kato K, Satoh H, Endo Y, et al. Thiazolidinediones down-regulate plasminogen activator inhibitor type 1 expression in human vascular endothelial cells: A possible role for PPARgamma in endothelial function. Biochem Biophys Res Commun 1999;258(2):431–5.

[64] Kruszynska YT, Yu JG, Olefsky JM, et al. Effects of troglitazone on blood concentrations of plasminogen activator inhibitor 1 in patients with type 2 diabetes and in lean and obese normal subjects. Diabetes 2000;49(4):633–9.

[65] Zirlik A, Leugers A, Lohrmann J, et al. Direct attenuation of plasminogen activator inhibitor type-1 expression in human adipose tissue by thiazolidinediones. Thromb Haemost 2004;91(4):674–82.

[66] Nordt TK, Peter K, Bode C, et al. Differential regulation by troglitazone of plasminogen activator inhibitor type 1 in human hepatic and vascular cells. J Clin Endocrinol Metab 2000;85(4):1563–8.

[67] Haffner SM. Insulin resistance, inflammation, and the prediabetic state. Am J Cardiol 2003; 92(4A):18J–26J.

[68] Desouza CV, Murthy SN, Diez J, et al. Differential effects of peroxisome proliferator activator receptor-alpha and gamma ligands on intimal hyperplasia after balloon catheter-induced vascular injury in Zucker rats. J Cardiovasc Pharmacol Ther 2003;8(4): 297–305.

[69] Yue TL, Chen J, Bao W, et al. In vivo myocardial protection from ischemia/reperfusion injury by the peroxisome proliferator-activated receptor-gamma agonist rosiglitazone. Circulation 2001;104(21):2588–94.

[70] Khandoudi N, Delerive P, Berrebi-Bertrand I, et al. Rosiglitazone, a peroxisome proliferator-activated receptor-gamma, inhibits the Jun NH(2)-terminal kinase/activating protein 1 pathway and protects the heart from ischemia/reperfusion injury. Diabetes 2002; 51(5):1507–14.

[71] Ridker PM, Rifai N, Rose L, et al. Comparison of C-reactive protein and low-density lipoprotein cholesterol levels in the prediction of first cardiovascular events. N Engl J Med 2002;347(20):1557–65.

[72] Fuell DL, Free MI, Greenberg AS, et al. The effect of treatment with rosiglitazone on C-reactive protein and interleukin-6 in patients with type 2 diabetes. Diabetes 2001; 50(Suppl 2):A435.

[73] Haffner SM, Greenberg AS, Weston WM, et al. Effect of rosiglitazone treatment on nontraditional markers of cardiovascular disease in patients with type 2 diabetes mellitus. Circulation 2002;106(6):679–84.

[74] Satoh N, Ogawa Y, Usui T, et al. Antiatherogenic effect of pioglitazone in type 2 diabetic patients irrespective of the responsiveness to its antidiabetic effect. Diabetes Care 2003; 26(9):2493–9.

[75] Dandona P, Aljada A, Mohanty P. The anti-inflammatory and potential anti-atherogenic effect of insulin: a new paradigm. Diabetologia 2002;45(6):924–30.

[76] Chandran M, Phillips SA, Ciaraldi T, et al. Adiponectin: more than just another fat cell hormone? Diabetes Care 2003;26(8):2442–50.

[77] Arita Y, Kihara S, Ouchi N, et al. Paradoxical decrease of an adipose-specific protein, adiponectin, in obesity. Biochem Biophys Res Commun 1999;257(1):79–83.

[78] Adamczak M, Wiecek A, Funahashi T, et al. Decreased plasma adiponectin concentration in patients with essential hypertension. Am J Hypertens 2003;16(1):72–5.

[79] Hotta K, Funahashi T, Arita Y, et al. Plasma concentrations of a novel, adipose-specific protein, adiponectin, in type 2 diabetic patients. Arterioscler Thromb Vasc Biol 2000;20(6): 1595–9.

[80] Yamauchi T, Kamon J, Waki H, et al. The fat-derived hormone adiponectin reverses insulin resistance associated with both lipoatrophy and obesity. Nat Med 2001;7(8):941–6.

[81] Combs TP, Wagner JA, Berger J, et al. Induction of adipocyte complement-related protein of 30 kilodaltons by PPARgamma agonists: a potential mechanism of insulin sensitization. Endocrinology 2002;143(3):998–1007.

[82] Esposito K, Pontillo A, Di Palo C, et al. Effect of weight loss and lifestyle changes on vascular inflammatory markers in obese women: a randomized trial. JAMA 2003;289(14): 1799–804.

[83] Ouchi N, Kihara S, Funahashi T, et al. Reciprocal association of C-reactive protein with adiponectin in blood stream and adipose tissue. Circulation 2003;107(5):671–4.

[84] Mattock MB, Morrish NJ, Viberti G, et al. Prospective study of microalbuminuria as predictor of mortality in NIDDM. Diabetes 1992;41(6):736–41.

[85] Imano E, Kanda T, Nakatani Y, et al. Effect of troglitazone on microalbuminuria in patients with incipient diabetic nephropathy. Diabetes Care 1998;21(12):2135–9.

[86] Bakris G, Viberti G, Weston WM, et al. Rosiglitazone reduces urinary albumin excretion in type II diabetes. J Hum Hypertens 2003;17(1):7–12.

[87] Nicholas SB, Kawano Y, Wakino S, et al. Expression and function of peroxisome proliferator-activated receptor-gamma in mesangial cells. Hypertension 2001;37(2 Part 2): 722–7.

[88] St John SM, Rendell M, Dandona P, et al. A comparison of the effects of rosiglitazone and glyburide on cardiovascular function and glycemic control in patients with type 2 diabetes. Diabetes Care 2002;25(11):2058–64.

[89] Nichols GA, Hillier TA, Erbey JR, et al. Congestive heart failure in type 2 diabetes: prevalence, incidence, and risk factors. Diabetes Care 2001;24(9):1614–9.

[90] Nesto RW, Bell D, Bonow RO, et al. Thiazolidinedione use, fluid retention, and congestive heart failure: a consensus statement from the American Heart Association and American Diabetes Association. Diabetes Care 2004;27(1):256–63.

[91] Masoudi FA, Wang Y, Inzucchi SE, et al. Metformin and thiazolidinedione use in Medicare patients with heart failure. JAMA 2003;290(1):81–5.

[92] Einhorn D, Rendell M, Rosenzweig J, et al. Pioglitazone hydrochloride in combination with metformin in the treatment of type 2 diabetes mellitus: a randomized, placebo-controlled study. The Pioglitazone 027 Study Group. Clin Ther 2000;22(12):1395–409.

[93] Fonseca V, Rosenstock J, Patwardhan R, et al. Effect of metformin and rosiglitazone combination therapy in patients with type 2 diabetes mellitus: a randomized controlled trial. JAMA 2000;283(13):1695–702.

[94] Suzuki M, Odaka H, Suzuki N, et al. Effects of combined pioglitazone and metformin on diabetes and obesity in Wistar fatty rats. Clin Exp Pharmacol Physiol 2002;29(4):269–74.

[95] Lebovitz HE. Rationale for and role of thiazolidinediones in type 2 diabetes mellitus. Am J Cardiol 2002;90(5A):34G–41G.

[96] Pradhan AD, Manson JE, Rifai N, et al. C-reactive protein, interleukin 6, and risk of developing type 2 diabetes mellitus. JAMA 2001;286(3):327–34.

[97] Viberti G, Kahn SE, Greene DA, et al. A diabetes outcome progression trial (ADOPT): an international multicenter study of the comparative efficacy of rosiglitazone, glyburide, and metformin in recently diagnosed type 2 diabetes. Diabetes Care 2002;25:1737–43.

[98] Sobel BE, Frye R, Detre KM. Bypass Angioplasty Revascularization Investigation 2 Diabetes Trial. Burgeoning dilemmas in the management of diabetes and cardiovascular disease: rationale for the Bypass Angioplasty Revascularization Investigation 2 Diabetes (BARI 2D) Trial. Circulation 2003;107:636–42.

[99] Gerstein HC, Yusuf S, Holman R, et al. Rationale, design and recruitment characteristics of a large, simple international trial of diabetes prevention: the DREAM trial. Diabetologia 2004;47:1519–27.

[100] Charbonnel B, Dormandy J, Erdmann E, et al. The Prospective Pioglitazone Clinical Trial in Microvascular Events (PROactive): can pioglitazone reduce cardiovascular events in diabetes? Study design and baseline characteristics in 5238 patients. Diabetes Care 2004;27: 1647–53.

ELSEVIER
SAUNDERS

Endocrinol Metab Clin N Am
34 (2005) 137–154

ENDOCRINOLOGY
AND METABOLISM
CLINICS
OF NORTH AMERICA

Insulin Therapy in People Who Have Dysglycemia and Type 2 Diabetes Mellitus: Can It Offer Both Cardiovascular Protection and Beta-Cell Preservation?

Hertzel C. Gerstein, MD, MSc[a],*,
Julio Rosenstock, MD[b,c]

[a]*Division of Endocrinology and Metabolism and the Population Health Research Institute,
Department of Medicine, McMaster University and Hamilton Health Sciences,
Room 3V38, 1200 Main Street West,
Hamilton, ON L8N 3Z5, Canada*
[b]*Dallas Diabetes and Endocrine Center,
7777 Forest Lane, C-618, Dallas, TX 75230, USA*
[c]*University of Texas Southwestern Medical School, Dallas, TX, USA*

There is growing recognition that the rapid rise in the prevalence of diabetes mellitus and lesser degrees of dysglycemia, in concert with the high levels of associated risk factors for cardiovascular (CV) disease, presages a global epidemic of CV disease, especially in western societies. Dysglycemia occurs when there is insufficient insulin action because of either insulin resistance with relative insulin deficiency, or absolute insulin deficiency. The possible mechanisms underlying the relationship among glucose, insulin effects, and CV disease coupled with the emerging interventional clinical data suggest that early insulin replacement may mitigate CV risk. This article explores these data and hypotheses.

Diabetes mellitus as a risk factor for cardiovascular disease

Diabetes mellitus is a strong risk factor for CV disease and atherosclerosis. People who have diabetes mellitus are two to three times more likely

Dr. Gerstein holds the McMaster University Population Health Institute Chair in Diabetes Research (sponsored by Aventis).

* Corresponding author.
E-mail address: gerstein@mcmaster.ca (H.C. Gerstein).

0889-8529/05/$ - see front matter © 2005 Elsevier Inc. All rights reserved.
doi:10.1016/j.ecl.2004.11.002

to die from CV disease than people with no history of diabetes mellitus; diabetes mellitus therefore is associated with a CV mortality rate that exceeds 70% [1]. This relationship between CV disease risk and diabetes mellitus is independent of the coexistence of many other traditional and emerging CV disease risk factors [1].

Dysglycemia as a risk factor for cardiovascular disease

Most of the literature dealing with CV disease risk and hyperglycemia has focused on people who have diabetes mellitus. The glucose thresholds used to diagnose diabetes mellitus, however, are well above the normal fasting and 2-hour postload mean physiologic levels of 92 mg/dL (5.1 mmol/L) and 97 mg/dL (5.4 mmol/L), respectively (Table 1) [2]. Because the diagnostic fasting (126 mg/dL; 7 mmol/L) and 2-hour postload (200 mg/dL; 11.1 mmol/L) glucose levels were chosen to identify people at risk for retinal disease [3], there is no a priori reason that they must be the same for CV disease risk. Several recent reviews and analyses of prospective data have shown that they are not, and that the risk for CV disease extends well below these levels [4–7].

These data are supported by a greater than 60% prevalence of impaired glucose tolerance or diabetes mellitus in people with double- or triple-artery coronary disease [8] and that at least two thirds of all individuals who present with a myocardial infarction have persistent evidence of either diabetes mellitus, impaired glucose tolerance, or a fasting glucose level of 110 mg/dL (6.1 mmol/L) or higher [9,10]. They also are supported by the direct relationship between the glucose level measured at the time of a myocardial infarction, acute coronary insufficiency, or stroke [11–15] and the subsequent risk for death or disability (regardless of antecedent diabetes mellitus status).

Therefore, any consistent rise of glucose above normal predicts an increase in the risk for CV events [16]. The recent lowering of the diagnostic threshold for an abnormal fasting plasma glucose recognizes this association; using 100 mg/dL (5.5 mmol/L) [17] as the cutoff is much closer to the normal levels.

Public health implications of the glucose–cardiovascular relationship

In the United States, approximately 8% of the adult population has either established or undetected diabetes mellitus, with higher rates

Table 1
Normal plasma glucose levels in individuals with no evidence of diabetes or impaired glucose tolerance

Plasma glucose level	Mean	75th percentile
Fasting	92 mg/dL (5.1 mmol/L)	97 mg/dL (5.4 mmol/L)
2 h after a 75-g glucose load	97 mg/dL (5.4 mmol/L)	122 mg/dL (6.8 mmol/L)

observed in middle-aged and elderly adults [18]. Similar rates have been reported from other western countries [19]. Moreover, the rate of diabetes mellitus is rising, most rapidly in the developing world [19]. This high prevalence and the adverse health consequences of diabetes mellitus accounted for over $130 billion of direct and indirect health care costs in the United States in 2000 [20]. CV disease accounted for the largest proportion of this cost.

Unfortunately, these alarming statistics pertain only to people who have diabetes mellitus, who represent the tip of the "dysglycemic iceberg" (Fig. 1). When the higher prevalence of nondiabetic glucose elevation is considered in light of its association with CV disease, the present and future health and economic costs of dysglycemia are likely to be staggering. These considerations highlight the need for further research to better understand the reasons for this relationship.

Explanation for the relationship between dysglycemia and cardiovascular disease

Potential reasons for the link between an elevated glucose level and CV disease include vascular toxicity secondary to (1) the elevated fasting or postprandial glucose level, (2) a relative lack of insulin effect or insulin resistance, (3) a reduced ability of insulin to mediate its biochemical and metabolic effects, (4) a relative or absolute reduction of insulin secretion, and (5) an underlying genetic or environmental abnormality that predisposes individuals to diabetes mellitus and CV disease [21,22]. The close link among these factors suggests that some combination of these factors is at play, and that they may interact with each other. Regardless, this strong epidemiologic relationship supports the hypothesis that interventions that normalize glucose may reduce risk for CV disease.

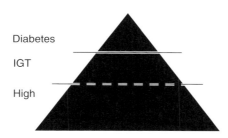

Fig. 1. People who have diabetes mellitus represent the clinically apparent minority of dysglycemic individuals who are at higher risk for cardiovascular events. People who have diabetes mellitus are at risk for eye, kidney, nerve, cardiovascular, and other consequences. People with lesser degrees of dysglycemia are at risk for future diabetes mellitus as well as cardiovascular disease.

Consequences of an elevated glucose level

Several explanations may account for the relationship between minor degrees of dysglycemia and CV risk. Several mechanisms likely are involved. First, an elevated glucose level may activate at least four metabolic pathways that can damage blood vessels in general and endothelial cells in particular [23]: (1) high levels of glucose lead to an increased flux through the polyol pathway (with conversion of excess glucose to sorbitol and fructose) and a concomitant decrease in the level of the intracellular antioxidant-reduced glutathione; (2) high levels of fructose-6-phosphate formed from glucose metabolism in the glycolytic pathway can activate the hexosamine pathway, and intermediates in this pathway (glucosamine-6-phosphate and acetylglucosamine) can promote transcription of proinflammatory and procoagulatory genes in the nucleus; (3) high levels of dihyydroxyacetone phosphate (DHAP) formed from further glucose metabolism in the glycolytic pathway increase production of diacylglycerol and subsequently protein kinase C (PKC), which activates various processes that reduce nitric oxide synthetase (NOS) and fibrinolysis, and increases endothelin, vascular permeability, inflammatory gene expression, and the generation of reactive oxygen species (ROS); and (4) glucose-induced intracellular and extracellular formation of advanced glycation endproducts (AGEs) leads to defective intracellular, membrane, and plasma proteins (eg, transcription factors, collagen, and lipoproteins), and promotes macrophage/scavenger cell activity and secretion of growth factors and cytokines. It has been suggested recently that these four processes may be mediated by an initial hyperglycemia-induced increase in mitochondrial superoxide molecules that inhibit the glycolytic pathway and lead to the intracellular accumulation of glucose and glycolytic intermediates (Fig. 2) [23].

Second, growing evidence suggests that these harmful effects of an elevated glucose are toxic to the beta cell, which seems to be particularly susceptible to oxidative stresses [24]. The resulting decline in beta-cell capacity from this glucose toxicity supports the observation that hyperglycemia begets hyperglycemia and the progressive and irreversible reduction in beta-cell function seen clinically [25]. Thus, if not normalized, minor degrees of dysglycemia may lead to cumulative beta-cell damage (and possible apoptosis) and initiate the set of processes described above.

Third, the hyperglycemia-related chronic oxidative stress seems to cause permanent changes in cellular function. These changes can lead to vascular damage even if euglycemia is restored, perhaps as a consequence of permanent damage to mitochondrial or nuclear DNA [23,24]. This possibility is supported directly by the posttrial follow-up of the Diabetes Control and Complications Trial (DCCT) cohort. Participants who were in the intensive control group (whose mean hemoglobin A1c [HbA1c] level was 7.2% during the 6.5-year trial) had a lesser progression of carotid atherosclerosis during 6 years of follow-up than the conventional group

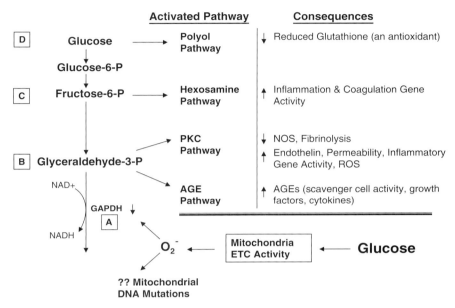

Fig. 2. Elevated intracellular glucose is metabolized through the cytoplasmic glycolytic pathway and then the mitochondrial tricarboxylic acid cycle. The resulting high levels of NADH and reduced FAD (FADH$_2$) interact with the mitochondrial electron transport chain (ETC) to generate superoxide (O$_2^-$) that inhibits the activity of glyceraldehyde-3-phosphate dehydrogenase, GAPDH (*A*). This leads to accumulation of the glycolytic intermediates glyceraldehyde-3-phosphate (*B*) and fructose-6-phosphate (*C*). Higher levels of these metabolites as well as glucose (*D*) activate the AGE, PKC, hexosamine, and polyol pathways, which in turn promote vascular damage. O$_2^-$ also may damage mitochondrial DNA. (*Adapted from* Brownlee M. Biochemistry and molecular cell biology of diabetic complications. Nature 2002;414(6865):813–20, with permission.)

participants (whose mean HbA1c level was 9% during the trial). This occurred despite subsequent convergence of glycemic control in both groups and minimal residual differences in HbA1c (in the low 8% range) during the posttrial period [26].

Thus, limited exposure to elevated glucose levels may lead to a "metabolic memory" or a "vascular imprint" with permanent progressive vascular disease, even after glucose levels have fallen. This also may explain why it has been difficult to detect a beneficial CV effect of glucose lowering in people who have established diabetes mellitus. Either the glucose lowering was not aggressive enough to stop continuing vascular damage by the persistently elevated (albeit lower) glucose levels, or the optimal window for successful intervention may have been missed.

Fourth, different degrees of elevated glucose may lead to secretion of various stress hormones that may damage vascular tissue by raising blood pressure, activating the renin-angiotensin system, increasing plasminogen activator inhibitor-1 (PAI-1), or increasing inflammatory markers and procoagulant molecules [27,28].

Consequences of absolute or relative insulin deficiency

Because insulin is the key hormone involved in glucose homeostasis, any deficiency in the amount or activity of insulin at its key target organs (muscle, fat, and liver) will lead to some degree of glucose elevation and its metabolic consequences. Even "normoglycemic" individuals with substantial insulin resistance have some elevation in glucose, and this elevation may be required to drive the hyperinsulinemia needed to overcome most of the insulin resistance effect [29]. Thus absolute and relative insulin deficiencies (ie, insulin resistance) are associated with elevated glucose level.

Deficient insulin action may promote CV disease through other mechanisms. First, insulin is a powerful inhibitor of lipolysis and of the lipolytic effect of stress hormones (especially cortisol and catecholamines). The increased free fatty acid (FFA) flux resulting from deficient insulin effect can (1) promote insulin resistance [30], (2) lead to ectopic fat deposition in islet cells [31] and subsequent beta-cell damage (thereby magnifying insulin deficiency), (3) stimulate the synthesis of atherogenic lipoproteins [30], and (4) inhibit glycolytic metabolism and anaerobic energy production in ischemic cardiac muscle, thereby increasing the damage done by an ischemic insult [32–34].

Second, the observation that insulin reduces inflammation by reducing tumor necrosis factor α, intercellular adhesion molecule–1, and monocyte and macrophage cytokines [35,36], as well as superoxide anion, suggests that insulin deficiency may be proinflammatory. Third, insulin reduces PAI-1 levels; insufficient insulin therefore represents a procoagulatory stimulus. Fourth, insulin deficiency may reduce ischemic preconditioning, making cardiac muscle more susceptible to ischemic damage [35,37]. Finally, lack of insulin reduces endothelial nitric oxide synthesis and vasodilation, especially in response to ischemia [35,37], and insulin may improve endothelial function [38].

These observations suggest that normalizing insulin action by either supplying sufficient insulin or reducing insulin resistance sufficiently to restore normal glucose homeostasis is likely to have beneficial CV effects.

A common risk factor for dysglycemia and cardiovascular disease

The possibility that dysglycemia and CV disease could be related to some antecedent and independent determinant is difficult to study. One obvious candidate is insulin resistance. Various risk factors for diabetes mellitus, such as hypertension [39], are CV risk factors; they also are associated with insulin resistance, defined as a reduced ability of insulin to facilitate glucose uptake into peripheral tissues and to suppress hepatic glucose production.

Individuals who are insulin-resistant, however, already have a somewhat higher glucose level than insulin-sensitive individuals [29]. Alternatively, prolonged insulin resistance may lead to beta-cell dysfunction and apoptosis in genetically predisposed individuals, causing subsequent elevated glucose levels [24]. Because insulin resistance is confounded so tightly with dysglycemia, it may be impossible to separate clearly its effect on CV disease risk from that of subsequent dysglycemia. Finally, environmental toxins represent another candidate risk factor for diabetes mellitus and CV disease. These include cadmium [40], arsenic [41], and smoking [42].

Possible cardiovascular benefits of insulin therapy

The foregoing supports the hypothesis that an intervention that safely provides sufficient insulin to normalize glucose levels and other metabolic disturbances may prevent CV disease (as well as diabetes mellitus). Insulin is an attractive candidate for such an intervention for several reasons: (1) there is no maximum dose and it can be titrated until normoglycemia is achieved; (2) new insulin preparations are available that maximize the predictability of its effect, reducing the risks for hypoglycemia; (3) there are no contra-indications to insulin therapy; and (4) prolonged ambulatory insulin therapy has been used safely in nondiabetic children [43] and newly diagnosed diabetic adults [44]. Finally, evidence from clinical trials in people who have diabetes mellitus provides preliminary support for the hypothesis that ambulatory insulin provision will reduce CV disease.

Results of insulin therapy in large clinical trials

Cardiovascular outcomes in clinical trials involving insulin therapy in type 2 diabetes mellitus

Table 2 lists all of the ambulatory clinical trials in which CV outcomes in response to initial or primary therapy with insulin were reported. None of these trials were designed or powered to detect a CV benefit of insulin. Nevertheless, taken together, they support the hypothesis that insulin therapy may reduce the risk for CV events.

The United Kingdom Prospective Diabetes Study (UKPDS) [44] included 3867 individuals with no previous history of diabetes mellitus who presented with newly diagnosed diabetes mellitus or who had a fasting plasma glucose (FPG) level $\geq$ 108 mg/dL ($\geq$ 6 mmol/L). Participants were allocated randomly to either conventional therapy, targeting FPG levels < 270 mg/dL (< 15 mmol/L) with no symptoms (N = 1138), or an intensive monotherapy regimen (N = 2729) that targeted a FPG < 108 mg/dL (< 6 mmol/L). Participants randomized to intensive therapy were allocated further to initial monotherapy either with insulin (N = 1156) or with sulfonylureas

Table 2
Effect of insulin therapy on incident cardiovascular events in clinical trials of glucose lowering

| Study [Ref.] | N | Years | HbA1c (%) | | | Event | RRR (95% CI) |
			Intensive group	Control group	Contrast (Delta)		
UKPDS [44]	3867	10	7.0	7.9	0.9	MI	13% (−9–30)
Kumamoto [45]	110	8	7.1	9.4	2.3	CV	44% (N/A; NS)
VACSDM [46]	153	2.3	7.1	9.3	2.2	CV	−40%[b] (N/A; NS)
DIGAMI [48]	620	1	7.1	7.9	0.8	Death	28% (8–45)
UGDP [47]	409	12.5	FPG~138[a]	FPG~178[a]	N/A	CV (death)	9% (N/A; NS)

Abbreviations: DIGAMI, Diabetes, Insulin and Glucose in Acute MI; FPG, fasting plasma glucose; N/A, not available; NS, not significant; RRR, relative risk reduction; UGDP, University Group Diabetes Program (Variable Insulin Dose); UKPDS, United Kingdom Prospective Diabetes Study; VACSDM, Veterans Affairs Cooperative Study in Type 2 Diabetes.

[a] HbA1c was not measured. Reported units are for the fasting plasma glucose in mg/dL (7.7–9.9 mmol/L).

[b] The minus represents an inverse relationship of increased relative risk.

(N = 1573). As shown in Table 2, after 10 years of follow-up the participants who were randomized to insulin therapy had a nonsignificant 13% reduction in myocardial infarction (MI) (95% confidence interval [CI] −9%–30%); no CV composite was analyzed.

The Kumamoto study randomized 110 people who had type 2 diabetes mellitus to either intensive or conventional monotherapy with insulin and achieved HbA1c levels of 7.1% and 9.4% in each group, respectively (see Table 2) [45]. After 8 years of follow-up, participants in the intensive group experienced reduced microvascular events. Although not powered for CV outcomes, a nonsignificant 44% reduction in CV events was reported. By contrast, the similarly sized 2.3-year Veterans Administration feasibility trial (N = 153) in the United States reported that high–CV risk individuals allocated to intensive glycemic therapy with insulin in combination with oral agents (who achieved a HbA1c level of 7.1%) experienced a nonsignificant 40% higher rate of CV events than control individuals who achieved a HbA1c level of 9.3% (see Table 2) [46].

The only other ambulatory trial data regarding insulin therapy and CV disease clinical outcomes in type 2 diabetes mellitus are found in the University Group Diabetes Program trial (UGDP) [47]. In that study, 409 individuals were allocated to either variable insulin therapy (achieving a FPG level of 138 mg/dL or 7.7 mmol/L) or fixed insulin therapy (achieving a FPG level of 178 mg/dL or 9.9 mmol/L) for 12.5 years; those allocated to the variable insulin group had a nonsignificant 9% lower risk for CV death.

Finally, in the Diabetes, Insulin and Glucose in Acute Myocardial Infarction (DIGAMI) trial of 620 individuals presenting with an acute MI, a 24-hour infusion of insulin followed by ambulatory subcutaneous insulin for at least 3 months reduced CV death by 28% compared with standard approaches to glycemic therapy [48]. This benefit was noted despite only modest differences in HbA1c levels between the two groups at 1 year and may have been caused by the acute effects of insulin on cardiac myocyte metabolism [49,50], including (1) an increase in the ability of the ischemic myocardium to generate ATP anaerobically, (2) the reduction in FFA (which promotes arrhythmias), and (3) membrane stabilization. Nevertheless, when these data are considered in the light of the other studies in Table 2, they support the hypothesis that insulin therapy may reduce CV events in people who have type 2 diabetes mellitus.

Cardiovascular outcomes in clinical trials of insulin therapy in type 1 diabetes mellitus

Several large clinical trials of intensive versus conventional insulin therapy have been completed in people who have type 1 diabetes mellitus. These studies convincingly demonstrated that intensive glycemic control reduces the risk of eye, kidney, and nerve disease in people who have type 1 diabetes mellitus. Because they all enrolled young individuals at low absolute risk for CV events, they were not designed or powered to detect an effect on these outcomes. Nevertheless, most measured CV outcomes and a recent meta-analysis [51] supported a consistent trend toward benefit from improving glycemic control.

The largest trial included in this meta-analysis is the DCCT, in which 1441 people who had type 1 diabetes mellitus (mean age 27 years) were allocated to intensive versus conventional insulin therapy and achieved a mean HbA1c level of 7.2% and 9.1%, respectively, for 6.5 years [52,53]. A trend favoring a CV benefit for the intensive versus the conventional group was noted [53]. Moreover, in the DCCT follow-up study [26], allocation to the intensive group reduced posttrial development of carotid atherosclerosis, a marker for the risk for CV events.

Cardiovascular outcomes in clinical trials of insulin therapy in people without diabetes mellitus

No clinical trials of the effect of insulin on CV outcomes have been done in ambulatory people without diabetes mellitus. Recent reports and an older meta-analysis [54] of the effect of intravenous insulin in individuals who have had an acute MI [55] or during cardiac surgery [56], however, generally have supported a trend toward reduced CV mortality and justify continuing international trials.

One study in 1548 individuals (13% had established diabetes mellitus) assessed the effect of an intravenous insulin infusion targeting a plasma glucose level $\leq$ 110 mg/dL ($\leq$ 6.1 mmol/L) versus standard care in postoperative individuals admitted to an intensive care unit [57]. The insulin-treated group had a 32% (95% CI 2%–55%) reduction in all-cause death, mainly from sepsis and general organ failure. No clear CV benefit per se was detected, however.

Safety of insulin therapy in large clinical outcome trials

The only established adverse effects associated with insulin therapy are hypoglycemia and moderate weight gain. Hypoglycemia occurs as a consequence of the mismatching of insulin provision with insulin need. Such mismatching may occur for many reasons, including unpredictable food intake or physical activity, variable insulin absorption, unpredictable insulin peaks, dose errors, and variable injection techniques. Recently, insulin analogs have helped to reduce significantly this mismatching by increasing the predictability of insulin absorption; thus less hypoglycemia occurs for the same degree of glycemic control achieved [58]. The better safety profile of these newer insulin preparations is allowing more aggressive targeting of lower glucose levels in more people who have diabetes mellitus. It also may facilitate their use in CV studies of nondiabetic individuals. Moderate weight gain also may occur because of improved glycemic control, reduced glycosuria, and imperfect matching of insulin supply to insulin needs.

No clinical trial evidence supports any other adverse effect of insulin therapy. Most trial evidence suggests either a benefit or neutral effect on clinically important outcomes such as eye, kidney, nerve, and CV disease as well as atherosclerosis. These trial data relating to exogenous insulin therapy need to be distinguished from epidemiologic data showing an association between high endogenous insulin levels and CV risk. In the latter instance, the insulin level is high to overcome underlying insulin resistance and, in many cases, mild dysglycemia; the high levels thus may be considered a reflection of a disordered gluco-metabolic state. Thus, the provision of exogenous insulin to these people may be understood as a therapy targeting this disordered state. In this therapeutic context, the important question is not whether insulin levels are high or low; in trials of intensive therapy, insulin levels in the intensive group are most likely higher than levels in the conventional group. Instead, the key issue is the degree to which the underlying metabolic lesion has been corrected.

Possible benefits of insulin therapy on beta-cell function

Growing evidence suggests that exogenous insulin therapy also may improve or preserve residual beta-cell function. Insulin secretion declines with time [25,59,60], presumably because of a toxic effect of hyperglycemia (glucotoxicity) and fatty acids (lipotoxicity) on pancreatic beta-cell function and structure [61–66]. By lowering glucose and FFA levels, exogenous insulin therapy may maintain the ability of the beta cell to secrete appropriate amounts of insulin in response to a glucose stimulus [67]. If this is true, the preserved beta-cell mass can help maintain normoglycemia through physiologic mechanisms, thus magnifying the direct effects of insulin on glucose metabolism.

Evidence for progressive beta-cell dysfunction and beta-cell loss

Data collected from people who had newly diagnosed type 2 diabetes mellitus in the UKPDS show that the ability to secrete insulin decreases with time. Initial therapy with sulfonylurea, metformin, or basal insulin versus diet alone more than doubled the proportion of patients who initially achieved glycemic targets [68]. After 3 years, however, nearly 50% of subjects on monotherapy were unable to maintain an HbA1c level $\leq$ 7%, and by 9 years only approximately 25% were able to do so [69]. Moreover, measurements of beta-cell function using the Homeostasis Model Assessment (HOMA) revealed an estimated 50% loss of beta-cell function at the time of diagnosis with an inexorable decline with time of about 5% per year [25].

These findings are supported by a careful analysis of pancreatic tissue obtained during 124 autopsies of obese and lean individuals with (1) no diabetes mellitus, (2) impaired fasting glucose, or (3) type 2 diabetes mellitus [70]. Compared with nondiabetic age and weight-matched controls, obese individuals with impaired fasting glucose had 40% less beta-cell volume and those with diabetes mellitus had a 63% deficit. Lean individuals who had type 2 diabetes mellitus exhibited a 41% deficit. Moreover, the frequency of beta-cell apoptosis was increased tenfold in lean subjects and threefold in obese subjects who had type 2 diabetes mellitus. Clearly, beta-cell loss is an early feature of the pathogenesis of type 2 diabetes mellitus. Whether or not aggressive glucose control with early insulin therapy can reduce this beta-cell loss in addition to enhancing endogenous insulin secretion requires further study.

Does early insulin use preserve beta-cell function?

Emerging evidence suggests that early insulin use may preserve beta-cell function, possibly by correcting glucotoxicity/lipotoxicity and "resting" the beta cell (Fig. 3); indeed, experimental evidence suggests that beta-cell defects could be reversible up to a certain point and irreversible thereafter [71]. For example, several studies of short-term intensive insulin therapy in people who have type 2 diabetes mellitus have demonstrated improved insulin action and secretion [72–76]. In addition, at least three uncontrolled studies showed that temporarily achieving normoglycemia with intensive insulin therapy in people who have newly diagnosed or early type 2 diabetes mellitus leads to a prolonged period of posttreatment normoglycemia. In these studies, after the initial insulin treatment was stopped, significant numbers of patients did not require pharmacotherapy to control fasting and postprandial glucose levels and had evidence of preserved C-peptide or insulin secretion [77–79].

These data were supported by a recent Scandinavian trial of 39 people who had newly diagnosed type 2 diabetes mellitus who were randomized to either two daily injections of insulin 70/30 or glyburide (3.5–10.5 mg/d) [80]. By the end of the second year, the HbA1c levels had deteriorated in the

Early Insulin Replacement In Type 2 DM
May Preserve β-Cell Function

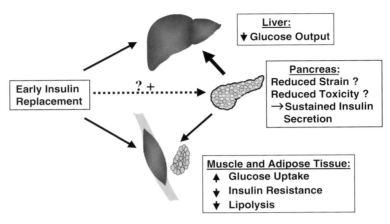

Fig. 3. Early insulin replacement: (1) corrects hyperglycemia by increasing peripheral glucose uptake and by suppressing hepatic glucose production; and (2) reduces FFAs by suppressing fat cell lipolysis. The reduced glucose and fatty acid levels may reduce demand on the beta cell as well as glucotoxicity and lipotoxicity, leading to enhanced insulin secretion. This "beta-cell rest" may preserve beta-cell integrity or delay progressive beta-cell loss, which can alter the course of type 2 diabetes mellitus and lead to more sustained glycemic control.

glyburide group, but not in the insulin-treated group. Moreover, at study end and at 1 year the glucagon-stimulated C-peptide response had increased in the insulin-treated group and decreased in the sulfonylurea group. After withdrawal of 2 years of therapy, fasting insulin levels were higher in the insulin-treated group compared with the sulfonylurea-treated group. This supports either a protective effect of insulin, a harmful effect of sulfonylureas or a combination of both possibilities.

These data suggest that early insulin treatment might slow or halt disease progression in people who have type 2 diabetes mellitus and lead to a durable glycemic response and sustained target HbA1c levels. It is tempting to speculate, therefore, that even earlier insulin therapy, perhaps from the outset of the disease, might be a more effective way to preserve beta-cell function.

New insulin replacement strategies

Most patients who have type 2 diabetes mellitus eventually will require insulin to attain and sustain glycemic targets. In the past, however, its use was delayed until 10 to 15 years had elapsed, and a traditional stepwise approach of lifestyle intervention followed by a combination of oral agents [81] had failed to maintain adequate glycemic control. This traditional and conservative approach was supported by (1) concerns regarding the risk for hypoglycemia and the pharmacokinetic limitations with the available insulin preparations [82,83], and (2) previous uncertainty regarding whether or not targeting lower glucose levels reduced eye, nerve, and kidney disease. The results of the UKPDS, together with trials reporting lower hypoglycemia rates when newer insulin preparations are used to target HbA1c levels recommended by current guidelines [58,84–86] are changing this approach. It is becoming unacceptable to delay insulin replacement as a last resort and the emerging consensus is to add insulin replacement early [83,87,88]. Nevertheless, hypoglycemia remains the biggest obstacle to achieving these recommended glycemic targets safely, and needs to be considered when setting individual treatment goals [83].

Current and future insulin recommendations for type 2 diabetes mellitus

The evolving treatment paradigm for early insulin therapy in type 2 diabetes mellitus is to use more physiologic replacement regimens, designed to achieve safely near-normal 24-hour fasting and postprandial glucose profiles, as a supplement to maximized oral combination agents if the HbA1c level consistently remains above 7%.

Basal insulin replacement provides a simple approach to the timely initiation of insulin in clinical practice. Basal insulin can be titrated easily and combined with oral agents [87]. Moreover, a single injection of a long-acting basal insulin can suppress effectively overnight hepatic glucose production and normalize fasting glucose levels. Thus, it is possible that early basal insulin supplementation (ie, when there is greater pancreatic beta-cell reserve) may facilitate the ability of the pancreas to secrete sufficient prandial insulin to normalize HbA1c levels [87]. The use of insulin from the onset of type 2 diabetes mellitus might theoretically halt or slow disease progression and permit the long-term maintenance of normal blood glucose levels with insulin either alone or in combination with oral agents.

The need for trials of insulin-based approaches to cardiovascular risk reduction

The clinical trials, epidemiologic, and physiologic evidence supports the hypotheses that insulin replacement may reduce the risk for CV events and preserve beta-cell function in high-risk dysglycemic individuals (ie, who have diabetes mellitus and nondiabetic degrees of hyperglycemia). These hypotheses are testable within the context of clinical trials, which can provide key information regarding the risks and benefits of such an approach.

Several large trials are underway in which aggressive insulin therapy is included as part of either (1) an acute intravenous intervention at the time of an MI or stroke or (2) an ambulatory subcutaneous intervention in high CV disease–risk individuals (Table 3). For example, the ORIGIN (Outcome

Table 3
Ongoing ambulatory trials of glucose lowering

Name	N	Population	Outcome tested
ACCORD	10,000	DM	Lower vs. higher HbA1c
VA DT	~1800	DM	Lower vs. higher HbA1c
RECORD	4400	DM	Rosiglitazone vs. placebo
BARI 2D	2800	DM	Sensitizers vs. secretagogues + insulin
PROACTIVE	5000	DM	Pioglitazone vs. placebo
NAVIGATOR	9541	IGT	Valsartan and/or nateglinide vs. placebo
ADVANCE	11,140	DM	Lower vs. higher HbA1c with Gliclazide
HEART 2D	1355	DM	Basal ± premeal insulin post-MI
DREAM	5269	IFG/IGT	Ramipril and/or rosiglitazone vs. placebo
ORIGIN	10,000	IFG/IGT/DM	Glargine insulin vs. guideline care

Abbreviations: ACCORD, Action to Control Cardiovascular Risk in Diabetes; ADVANCE, Action in Diabetes and Vascular Disease; BARI 2D, Bypass Angioplasty Revascularization Investigation 2 Diabetes; DM, diabetes mellitus; DREAM, Diabetes Reduction Assessment with Ramipril and Rosiglitazone Medication; HEART 2D, Hyperglycemia and its Effect after Acute Myocardial Infarction on Cardiovascular Outcomes in Type 2 Diabetes; IFG, impaired fasting glucose; IGT, impaired glucose tolerance; NAVIGATOR, Nateglinide and Valsartan in Impaired Glucose Tolerance Outcomes Research; ORIGIN, Outcome Reduction with Initial Glargine Intervention; PROACTIVE, Prospective Pioglitazone Clinical Trial in Macrovascular Events; RECORD, Rosiglitazone Evaluated for Cardiac Outcomes and Regulation of Glycaemia in Diabetes; VA DT, Veterans Administration Diabetes Trial.

Reduction with Initial Glargine Intervention) trial is assessing the CV benefits of early treatment with insulin glargine in high-risk individuals who have impaired glucose tolerance, impaired fasting glucose, or early type 2 diabetes mellitus. The results of these trials should be available within the next 3 to 5 years and will provide further insight into the role of insulin therapy in the prevention of CV disease in diabetic and nondiabetic individuals with an elevated glucose level.

Summary

Mounting evidence suggests that insulin therapy may reduce risk for CV events while preserving beta-cell function, and several continuing long-term CV trials are testing these hypotheses explicitly.

References

[1] Gerstein HC, Malmberg K, Capes S, et al. Cardiovascular diseases. In: Gerstein HC, Haynes RB, editors. Evidence-based diabetes care. Hamilton (Ontario): BC Decker Inc.; 2001. p. 488–514.
[2] Cowie CC, Harris MI. Physical and metabolic characteristics of persons with diabetes. In: Harris MI, Cowie CC, Stern MS, et al, editors. Diabetes in America. NIH Publication No. 95–1468. Bethesda (MD): National Institutes of Health; 1995. p. 117–64.
[3] Expert Committee on the Diagnosis and Classification of Diabetes Mellitus. Report of the Expert Committee on the Diagnosis and Classification of Diabetes Mellitus. Diabetes Care 1997;20(7):1183–97.

[4] Coutinho M, Gerstein HC, Wang Y, et al. The relationship between glucose and incident cardiovascular events. A metaregression analysis of published data from 20 studies of 95,783 individuals followed for 12.4 years. Diabetes Care 1999;22(2):233–40.

[5] DECODE Study Group EDEG. Is the current definition for diabetes relevant to mortality risk from all causes and cardiovascular and noncardiovascular diseases? Diabetes Care 2003; 26(3):688–96.

[6] Khaw KT, Wareham N, Luben R, et al. Glycated haemoglobin, diabetes, and mortality in men in Norfolk cohort of European Prospective Investigation of Cancer and Nutrition (EPIC-Norfolk). BMJ 2001;322(7277):1–6.

[7] Meigs JB, Nathan DM, D'Agostino RB Sr, et al. Fasting and postchallenge glycemia and cardiovascular disease risk: the Framingham Offspring Study. Diabetes Care 2002;25(10): 1845–50.

[8] Kowalska I, Prokop J, Bachorzewska-Gajewska H, et al. Disturbances of glucose metabolism in men referred for coronary arteriography. Postload glycemia as predictor for coronary atherosclerosis. Diabetes Care 2001;24(5):897–901.

[9] Norhammar A, Tenerz A, Nilsson G, et al. Glucose metabolism in patients with acute myocardial infarction and no previous diagnosis of diabetes mellitus: a prospective study. Lancet 2002;359(9324):2140–4.

[10] Gerstein HC, Pais P, Pogue J, et al. Relationship of glucose and insulin levels to the risk of myocardial infarction: a case-control study. J Am Coll Cardiol 1999;33(3):612–9.

[11] Capes SE, Hunt D, Malmberg K, et al. Stress hyperglycaemia and increased risk of death after myocardial infarction in patients with and without diabetes: a systematic overview. Lancet 2000;355(9206):773–8.

[12] Foo K, Cooper J, Deaner A, et al. A single serum glucose measurement predicts adverse outcomes across the whole range of acute coronary syndromes. Heart 2003;89(5): 512–6.

[13] Sala J, Masia R, Gonzalez de Molina FJ, et al. Short-term mortality of myocardial infarction patients with diabetes or hyperglycaemia during admission. J Epidemiol Community Health 2002;56(9):707–12.

[14] Norhammar AM, Ryden L, Malmberg K. Admission plasma glucose. Independent risk factor for long-term prognosis after myocardial infarction even in nondiabetic patients. Diabetes Care 1999;22(11):1827–31.

[15] Weir CJ, Murray GD, Dyker AG, et al. Is hyperglycaemia an independent predictor of poor outcome after acute stroke? Results of a long-term follow up study. BMJ 1997;314(7090): 1303–6.

[16] Gerstein HC, Capes SE. Dysglycemia: a key cardiovascular risk factor. Semin Vasc Med 2002;2(2):165–74.

[17] Genuth S, Alberti KG, Bennett P, et al. Follow-up report on the diagnosis of diabetes mellitus. Diabetes Care 2003;26(11):3160–7.

[18] Harris MI, Flegal KM, Cowie CC, et al. Prevalence of diabetes, impaired fasting glucose and impaired glucose tolerance in US adults. The third National Health and Nutrition Examination Survey, 1988–1994. Diabetes Care 1998;21(4):518–24.

[19] Wild S, Roglic G, Green A, et al. Global prevalence of diabetes: estimates for the year 2000 and projections for 2030. Diabetes Care 2004;27(5):1047–53.

[20] Hogan P, Dall T, Nikolov P. American Diabetes Association. Economic costs of diabetes in the US in 2002. Diabetes Care 2003;26(3):917–32.

[21] Ceriello A, Motz E. Is oxidative stress the pathogenic mechanism underlying insulin resistance, diabetes, and cardiovascular disease? The common soil hypothesis revisited. Arterioscler Thromb Vasc Biol 2004;24(5):816–23.

[22] Stern MP. Diabetes and cardiovascular disease: the "common soil" hypothesis. Diabetes 1995;44(4):369–74.

[23] Brownlee M. Biochemistry and molecular cell biology of diabetic complications. Nature 2001;414(6865):813–20.

[24] Robertson RP, Harmon J, Tran PO, et al. Glucose toxicity in beta-cells: type 2 diabetes, good radicals gone bad, and the glutathione connection. Diabetes 2003;52(3):581–7.

[25] UK prospective diabetes study 16. Overview of 6 years' therapy of type II diabetes: a progressive disease. UK Prospective Diabetes Study Group. Diabetes 1995;44(11):1249–58.

[26] Nathan DM, Lachin J, Cleary P, et al. Intensive diabetes therapy and carotid intima-media thickness in type 1 diabetes mellitus. N Engl J Med 2003;348(23):2294–303.

[27] Eckel RH, Wassef M, Chait A, et al. Prevention Conference VI: Diabetes and Cardiovascular Disease: Writing Group II: pathogenesis of atherosclerosis in diabetes. Circulation 2002;105(18):e138–43.

[28] Beckman JA, Creager MA, Libby P. Diabetes and atherosclerosis: epidemiology, pathophysiology, and management. JAMA 2002;287(19):2570–81.

[29] Stumvoll M, Tataranni PA, Stefan N, et al. Glucose allostasis. Diabetes 2003;52(4):903–9.

[30] Lewis GF, Carpentier A, Adeli K, et al. Disordered fat storage and mobilization in the pathogenesis of insulin resistance and type 2 diabetes. Endocr Rev 2002;23(2):201–29.

[31] Dubois M, Kerr-Conte J, Gmyr V, et al. Non-esterified fatty acids are deleterious for human pancreatic islet function at physiological glucose concentration. Diabetologia 2004;47(3):463–9.

[32] Diaz R. Metabolic modulation of acute myocardial infarction. Crit Care Clin 2001;17(2):469–76.

[33] Wolff AA, Rotmensch HH, Stanley WC, et al. Metabolic approaches to the treatment of ischemic heart disease: the clinicians' perspective. Heart Fail Rev 2002;7(2):187–203.

[34] Lopaschuk GD. Metabolic abnormalities in the diabetic heart. Heart Fail Rev 2002;7(2):149–59.

[35] Das UN. Is insulin an endogenous cardioprotector? Crit Care 2002;6(5):389–93.

[36] Hansen TK, Thiel S, Wouters PJ, et al. Intensive insulin therapy exerts antiinflammatory effects in critically ill patients and counteracts the adverse effect of low mannose-binding lectin levels. J Clin Endocrinol Metab 2003;88(3):1082–8.

[37] Das UN. Insulin: an endogenous cardioprotector. Curr Opin Crit Care 2003;9(5):375–83.

[38] Vehkavaara S, Makimattila S, Schlenzka A, et al. Insulin therapy improves endothelial function in type 2 diabetes. Arterioscler Thromb Vasc Biol 2000;20(2):545–50.

[39] Gress TW, Nieto FJ, Shahar E, et al. Hypertension and antihypertensive therapy as risk factors for type 2 diabetes mellitus. Atherosclerosis Risk in Communities Study. N Engl J Med 2000;342(13):905–12.

[40] Schwartz GG, Il'yasova D, Ivanova A. Urinary cadmium, impaired fasting glucose, and diabetes in the NHANES III. Diabetes Care 2003;26(2):468–70.

[41] Longnecker MP, Daniels JL. Environmental contaminants as etiologic factors for diabetes. Environ Health Perspect 2001;109(Suppl 6):871–6.

[42] Hu FB, Manson JE, Stampfer MJ, et al. Diet, lifestyle, and the risk of type 2 diabetes mellitus in women. N Engl J Med 2001;345(11):790–7.

[43] Diabetes Prevention Trial–Type 1 Diabetes Study Group. Effects of insulin in relatives of patients with type 1 diabetes mellitus. N Engl J Med 2002;346(22):1685–91.

[44] Prospective Diabetes Study UK (UKPDS) Group. Intensive blood-glucose control with sulphonylureas or insulin compared with conventional treatment and risk of complications in patients with type 2 diabetes (UKPDS 33). Lancet 1998;352:837–53.

[45] Ohkubo Y, Kishikawa H, Araki E, et al. Intensive insulin therapy prevents the progression of diabetic microvascular complications in Japanese patients with non-insulin-dependent diabetes mellitus: a randomized prospective 6-year study. Diab Res Clin Pract 1995;28:103–17.

[46] Abraira C, Colwell JA, Nuttall F, et al. Cardiovascular events and correlates in the veterans affairs diabetes feasibility trial. Arch Intern Med 1997;157:181–8.

[47] Genuth S. Exogenous insulin admininstration and cardiovascular risk in NIDDM and IDDM. Ann Intern Med 1996;124(1 pt 2):104–9.

[48] Malmberg K. Prospective randomised study of intensive insulin treatment on long-term survival after acute myocardial infarction in patients with diabetes mellitus. DIGAMI (Diabetes Mellitus, Insulin Glucose Infusion in Acute Myocardial Infarction) Study Group. BMJ 1997;314(7093):1512–5.

[49] Apstein CS. Increased glycolytic substrate protection improves ischemic cardiac dysfunction and reduces injury. Am Heart J 2000;139(2 Pt 3):S107–14.

[50] Quinones-Galvan A, Ferrannini E. Metabolic effects of glucose-insulin infusions: myocardium and whole body. Curr Opin Clin Nutr Metab Care 2001;4(2):157–63.

[51] Lawson M, Gerstein HC, Tsui E, et al. Effect of intensive therapy on early macrovascular disease in young individuals with type 1 diabetes. A systematic review and meta-analysis. Diabetes Care 1999;22(Suppl.2):B35–9.

[52] Diabetes Control and Complications Trial Research Group. The effect of intensive treatment of diabetes on the development and progression of long-term complications in insulin-dependent diabetes mellitus. N Engl J Med 1993;329:977–86.

[53] Diabetes Control and Complications Trial (DCCT) Research Group. Effect of intensive diabetes management on macrovascular events and risk factors in the diabetes control and complications trial. Am J Cardiol 1995;75:894–903.

[54] Fath-Ordoubadi F, Beatt KJ. Glucose-insulin-potassium therapy for treatment of acute myocardial infarction: an overview of randomized placebo-controlled trials. Circulation 1997;96(4):1152–6.

[55] Diaz R, Paolasso EA, Piegas LS, et al. Metabolic modulation of acute myocardial infarction. The ECLA (Estudios Cardiologicos Latinoamerica) Collaborative Group. Circulation 1998; 98(21):2227–34.

[56] Furnary AP, Gao G, Grunkemeier GL, et al. Continuous insulin infusion reduces mortality in patients with diabetes undergoing coronary artery bypass grafting. J Thorac Cardiovasc Surg 2003;125(5):1007–21.

[57] van den Berghe G, Wouters P, Weekers F, et al. Intensive insulin therapy in critically ill patients. N Engl J Med 2001;345(19):1359–67.

[58] Riddle MC, Rosenstock J, Gerich J. The treat-to-target trial: randomized addition of glargine or human NPH insulin to oral therapy of type 2 diabetic patients. Diabetes Care 2003;26(11):3080–6.

[59] Weyer C, Bogardus C, Mott DM, et al. The natural history of insulin secretory dysfunction and insulin resistance in the pathogenesis of type 2 diabetes mellitus. J Clin Invest 1999; 104(6):787–94.

[60] Bogardus C, Tataranni PA. Reduced early insulin secretion in the etiology of type 2 diabetes mellitus in Pima Indians. Diabetes 2002;51(Suppl 1):S262–4.

[61] Robertson RP, Harmon J, Tran PO, et al. Beta-cell glucose toxicity, lipotoxicity, and chronic oxidative stress in type 2 diabetes. Diabetes 2004;53(Suppl 1):S119–24.

[62] Unger RH. Lipotoxic diseases. Annu Rev Med 2002;53:319–36.

[63] Leibowitz G, Yuli M, Donath MY, et al. Beta-cell glucotoxicity in the Psammomys obesus model of type 2 diabetes. Diabetes 2001;50(Suppl 1):S113–7.

[64] Leahy JL, Bonner-Weir S, Weir GC. Minimal chronic hyperglycemia is a critical determinant of impaired insulin secretion after an incomplete pancreatectomy. J Clin Invest 1988;81(5):1407–14.

[65] Rossetti L, Shulman GI, Zawalich W, et al. Effect of chronic hyperglycemia on in vivo insulin secretion in partially pancreatectomized rats. J Clin Invest 1987;80(4):1037–44.

[66] Bonner-Weir S, Trent DF, Weir GC. Partial pancreatectomy in the rat and subsequent defect in glucose-induced insulin release. J Clin Invest 1983;71(6):1544–53.

[67] McGarry JD. Banting lecture 2001: dysregulation of fatty acid metabolism in the etiology of type 2 diabetes. Diabetes 2002;51(1):7–18.

[68] Prospective Diabetes Study UK. (UKPDS) Group. Effect of intensive blood glucose control with metformin on complications in overweight patients with type 2 diabetes (UKPDS 34). Lancet 1998;352:854–65.

[69] Turner RC, Cull CA, Frighi V, et al. Glycemic control with diet, sulfonylurea, metformin, or insulin in patients with type 2 diabetes mellitus: progressive requirement for multiple therapies (UKPDS 49). UK Prospective Diabetes Study (UKPDS) Group. JAMA 1999; 281(21):2005–12.

[70] Butler AE, Janson J, Bonner-Weir S, et al. Beta-cell deficit and increased beta-cell apoptosis in humans with type 2 diabetes. Diabetes 2003;52(1):102–10.

[71] Gleason CE, Gonzalez M, Harmon JS, et al. Determinants of glucose toxicity and its reversibility in the pancreatic islet beta-cell line, HIT-T15. Am J Physiol Endocrinol Metab 2000;279(5):E997–1002.

[72] Kosaka K, Kuzuya T, Akanuma Y, et al. Increase in insulin response after treatment of overt maturity-onset diabetes is independent of the mode of treatment. Diabetologia 1980;18(1): 23–8.

[73] Scarlett JA, Gray RS, Griffin J, et al. Insulin treatment reverses the insulin resistance of type II diabetes mellitus. Diabetes Care 1982;5(4):353–63.

[74] Andrews WJ, Vasquez B, Nagulesparan M, et al. Insulin therapy in obese, non-insulin-dependent diabetes induces improvements in insulin action and secretion that are maintained for two weeks after insulin withdrawal. Diabetes 1984;33(7):634–42.

[75] Garvey WT, Olefsky JM, Griffin J, et al. The effect of insulin treatment on insulin secretion and insulin action in type II diabetes mellitus. Diabetes 1985;34(3):222–34.

[76] Pratipanawatr T, Cusi K, Ngo P, et al. Normalization of plasma glucose concentration by insulin therapy improves insulin-stimulated glycogen synthesis in type 2 diabetes. Diabetes 2002;51(2):462–8.

[77] Ilkova H, Glaser B, Tunckale A, et al. Induction of long-term glycemic control in newly diagnosed type 2 diabetic patients by transient intensive insulin treatment. Diabetes Care 1997;20(9):1353–6.

[78] Park S, Choi SB. Induction of long-term normoglycemia without medication in Korean type 2 diabetes patients after continuous subcutaneous insulin infusion therapy. Diabetes Metab Res Rev 2003;19(2):124–30.

[79] Ryan EA, Imes S, Wallace C. Short-term intensive insulin therapy in newly diagnosed type 2 diabetes. Diabetes Care 2004;27(5):1028–32.

[80] Alvarsson M, Sundkvist G, Lager I, et al. Beneficial effects of insulin versus sulphonylurea on insulin secretion and metabolic control in recently diagnosed type 2 diabetic patients. Diabetes Care 2003;26(8):2231–7.

[81] Inzucchi SE. Oral antihyperglycemic therapy for type 2 diabetes: scientific review. JAMA 2002;287(3):360–72.

[82] Rosenstock J. Insulin therapy: optimizing control in type 1 and type 2 diabetes. Clin Cornerstone 2001;4(2):50–64.

[83] Rosenstock J, Riddle MC. Insulin therapy in type 2 diabetes. The CADRE handbook of diabetes management. New York: Medical Information Press; 2004.

[84] American Diabetes Association. Standards of medical care for patients with diabetes mellitus. Diabetes Care 2004;27(S1):S15–35.

[85] Yki-Jarvinen H, Dressler A, Ziemen M. Less nocturnal hypoglycemia and better post-dinner glucose control with bedtime insulin glargine compared with bedtime NPH insulin during insulin combination therapy in type 2 diabetes. HOE 901/3002 Study Group. Diabetes Care 2000;23(8):1130–6.

[86] Rosenstock J, Schwartz SL, Clark CM Jr, et al. Basal insulin therapy in type 2 diabetes: 28-week comparison of insulin glargine (HOE 901) and NPH insulin. Diabetes Care 2001;24(4): 631–6.

[87] Rosenstock J, Wyne K. Insulin treatment in type 2 diabetes. In: Goldstein BJ, Muller-Wieland D, editors. Textbook of type 2 diabetes. London: Martin Dunitz; 2003. p. 131–54.

[88] Canadian Diabetes Association Clinical Practice Guidelines Expert Committee. Canadian Diabetes Association 2003 clinical practice guidelines for the prevention and management of diabetes in Canada. Can J Diabetes 2003;23(Supp 2):S1–S152.

ELSEVIER
SAUNDERS

Endocrinol Metab Clin N Am
34 (2005) 155–197

ENDOCRINOLOGY
AND METABOLISM
CLINICS
OF NORTH AMERICA

Novel Pharmacologic Agents
for Type 2 Diabetes

Gabriel I. Uwaifo, MD[a,b], Robert E. Ratner, MD[c,*]

[a]*Georgetown University College of Medicine, Washington DC 20003, USA*
[b]*MedStar Research Institute, 650 Pennsylvania Avenue Southeast, Suite 50, Washington DC
20003, USA*
[c]*MedStar Research Institute, 6495 New Hampshire Avenue, Suite 201, Hyattsville, MD,
20783, USA*

Introduction and background

Since the discovery of insulin by Banting and Best in the early 20th
century, the clinical management of diabetes has undergone significant
changes. The last decade has been associated with an explosion in
therapeutic options for management of type 2 diabetes that has significantly
increased the pharmacologic options available to clinicians. Largely driven
by advances in recombinant DNA technology and other advanced methods
of molecular biology and clinical chemistry, human recombinant insulin and
insulin analogs have replaced animal insulins and may soon displace NPH,
regular, lente, and ultralente. Analogs such as insulin glargine, insulin lispro,
insulin aspart, and soon insulin glulisine, are becoming part of mainstream
diabetes management. Beyond these, there are several other promising
agents (insulin analogs and noninsulin antidiabetics) in various stages of
development, which may become clinically available for the management of
type 2 diabetes within the next decade. Among these, the incretin analogs,
amylin analogs, combined PPAR-α and -γ agonists, and islet neogenesis
gene-associated protein (INGAP) are among the most prominent. This
review aims to discuss these novel pharmocotherapeutic options for diabetes
management. Agents for diabetes management can be broadly classified into
two major categories: antihyperglycemics and hypoglycemics. The distinction is crucial because hypoglycemic agents are capable of inducing more
clinical hypoglycemia—the major adverse event that limits near-normal
glycemic control by most of the agents presently available.

* Corresponding author.
E-mail address: RatnerMRI@aol.com (R.E. Ratner).

0889-8529/05/$ - see front matter © 2005 Elsevier Inc. All rights reserved.
doi:10.1016/j.ecl.2004.11.006   *endo.theclinics.com*

Another method of classification is based on the modes and sites of action of medications. Whereas this is helpful conceptually, it is limited by the site(s) and mode(s) of action of some of the agents are unknown: other agents have multiple sites and modes of action. Such a classification scheme may appear as in Box 1:

This review discusses those agents furthest along in the process of development for clinical use in type 2 diabetes. There are a host of other agents in various stages of development which also show promise, but not discussed in detail here primarily because their potential for clinical use in

---

Box 1. Modes and sites of action of medications

Intestinal agent
- Inhibitors of carbohydrate digestion
- Inhibitors of glucose absorption
- Modulators of incretin hormones

Insulin and insulin-modulating strategies
- Insulin analogs with designer pharmacokinetics
- Alternative insulin delivery methods and routes
- Endogenous insulin secretagogues
- Agents for regeneration of pancreatic β-cells
- Insulin mimetics which, though structurally different, act on the insulin receptor

Insulin sensitizers
- Systemic insulin sensitizers
- Hepatic insulin sensitizers
- Global insulin sensitizers (which have systemic and hepatic insulin sensitization properties)

Incretins
- Amylin analogs
- Glucagons-like peptide-1 (GLP-1) agonists and related analogues
- Dipeptidyl peptidase IV inhibitors

Other agents
- Inhibitors of counter-regulatory hormones
- Antilipolytic agents
- Fatty acid–oxidation inhibitors
- Inhibitors of gluconeogenesis
- Very-low-density lipoprotein synthesis inhibitors
- Glycogenolysis inhibitors
- Antiobesity agents

type 2 diabetes in the near future is still unclear. The agents detailed are (1) amylin analogs; (2) exendin and other GLP-1 agonists; (3) dipeptidyl peptidase IV inhibitors; (4) combined α- and γ-peroxisome proliferator activator receptor (PPAR) agonists, also known as the glitazars; (5) insulin detemir; (6) inhaled insulins; (7) oral insulins; and (8) INGAP.

Pramlintide

Rationale and background

Amylin is a naturally occurring 37–amino acid peptide that is normally cosecreted in equimolar amounts with insulin from the pancreatic β-cells [1]. Amylin secretion has been shown to be delayed and diminished in more advanced cases of type 2 diabetes and markedly reduced to absent in people who have type 1 diabetes [2]. In addition amylin secretion in gestational diabetes is also impaired and characterized by inappropriately exaggerated secretion during pregnancy followed by impaired poststimulatory secretion in the puerperium compared with pregnant women who do not have gestational diabetes [3]. Though initially presumed to be related to the islet amyloid in the pathogenesis and progression of type 2 diabetes, the physiologic role of amylin in postprandial glycemic control is now fairly well established and different from the amyloid [4–6].

Description of agent

Among the identified metabolic effects of amylin and its synthetic analog, pramlintide, are (1) suppression of endogenous glucagon production, especially in the postprandial state; (2) consequent reduction of postprandial hepatic glucose production; (3) reduction in gastric emptying time; (4) centrally-mediated induction of satiety; and (5) reduction in postprandial glucose levels [1,2,7–13]. Because of the innate tendency of the amylin compound to aggregate and adhere to surfaces and its instability in solution, it is difficult to store, mass manufacture, and formulate as a pharmaceutical. What was needed was an analog with better physical properties but similar clinical efficacy [2]. Pramlintide has these beneficial properties [14–16].

Pramlintide has been extensively investigated in doses ranging from 30 to 120 mcg three times daily given subcutaneously, and shown to have modest effects on glycemic control in type 1 and 2 diabetic subjects, especially when administered at or just before meals [17,18]. The same physiologic effects associated with amylin in normal subjects, such as suppression of postmeal-glucagon levels and slowing of gastric emptying have been described in type 1 and 2 diabetes [10,19–23]. It has been observed that in subjects who have type 1 and insulin deficient type 2 diabetes, postprandial hyper-glucagonemia and hepatic glucose production are exaggerated [24,25]. Thompson and colleagues [14] gave pramlintide to 203 insulin-requiring patients who had type 2 diabetes and documented significant improvements in fructosamine, with concomitant reduction in the frequency and severity of hypoglycemic episodes over a 4-week trial period. There is now data that indicates that amylin (and thus presumably pramlintide) potently inhibits the orexogenic (appetite-stimulating) stomach hormone ghrelin, which could explain some of the amylin claims of having some appetite suppressant effect [26]. The long-term efficacy of pramlintide as an adjunct to insulin has been established in subjects who have type 1 and 2 diabetes [17,18,27–30]. In cohorts, the addition of amylin to insulin resulted in significant reductions in hemoglobin A1c (HbA1c) (of between 0.6%–0.9%) with mean weight loss of ~2 kg, without concomitant increases in insulin doses or frequency of hypoglycemic episodes [2,27,30]. These findings have been sustained over 2 years in uncontrolled open-label extension studies [2,28,31]. Also of note is that the HbA1c improvement in subjects treated with pramlintide occurred in the setting of weight loss rather than weight gain, which is typical of intensive insulin-based therapeutic regimens [2,30]. These beneficial effects have also been demonstrated in a small study with subjects using insulin pumps to whom pramlintide was added as adjunctive therapy [32]. Pramlintide has also been demonstrated to be an adjunct for reducing postprandial glycemic surges even in subjects already being treated with regular insulin or insulin lispro [17,18]. Weyer and colleague's study [17,18] demonstrated a 75% reduction in the postprandial glucose area under the curve for subjects treated with pramlintide combined with insulin lispro compared with subjects treated with insulin lispro alone and a 100% reduction compared with subjects treated with regular insulin alone. Similar preliminary studies in adolescents have replicated the findings from adult diabetic cohorts [33]. Pramlintide has also been shown to be associated with reduction of postprandial glucagon and triglyceride excursions and reduction in overall daily glycemic flux in type 1 diabetic patients on insulin pumps [32]. Other studies [34] have demonstrated that, despite minimal differences in pharmacokinetics, there are no clinically significant differences in pramlintide's clinical efficacy irrespective of site of injection, needle length, and subject body size. There is also considerable data [35] regarding the safety and tolerability of pramlintide-use over extended periods. Want and colleagues [35] prospectively followed 27 subjects using pramlintide for 2 to 7 years continuously; they showed improvements in the proportion of subjects achieving target glycemic control (HbA1c < 7%) but, remarkably, without weight gain. Of particular interest was the finding that subjects who have a baseline body mass index (BMI) greater than 25 at enrollment on average lost ~4 kg over the follow up period [35]. This study, however, was not randomized but a report of a selected population of *responders* who were chosen because they best tolerated the medication with minimal-to-no side effects. Chapman and colleagues [36] report on a small, double-blind, placebo, control crossover meal study of 11 subjects who had type 2 diabetes and obesity, and an additional 15 nondiabetic obese subjects treated with pramlintide showed significant reductions in total caloric intake with equivalent reductions in fat, carbohydrate, and protein intake. This acute feeding study demonstrated a 19% reduction in caloric intake following a single dose of 120 mcg of pramlintide, the result of equivalent reductions in meal derived fat, carbohydrate, and protein [36].

Because of concerns regarding the need for additional injections to use pramlintide, there have been studies to evaluate perceptions and quality of life measures in patients using pramlintide. Since the medication is administered preprandially and cannot be mixed with insulin products as presently constituted, this does amount to at least three additional subcutaneous injections. Data from 266 such patients reported by Marrero and colleagues [37] indicate that pramlintide use was associated with significant improvements in quality of life measures (such as perception of better glucose control, better functional ability at work, home and school and better self confidence in diabetes self management), though the patients were aware of more side effects than in the insulin alone treated study arm. Subjects indicated that the benefits of pramlintide outweighed the need for additional injections. This study involved using a 14-item well-validated satisfaction survey measured on a 6-point Likert scale. Among the items included in the survey were perception of glycemic control; perception of weight control; perception of appetite control; ability to function independently at home, work, and school; and an overall feeling of well-being [37].

Pramlintide summary

Pramlintide has been extensively studied in phase 2 and 3 trials demonstrating the utility of pramlintide in management of type 1 and 2 diabetes with improvements in glycemic swings and a weight-neutral profile. Pramlintide currently has an approvable letter from the U.S. Food and Drug Administration (FDA) as an adjunct for diabetic pharmacotherapy, however, since it represents an entirely new class of antidiabetic agent and the first injectable since insulin this process has been approached with caution by the regulatory bodies. The initial application to the FDA for Pramlintide was rejected because of safety concerns related to hypoglycemic episodes and related to the FDA requirement at that time that in testing adjunctive medications the prior insulin dose not be adjusted. Consequently, though HbA1c levels declined in pramlintide treated subjects, incidence of hypoglycemia also increased. Later trials [33,38,39] have allowed the down titration of insulin doses with pramlintide use, which has resulted in attenuation of hypoglycemia.

Potential niche

Pramlintide may have a useful place in the management of individuals who have wide glycemic swings and holds promise as a potential adjunct for use in insulin-resistant subjects who require large amounts of insulin and who are obese, but there are no data to substantiate this claim. Pramlintide may have a role in the management of subjects who have predominantly postprandial as opposed to fasting hyperglycemia. The requirement of 2 to 3 additional injections for administration does suggest that the use of pramlintide will be restricted to type 1 and 2 diabetics who already use insulin and are thus unlikely to be needle phobic and willing to accept a total of 5 to 6 injections a day.

Adverse reactions, problems, and concerns

The major side effects associated with pramlintide are gastrointestinal, including mild to moderate nausea; anorexia; early satiety; and less commonly, vomiting. Whereas nausea has been reported [29,32] to be twice as common in pramlintide users compared with placebo during the first few weeks of therapy, this nausea tends to resolve with continued use. The side effects tend to be dose dependent and tolerance tends to occur with continued use of the peptide. Hypoglycemia has been also described in the setting of pramlintide use as an insulin adjunct. This is generally mild to moderate and tends to resolve when insulin doses are appropriately reduced once pramlinitide is established in the individual.

Glucagons-like peptide-1 agonists

Rationale and background

The intestinal derived hormone GLP-1 appears to be the major mediator of the incretin effect. This effect results in the enhanced insulin secretion associated with caloric intake that is oral as opposed to intravenous or parenteral [40,41]. These hormones function in the so-called *ileal break system*, which inhibits upper gastrointestinal motility and bowel-associated secretions when nutrients reach the small intestines [41,42]. In addition, they induce satiety and promote insulin-mediated tissue glucose uptake partly by enhancing endogenous insulin release in response to oral caloric intake [39,40].

GLP-1 is estimated to account for 70%–80% of the endogenous incretin effect that has a role in maintenance of normoglycemia in nondiabetic individuals (especially following a caloric load) and has potential for use in the treatment of diabetes [43–46]. It has been shown [47–49] that diet-related GLP-1 surges in subjects who have type 2 diabetes are impaired compared with matched healthy controls. Among GLP-1's proposed effects are (1) glucose-dependent enhancement of endogenous insulin secretion and perhaps insulin sensitivity, (2) inhibition of endogenous glucagon secretion, (3) possible appetite suppression and satiety induction, (4) reduction in speed of gastric emptying, and (5) possible stimulation of islet growth, differentiation, and regeneration (apparently mediated by the transcription factor PDX-1) [40,50–52]. Furthermore, there is early experimental data [53–55] suggesting that GLP-1 and its analogues may also play a role in protection and preservation of β-cells from cytokine and free fatty acid–mediated injury and apoptosis. GLP-1 and the synthetic analog exendin-4 have also been demonstrated to ameliorate streptozotocin-induced diabetes in Wistar rats and induce β-cell neogenesis in islets with resultant improvement in glycemic profiles [56]. The GLP-1 analog liraglutide (NN2211) has also been shown to inhibit free fatty acid–induced apoptosis in rat β-cells [44]. Liraglutide normalized fasting and postprandial glucose tolerance, normalized measures of baseline insulin resistance, and reduced weight (predominantly due to reduced food intake) in diet-induced obesity-prone rats compared with control Sprague Dawley rats [57]. Some of these effects have been demonstrated with certain degree in healthy human subjects and in subjects who have type 1 and 2 diabetes [40]. The endogenous peptide is rapidly cleared in vivo by the action of the endoprotease dipeptidyl peptidase IV (DPP-IV), thus resistant analogs of the peptide/receptor agonists have been developed to exploit its favorable metabolic effects as a potential treatment for type 2 diabetes.

Description of agent

GLP-1 itself is a peptide hormone (molecular weight ∼3000 KD) produced by the endoprotease cleavage of the proglucagon precursor. GLP-1 is secreted by intestinal L cells. Based on the unfavorable pharmacokinetics of endogenous GLP-1 (the half-life of GLP-1 infused intravenously in humans is 4–11 minutes with a clearance rate of ∼13 mL/kg/min) [58,59], the development of analogs has become paramount.

While there are several GLP-1 agonists in various stages of development, the most advanced products are liraglutide (an acylated GLP-1 analog bound to albumin) and exendin 4 (whose synthetic analog, exenatide, is also known as AC-2993 and derived from the venom of the Gila monster, *Heloderma suspectum*). Exenatide is a 39–amino acid–GLP-1 receptor antagonist with a 53% homology to mammalian-derived GLP-1 [40].

Liraglutide is resistant to DPP-IV because of its albumin-binding acylated side chain. Liraglutide replicates all the metabolic activities of endogenous GLP-1 and has a half-life of 12 to 14 hours.

Available data

Early short-term studies [60,61] have shown that infusion of adequate doses of GLP-1 intravenously (sufficient to give a plasma GLP-1 concentration of 7–120 pmol/L) is associated with restoration of normo-glycemia in subjects who have type 2 diabetes. Peak GLP-1 concentrations following subcutaneous injections occur in about 30 minutes and, even with supraphysologic doses, basal levels are generally restored within 90 to 120 minutes [40]. GLP-1 levels above 500 pmol/L are generally the thresh-hold at which nausea and vomiting develop and these remain the major side effects of this group of medications. There have been several other human trials [62–66] of GLP-1 in normal controls and type 2 diabetics demonstrating its utility in intravenous and subcutaneous administration.

There have been several trials [67–69] of liraglutide (NN-2211) in which its ability to reduce fasting morning glucose and breakfast-related glycemic excursions have been demonstrated. Thus far no side effects beyond those known to be associated with native GLP-1, such as nausea and vomiting, have been identified. Matthews and colleagues [70] studied 193 subjects who have type 2 diabetes using five different dose regimens. The medication was administered as a single daily injection. The two lowest doses (0.045 mg/d and 0.225 mg/d) had no effect on glycemic control while the other three doses (0.45 mg/d, 0.6 mg/d, and 0.75 mg/d) were associated with glycemic control comparable to glimepiride monotherapy with minimal side effects, low risk for tight hypoglycemia, and a trend towards weight loss [70]. Most recently, Nauck and colleagues [71] studied a cohort of 144 subjects in which the utility of liraglutide as either monotherapy or add-on therapy to metformin as compared with either metformin monotherapy or combined metformin–glimepiride. The liraglutide dosage was titrated as required from 0.5 mg/day to 2 mg/day over a 5-week period and the liraglutide–metformin group had a 1.1% reduction in HbA1c with no episodes of hypoglycemia [71]. Nausea though, the most prominent side effect, was associated only with medication withdrawal in 4% of subjects. As compared with the glimepiride treatment groups (who gained ~0.9% over the study period), the liraglutide treatment groups were also associated with a 2.4% weight loss [71].

Exendin-4 (and the synthetic version AC 2993) has also been shown to have the whole spectrum of activity demonstrated for endogenous GLP-1 [72–75]. Doses between 5 mcg/day to 10 mcg/day or twice daily have been tried in various human clinical trials. The side effect profile is similar to GLP-1 mainly nausea and vomiting and the immunologic profile is still under investigation [40,60–62,65,66]. Recent data reported in only abstract form from the Amigo trials [76,77] have noted that exendin-4 injections in human subjects are associated with endogenous auto-antibody production but this has not been found thus far to be associated with any obvious clinical consequences (allergic reactions, serum sickness, etc), or any significant effect on glycemic response. Clinical trial data [74,75,78] indicate exendin-4's main potency and utility is in managing postprandial hyperglycemia with less of an effect on fasting hyperglycemia as adjunctive therapy to established oral agents. Because of some animal data suggesting that exendin-4 is capable of increasing β-cell mass by inducing β-cell neogenesis, there have been some concerns regarding potential association with nesidioblastosis, insulinomas, or other pancreatic islet proliferative disorders. Hiles and colleagues [79], however, found no significant associations or trends between use of exendin-4 for ~2 years of exposure in mice and rat populations.

Extensive phase 3 trials of exenatide have recently been completed (Amigo Trials) and presented in part and in abstract form [76,77]. In one uncontrolled study protocol with 120 subjects, open-label exenatide was subcutaneously administered at 5 mcg/twice daily for 4 weeks followed by 10 mcg/twice daily for an additional 20 weeks. HbA1c was reduced by a mean of 1.3%, whereas fasting glucose was reduced by ~28 mg/dL and weight by 3.4 kg. The incidence of nausea in subjects on exenatide reduced over time from a peak of ~22% in the first 4 weeks of therapy to just ~1% by 24 weeks of therapy.

The definitive phase 3 trials randomized subjects who have type 2 diabetes in three separate protocols; one for subjects on metformin monotherapy of at least 1500 mg/day, one for subjects who have maximally effective sulfonylurea therapy, and one with a combination of maximally effective sulfonyurea therapy and at least 1500 mg/day of metformin. The study design for each of the three protocols was a randomized double-blind placebo control design with two separate *active* exenatide dosing regimens. Patients received either 5 mcg/twice daily for 4 weeks followed by the same dose for the next 26 weeks or 5 mcg/twice daily for 4 weeks followed by a dose escalation to 10 mcg/twice daily for the next 26 weeks. Exenatide was associated with a significant reduction in HbA1c when used as an adjunct in these protocols with the higher dose regimens associated with greater HbA1c declines (−0.8% versus −0.4%). In addition, marked dose-dependent reductions in postprandial plasma glucose more than fasting hyperglycemia and body weight were demonstrated (−2.6 kg versus −1.6 kg). Nausea, vomiting, diarrhea, and upper respiratory symptoms were the most common adverse reactions. The incidence of hypoglycemia was ~5% and comparable with that in the placebo study arm among the metformin treated group of patients. Nausea and vomiting remain the major side effect concerns and are significantly influenced by dose and titration frequency. The open-label uncontrolled extension phases of these protocols, which now have over a year of accumulated data in preliminary analyses, show these findings to be sustained and replicated in the prior placebo groups once they were also exposed to exenatide adjunctive therapy. These results were consistent irrespective of the underlying adjunctive therapy (metformin, sulfonylureas or both) [76,77]. Buse and colleagues [80] recently reported on the sulfonylurea monotherapy group from the Amigo trials and demonstrated that after 30 weeks of treatment, the 10-mcg/twice-daily and 5-mcg/twice-daily groups had significant improvements in HbA1c (−0.86 ± 0.11 and −046 ± 0.12) compared with the placebo arm (+0.12±0.09). The treatment subjects also had significantly lower fasting glucose at the study end and dose-dependent weight loss. The 10-mcg group had the greatest weight loss; −1.6 ± 0.3kg compared with study baseline [80]. No severe hypoglycemic episodes were noted in the cohort. The observed nonsevere hypoglycemia episodes observed are probably due to concomitant sulfonyluria use.

Other similar agents have undergone clinical trials [81,82] in this class including the long acting analog developed by ConjuChem (CJC-1131) which is in the process of development and is based on binding the GLP-1 analog to a reactive moiety which binds to albumin on in vivo subcutaneous and/or intravenous injection thus giving a half-life similar to that of albumin (~2 weeks). CJC-1131 thus far has not been found to be associated with any significant cell or humoral-based immunogenicity [83]. Preliminary data using CJC-1131 in animal models and humans confirm this peptide's utility as an adjunct for improving glycemic control and that its efficacy persists up to 1 week following administration [84]. The exact dosing schedule, interval, and amount to use in humans are the subject of ongoing clinical trials. Guivarch and colleagues [85] recently reported on 22 patients treated with CJC-1131 over 2 weeks with variable doses of 2 mcg/kg, 4 mcg/kg, 8 mcg/kg, or 12 mcg/kg. The three dosing protocols were generally well tolerated with no signs of immunogenecity, however, nausea and vomiting occurred in a dose-dependent fashion. In addition, glycemic levels reduced in a dose-dependent fashion up to 35% by mean 7-point glucose reduction and up to 31% of mean fasting glucose. Body weight was reduced between 1.7 kg to 3 kg over the study period in a dose-dependent fashion. This report had no cases of hypoglycemia or local injection site irritation [85].

Another agent, Ly-307161, is also a DPP-IV-resistant GLP-1–agonist and has been removed from the growing list of candidates. Preliminary trial data [81–84,86–88] indicated that single daily doses as small as 4.5 mg/day may be associated with normalization of glycemic profiles and weight loss in subjects who have type 2 diabetes; however, nausea and injection site discomfort caused its withdrawal from further study.

Prospects

GLP-1 agonists in various stages of progress will likely become part of the therapeutic arsenal against diabetes in the next 1 to 5 years. Exenatide in particular has completed fairly extensive phase 3 trials and has a new drug application submitted to the FDA. Extended release formulations that may permit once-weekly intramuscular injection dosing schedules are also in development. Dose titration of these long acting formulations, however, remains problematic. The potential of oral (buccal) delivery systems for GLP-1 is also being investigated [89,90].

Potential niche

These agents effectively control postprandial hyperglycemia predominantly and have demonstrated efficacy in advanced type 2 diabetes. Their association with satiation and weight loss is also a highly attractive feature. The major draw back for this group of medications is the need for administration by subcutaneous injection (twice daily with exenatide and once daily with liraglutide), which could negatively impact compliance and willingness to use it among needle-naïve patients who have type 2 diabetics.

Despite this, it is reasonable to anticipate that GLP-1 agonists, when clinically available, will find a niche among obese patients who have type 2 diabetes inadequately controlled with multiple oral agents. The potential that these agents may also have β-cell neogenesis and antiapoptotic effects makes them attractive therapeutic and potentially disease-modifying agents; but besides some experimental data, there is no clinical evidence yet to support this hypothesis.

Adverse reactions, problems, and concerns

These agents have a favorable side effect profile except for nausea, fullness, bloating, and vomiting as major side effects, which, however, are generally dose-dependent and can be ameliorated by reducing doses and/or doing slow-dose escalation. GLP-1 agonists on their own do not cause clinically-significant hypoglycemia [40,61] except when associated with sulfonylureas.

Stage of development

Several advanced phase 2 and 3 trials of several agents in this class are ongoing, while the exenatide phase 3 trials have been recently completed making the potential of a GLP-1 agonist joining the diabetes therapeutic arsenal highly likely in the near future (possibly within the next 1–5 years).

The dipeptidyl peptidase–IV inhibitors

Rationale and background

Another therapeutic alternative to enhance the incretin system activity is the blocking of or interference with GLP-1 degradation. The duration of action of GLP-1 (the major incretin hormone) is limited by rapid enzymatic breakdown by the widespread endopeptidase, DPP-IV [91,92]. DPP-IV activity is increased in the fasting state in subjects who have type 2 diabetes compared with healthy controls [93]. This may be one of the reasons why type 2 diabetes is associated with impaired postprandial GLP-1 secretion [93]. One therapeutic strategy in type 2 diabetes has been to develop DPP-IV antagonists to enhance the natural incretin effects of these hormones [91,92].

DPP-IV knockout mice have a phenotype that is resistant to diet-induced obesity, insulin resistance, and thus, type 2 diabetes [94]. Furthermore, long-term DPP-IV inhibition in Wistar rats pretreated with streptozotocin injections (to induce a model of insulinopenic diabetes) revealed significant improvements in glycemic status and overall well-being. Similar findings have been described in C57 mice using three different DPP-IV inhibitors (LAF237, NVP728, and Compound BI-A) demonstrating acute antihyperglycemic effects [95]. Insulin sensitization (by improvements in the homeostasis model

assessment of insulin resistance [HOMA-IR]) and a capacity to reduce progression of insulinopenic diabetes were demonstrated in db/db mice administered a similar, but more potent DPP-IV inhibitor, BI-B, over a 31-day
period [95]. The insulinotropic effects of GLP-1 and glucose-dependent
insulinotropic polypeptide (GIP) are enhanced by use of DPP-IV inhibitors
[96,97]. The greatest potential advantage of DPP-IV inhibitors over GLP-1
agonists is that DPP-IV inhibitors can be given orally (Table 1). Preliminary
data from obese rat studies [98] suggest that compared with the GLP-1
agonist liraglutide, LAF237 is associated with significantly lower plasma
GLP-1 levels and a less-pronounced impact on weight and caloric intake.
While liraglutide-treated rats had weight loss and significant reductions in
candy-derived caloric intake, the LAF237 treated rats were weight neutral
with no observed changes in caloric intake [98]. The potential implications of
this with regards to the differential effects of DPP-IV agents versus GLP-1
agonists in humans vis-à-vis gastrointestinal side effects and weight loss are
yet to be investigated. It is conceivable that GLP-1 agonists, by causing
greater serum GLP-1 levels, may be associated with more gastrointestinal
side effects and more weight loss than DPP-IV inhibitors.

Description of agent

While there several different DPP-IV antagonists have been investigated
in animal models and human subjects, the most promising and advanced
products appear to be LAF237, which is undergoing phase 3 trials at present
[99–102]. There are also some preliminary data demonstrating the utility of
another DPP-IV inhibitor, MK-0431, in increasing endogenous GLP-1
levels and reducing post-oral glucose glycemic excursions [103].

Available data

Ahren and colleagues [101] studied NVP-DPP-728 over a 4-week period in
93 subjects who have type 2 diabetes in a double-blind, multicenter trial. The
oral 100-mg/three-times-daily and the 150-mg/twice-daily dose regimens
used in the trial were effective in reducing fasting glucose and prandial
glucose excursions, thus resulting in significant reduction in HBAIC from
7.4 ± 0.7% to 6.9 ± 0.7% [101]. Medication tolerability was good in both
treatment groups. Similar preliminary findings have been demonstrated using
LAF237 in subjects who have type 2 diabetes [104]. One such study [104]
demonstrated significant reductions in fasting and postprandial glucose with
preservation of first- and second-phase insulin secretion while associated with
reduction in postprandial glucagon secretion. More recent data [105] utilizing
LAF237 (50 mg/d) in a 12-week study in combination with metformin demonstrated significant reductions in fasting glucose, mean prandial glucose,
and peak prandial glucose. This cohort of patients who have type 2 diabetes
also demonstrated significant improvements in meal-related insulin excursion

Table 1
Comparison of dipeptidyl peptidase–IV antagonists with glucagons-like peptide-1 and glucagons-like peptide-1 agonists

Property	DPP-IV antagonists	GLP-1/agonists
Route of administration	Oral	Subcutaneous and intravenous. Oral preparations are in rudimentary stages of development
Effect on weight	Appears at least weight neutral. May be associated with mild weight loss	Clearly demonstrated to be associated with weight loss
Adverse effects	Pruritus, diarrhea, dizziness and diaphoresis are notable	Nausea, vomiting, anorexia, and early satiety are notable
Glycemic control	Has demonstrable efficacy in controlling fasting and postprandial hyperglycemia	Most dominant effect appears related to controlling prandial hyperglycemia. Long-acting analogues with greater effect on fasting hyperglycemia are also being tested
Dosing schedule	Twice daily and three times daily dosing schedules so far tested	Preprandial multiday dosing schedules well tested. Potential for less frequent dosing including once daily, 2–3 times weekly or even once weekly are the subject of ongoing trials.
Experience	Still limited. Multiple studies underway	Fairly extensive human experience from several different pharmaceutical groups
Mode of action	Inhibition of endogenous, ubiquitous plasma enzyme DPP-IV	Enhancement of endogenous incretin hormone effects
Patient compliance	Excellent, side effects infrequent and generally tolerable	Good, for subjects who are not needle phobic. The side effects are generally mild when present and largely tolerable
Natural homologues	None thus far identified	Exendin-4 from the Gila monster
Associated hypoglycemia when used as monotherapy	Probably no but even if so uncommon and generally mild	No
Lingering concerns	DPP-IV is a ubiquitous enzyme that in vivo degrades over 20 different endogenous human peptides. The consequences of inhibiting the degradation of all these peptides on a long-term basis in humans and even animals is yet unclear.	None but still unknown Physiologic effects and consequences of GLP-1 fairly well understood and extensively studied in animals and humans
Prospects for clinical utility	Good, two agents (from Novartis and Merck) in phase 2 and 3 trials	Good, several different agents in phase 2 and 3 trials

and insulin sensitivity (as estimated using the HOMA-IR) [105]. Only one episode of mild, predominantly exercise-related hypoglycemia was described in this cohort [105]. The initial 12-week randomized, double-blind, placebo controlled trial was followed by a 40-week extension study [106]. The cohort included 51 subjects on placebo and 56 subjects on the active treatment (LAF237, 50 mg/d). In the active treatment group, HbA1c decreased by $0.6 \pm 0.1\%$ from the baseline of $7.7 \pm 0.1\%$ by week 12 of treatment, whereas there was no significant change in the placebo group over the same period [106]. Mean prandial and fasting glucose were also significantly reduced in the active treatment group versus the placebo group over the 12-week period. Over the extension period of 40 weeks, mean prandial glucose and fasting glucose remained significantly lower than in the placebo group (with between group differences of $\sim$43 mg/dL and 20 mg/dL, in the treatment and placebo groups, respectively) as did the HbA1c (with a between group difference of $\sim$1.1 $\pm$ 0.2%) [106]. Pratley and colleagues [107] studied LAF237 in a medication-naïve cohort of patients who had type 2 diabetes over a 12-week period. They found a significant reduction in HBAIC (-0.6%) with 47% of LAF237 treated subjects achieving HbA1c values below 7% [107]. Fasting and 4-hour mean postprandial glucose values were also significantly reduced in the treatment group with associated signifcant increases in 4-hour mean postprandial insulin and C-peptide levels [107]. Hypoglycemia was described in 10% of subjects and was generally mild and often related to missed meals and/or strenous exercise [107].

The data on MK-0431 reported recently by Herman and colleagues [103] involved 56 patients who had medication-naïve type 2 diabetes in a three-period cross study design. All subjects received either 25 mg/day or 200 mg/day of the active agent, or placebo separated by 7-day washout periods. In this cohort, MK-0431 was associated with significantly reduced post-oral glucose glycemic excursions (22% versus 26% reductions in the 25- and 200-mg treatment groups compared with placebo) and roughly a twofold increase in plasma GLP-1 levels [103]. In addition, post-oral glucose C-peptide and insulin levels also significantly increased, while post-oral glucose and glucagon levels were significantly reduced [103].

Prospects

While still in early phase 2 and 3 trials, the prospects for NVP-DPP-728 (phase 2), LAF237, and MK-0431 (phases 2 and 3) are good. It is likely that the near future will see the development of other DPP-IV inhibitors.

Potential niche

DPP-IV antagonists hold considerable promise as oral agents that may have utility as adjuncts or monotherapy in subjects who have early onset type 2 diabetes. Their weight neutral/weight loss profile would make them particularly attractive for use in obese subjects while its oral means of administration would be appealing to patients who prefer to avoid injections required for GLP-1 agonists. Since DPP-IV antagonists have novel mechanisms of action and metabolism, they are additive to any current therapies.

Adverse reactions, problems and concerns

The long-term consequences of chronic inhibition of DPP-IV in humans are still unclear and are a cause of concern given the ubiquitous nature of the enzyme [41,108]. Of note is DPP-IV is the major means of degradation of over 20 different peptides including substance P, insulin-like growth factor-1, neuropeptide Y, GLP-2, and GIP [100,101,109,110]. The potential effects of chronically elevated levels of all these peptides, that could conceivably result from long standing DPP-IV use, is not known. The short-term trials [100,101,109] thus far have shown good tolerability, with the major reported side effects being pruritus, diarrhea, nausea, dizziness, and diaphoresis. Of particular importance, DPP-IV inhibitors as monotherapy do not appear to be associated with hypoglycemia though it may occur in extenuating circumstances such as heavy alcohol use [100,101,109].

Combined α- and γ-peroxisome proliferator activator receptor agonists (the glitazars)

Rationale and background

Thiazolidinediones were the first class of therapeutic agents developed that directly exploit the peroxisome proliferator activator receptor (PPAR)-γ receptors with a consequent direct effect on peripheral insulin sensitivity. It has been known that stimulation of the PPAR-α receptors, as demonstrated by the fibrates such as gemfibrozil, clofibrate, and fenofibrate, is associated with salutary modulation of lipids, especially triglycerides. Since dyslipidemia is such a common accompaniment of diabetes mellitus, there has been a desire to develop pharmaceuticals that have a significant combined α- and γ-PPAR agonist activity [111]. The combined PPAR-α and -γ agonists as a group are called the glitazars.

Description of agent

The glitazars can be broadly subclassified into thiazolidinedione variants (like DRF-2189 and KRP-297) and nonthiazolidinedione variants (like JTT-501, BMS-298585 [muraglitazar], AZ-242 [tesaglitazar], and NN-622 [ragaglitazar]).

Available data

Published data of human trials is scant. A group of glitazars, however, called the aryloxazolidinediones, has recently been identified as having efficacy in management of type 2 diabetes in db/db mice [112,113]. The efficacy of these agents as antidiabetics and in the amelioration of hypertriglyceridemia in this mouse model is suggested to be superior to that of the established thiazolidinedione rosiglitazone [108,109]. The preliminary data [114,115] on these agents also suggests a favorable side effect profile with no findings thus far of the cardiac hypertrophy noted in rats using selective PPAR-γ agonists. Other effects of these agents suggested by preliminary studies [116] include antiproliferative properties, angiotensin 2 antagonism, and antioxidant effects. Aryloxazolidinediones have beneficial vascular effects including reduction of blood pressure, correction of endothelial dysfunction, and amelioration of cardiac fibrosis associated with hypertension and myocardial infarctions [116–119]. Though promising, these findings are largely the result of in vitro and/or animal model studies and thus need confirmation in human populations before their ultimate clinical importance and relevance can be definitively ascertained. Other studies [120] in db/db and C57BL/6J mice suggest that the glitazar, KRP-297, may have better effect on glucose-stimulated pancreatic insulin secretion and less weight gain than the PPAR-γ agonist, pioglitazone, or even the combination of pioglitazone with the PPAR-α agonist, bezafibrate. Similar findings [121] have been described using tesaglitazar in ob/ob mice and obese Zucker rats. Data [122] on another glitazar, ragaglitazar in fat-fed rats showed potent improvement in insulin sensitivity, reduction in hepatic glucose output, reduced serum triglyceride levels, and reduced intramyocellular lipid accumulation to a degree superior to either rosiglitazone or the PPAR-α agonist, Wy-14643. Furthermore, and particularly noteworthy, ragaglitazar was associated with resolution of visceral adiposity and hepatic fatty infiltration without associated hepatomegaly [122]. Glitazars upregulate human macrophage lipoprotein lipase activity, which could have beneficial effects on the clinical course of atherosclerotic vascular disease [123]. *Pan*-PPAR agonists, like the amphipathic propylbenzisoxaoles, are also in development and show efficacy superior to rosiglitazone in the db/db mouse model [114].

Prospects

While the efficacy of the glitazars as adjuncts in the management of type 2 diabetes seems promising based on metabolic parameters, it is disturbing and somewhat discouraging that several agents have been abandoned because of unexpected clinically significant adverse events such as excessive peripheral edema, volume overload, heart failure, cardiomyopathy, and bone marrow hematopoietic changes. While there is no published data on carcinogenicity with the glitazars as a group, ragaglitazar and another experimental glitazar from Merck were found to be associated with soft tissue neoplasms in rodents administered these medications. As a result of these disturbing findings, the FDA has now required that prior to human trials of any medications in this class, at least 2 years of animal-based carcinogenicity data must be accumulated. Since the institution of this policy, TAK-559 and tesaglitazar have provided such data showing no carcinogenic potential and thus allowing ongoing human clinical trials. At present, a product from Takeda (TAK-559) is in phase 1 and 2 human trials and a product from Bristol-Myers-Squibb is undergoing phase 3 human trials while similar trials are planned in the near future for the Astra-Zeneca product, tesaglitazar. The most recent developments regarding TAK-559 indicate that further trials of the product are on hold following the findings of significant liver enzyme elevations in a proportion of study subjects taking the active agent. The ultimate disposition of the agent is presently unclear.

Potential niche

If and when the ideal glitazar is developed, it would fill the niche of potent insulin sensitizer with potent hypolipidemic effects and possible weight neutrality. The reports from animal studies suggest that such an agent would also have salutary effects on other aspects of the metabolic syndrome including visceral, hepatic, and myocellular fat accumulation. Such an agent would likely assume a prominent role as an adjunct or monotherapy for subjects who have early type 2 diabetes; especially in those who are obese and insulin-resistant, as long as they have a good adverse event profile. The potential of these agents for the management of the metabolic syndrome and prevention of diabetes could also make them attractive prospects that will need to be demonstrated in long-term controlled trials.

Stage of development

There are several glitazars in phase 1 and 2 trials, and BMS-298585, muraglitazar, is presently in the phase 3 trial stage which implies some of the agents of this class may become widely available for type 2 diabetes care in the future.

Insulin detemir

Rationale and background

The paradigm of using a combination of basal and bolus insulin delivery to simulate physiologic insulin dynamics in diabetic subjects has made popular the use of multiple mixed/split insulin injection regimens. Since there are several options available for short-acting bolus insulin delivery including regular human insulin, insulin lispro, aspart, and glulisine, there are relatively few options presently available for basal insulin delivery.

Insulin glargine is the only *peakless* long-acting insulin presently available. In order to provide other alternatives which attempt to address some of the limitations of glargine, such as miscibility, the drive to develop other long-acting peakless insulin analogs has been ongoing. Insulin detemir was developed to address this need.

Description of agent

Insulin detemir (NN-304) is a soluble long-acting insulin analog [124] with the structure; Lys (B29)-tetradecanoyl des (B30) human insulin. It is a fatty acid acylated insulin which binds reversibly to albumin in vivo, thus extending its pharmacodynamic profile. Clamp studies [125] have confirmed its efficacy in mediating insulin stimulated glucose uptake with a delayed onset of action and delayed tissue delivery.

Available data

Vague and colleagues [126] report on a 6-month study comparing detemir with NPH insulin in subjects who have type 1 diabetes found that despite comparable HbA1cs between the treatment groups, detemir-treated subjects had more predictable glycemic profiles, lower fasting glucose levels, and less episodes of hypoglycemia. This 6-month multinational study involved 448 patients randomized in a 2:1 fashion to either detemir or NPH insulin and demonstrated a significantly reduced within-subject variation of self-monitored fasting glucose (the standard deviation of self-measured blood glucose values in the detemir versus NPH-treated groups was 60.7 versus 68 mg/dL); 22% significantly lower risk of hypoglycemia compared with NPH and a 34% lower risk of nocturnal hypoglycemia (923 overall hypoglycemic events versus 689; 198 involved patients versus 110; and 0.64 events/subject month versus 0.96 with an overall relative risk of 0.66 [0.5–0.87 confidence interval]) [126]. The within-subject variation of blood glucose was computed over 7 days of treatment for each group and the two groups were then compared using variance component models. In addition, the coefficient of variation of nocturnal blood glucose values (between 11 PM and 7 AM) was lower in the detemir-treated group with nocturnal blood glucose values ranging between 140 mg/dL to 158 mg/dL in the detemir-treated group versus 126 mg/dL to 176 mg/dL in the NPH-treated group. Furthermore, the detemir-treated group had slighly lower body weight (70.9 ± 0.28 kg versus 71.8 ± 0.33 kg) at the end of the end of the 6-month study period [126]. These findings were previously observed by other investigators [127] in other populations. Hermansen and colleagues [127] compared detemir and NPH insulin in 59 subject who had type 1 diabetes in consecutive 6-week trial periods using either once-daily detemir or once-daily NPH in addition to meal-related bolus insulin. While the nocturnal glucose area under the curve amounts was similar in the two interventions, intrasubject fasting glucose during the last 4 days of therapy was significantly lower for detemir. In addition, hypoglycemia was significantly less common in the detemir-treated study arm (60% versus 77%) [127]. It appears that detemir has a decreased potency compared with NPH. Detemir does, however, appear to have a more predictable pharmacokinetic profile and smoothness of glycemic control [128,129]. It is important to note, however, that detemir insulin is constituted with higher molar concentrations than NPH thus enabling use of similar injection volumes, but different notation of units (U) rather than the typical international units (IU) utilized for other insulins [130]. Like native insulins, however, detemir exists predominantly as a hexamer in the presence of zinc or phenol. Only the monomeric form is biologically active and can only affect its biologic response when the 14-C fatty acyl moiety on position B29 is dissociated from plasma albumin [130]. The consequences of the relative hyperinsulinemia required to achieve equivalent glycemic control with detemir relative to NPH is still unclear [129]. Maximal concentrations following subcutaneous injection of detemir appear to be ~4 to 6 hours with a duration of action of ~12 hours. It does not, however, demonstrate the pronounced peak of activity associated with NPH, but a more plateaulike pharmacodynamic profile [131]. Detemir use is consistently associated with either weight neutral status or weight loss despite improvement in glycemic control [126,132]. The weight loss from these and other reports of detemir use have generally been in the order of 0.5 kg to 0.8 kg from baseline as compared with weight gains of ~0.5 kg to 1.5 kg in subjects similarly treated with NPH insulin [126,132]. This is distinctive and significantly different from NPH and other long acting insulin preparations. Available data including data presented at the 2004 American Diabetes Association scientific meeting also demonstrate this consistent trend of either weight neutrality or loss of ~0.7 kg as compared with NPH in type 1 and 2 diabetic cohorts [126,127,132–134]. The basis of this effect is at present unclear.

Prospects

Detemir insulin joins a sparse field of long-acting insulins with a predictable pharmacokinetic profile that makes for reliable basal insulin delivery. The problems with variable kinetics and variable peaks of activity have made NPH insulin, lente, and ultralente insulin much less popular leaving insulin glargine as the single reliable *peakless* insulin presently available. Detemir thus offers the prospect of another alternative for consistent, reliable, basal insulin delivery. The results of an ongoing head-to-head study [135] comparing add-on insulin glargine versus insulin detemir with oral agents in insulin-naïve patients with type 2 diabetes are awaited with great interest.

Like glargine, detemir as presently constituted is not approved to be mixed with short-acting analogs such as insulin aspart, lispro, or glulisine in premixed formulations. However, detemir has a neutral pH and is soluble (unlike glargine, which has an acidic pH) making the prospects for miscibility with other insulins much better. Definitive pharmacokinetic and pharmcodynamic mixing studies are yet to be completed, but their results are eagerly awaited.

Potential niche

When clinically available, detemir would likely be used as another option for basal insulin delivery in type 1 and 2 diabetes. It could be used as part of single-split insulin regimens or multisplit regimens in combination with short-acting insulins and/or analogs.

Adverse reactions, problems, and concerns

There are no reports to suggest any distinct or unique side effects or adverse reactions of detemir beyond those already well known and characterized for insulin in general. There do not appear to be any significant drug interactions affecting the interaction between detemir and plasma albumin binding [136,137].

Stage of development

Detemir has completed extensive phase 3 trials and a formal application for clinical approval has been filed with the FDA and in Canada. It has recently obtained approval for open-market use in several European countries. It is possible that detemir may gain such approval in the United States sometime in early 2005.

Inhaled insulins

Rationale and background

The development of inhaled insulins has been spurred by an attempt to provide an alternative route of insulin delivery that is more acceptable to patients than the traditional needle-based delivery systems. The highly vascular and easily accessible mucosal tissue beds of the lungs are exploited by these delivery systems.

Description of agent

Presently, there are several formulations of pulmonary insulin delivery systems in phase 2 and 3 trials. They have been demonstrated to be associated with significant improvements in patient satisfaction compared with subcutaneous insulin [138,139]. Bioavailability issues remain a concern and have necessitated the use of significantly higher molar insulin amounts by inhalation routes than by parenteral routes to achieve equivalent glycemic controlling effects. The pulmonary insulin delivery devices continue to be improved and are now of acceptable size with acceptable clinical efficacy though the delivery is still largely inefficient with ~90% of administered insulin being lost [140]. Effective insulin delivery is dependent on adequate aerosol generation, appropriate particle size (< 5 μm), and appropriate inhalation mechanics to ensure delivery of the particles to the alveolar bed [141,142].

Aerosols can be developed either by nebulization of insulin solutions or pulverization of solid insulin particles/crystals to form mists. Unlike other insulin products, the insulin molecule and the delivery system have to be studied as a unit to demonstrate clinical efficacy.

Available data

Aradigm (using the AERx inhaler; Aradigm) is a liquid. The other major pulmonary insulins; Exubera (using initially the Inhale Therapeutics inhaler that subsequently changed the name to Nektar pulmonary delivery system) and Lilly (from Alkermes) are dry powders [140]. The Mannkind product is a powder, but uses a novel particulate drug carrier called Technosphere to which the insulin is bound [140]. Technosphere is a diketopiperazine derivative, which is able to reversibly bind insulin and a host of other peptides. Technosphere self assembles in a spherical lattice array (spherules) at low pH and then dissolves as the neutral pH of the alveolus rapidly releases the bound insulin [143,144]. Of note, the Alkermes delivery system, which involves use of porous individual particles, can also be used for delivery of long-acting insulin products [145]. Other companies such as Alliance pharmaceuticals and Inhale Therapeutics (now known as Nektar therapeutics) are in the process of developing other artificial particles for pulmonary delivery of peptides such as insulin (Pulmospheres) [140]. The development of modern inhalers mainly driven by asthma care has enhanced the clinical development of pulmonary insulin delivery systems. Among the advantages of the newer inhaler systems are that they do not depend on achieving sufficient air-flow rates prior to inhalation, they are much smaller and thus more cosmetically acceptable, and they do not require spacer systems or patient actuation (patient initiation) of the aerosol before inhalation (Table 2).

Clinical trials [146–148] of all the major pulmonary insulin products consistently demonstrate a rapid onset of action, generally faster than subcutaneous regular insulin and in some cases even faster than rapid-acting insulin analogs. Inhaled insulin has been studied in comparison to regular insulin and lispro and found to have a more rapid onset of action than subcutaneous regular insulin and similar to lispro insulin with an intermediate duration of action between the two and with a biopotency of ~10 to 11 ± 4% compared with either [140,147,148]. In a 3-month study [149] of poorly controlled subjects who had type 2 diabetes Exubera improved glycemic control better than oral hypoglycemic agents alone (HbA1c was 1.2%–1.7%

Table 2
Comparison of oral-, nasal-, and pulmonary-inhaled insulin delivery systems

Product (company)	Route	Device	Energy supply	Aerosol actuation	Insulin formulation	Concerns and caveats	Phase of development
Generex	Buccal	Spray/simple metered dose inhaler	No	No	Liquid	Early in development	Early phase 1 and 2
Several different brands	Nasal	Simple nasal metered dose inhalers or nasal sprays	No	No	Liquid	Poor bioavailability with need for absorption enhancers	Presently halted trials
Astra	Pulm	Simple metered dose inhaler	No	No	Powder	Needs absorption enhancer	Presently halted trials
Mannkind (Technosphere insulin)	Pulm	Medtone inhaler	No	No	Powder with carrier molecule Technosphere	—	Phase 2 and early phase 3
Lilly (Alkermes)	Pulm		No	No	Powder	·	Phase 1
Aerogen (Becton Dickinson)	Pulm	Aerodose inhaler	Yes	Yes	Liquid	—	Phase 1
Aradigm (Novo Nordisk)	Pulm	AERx inhaler	Yes	Yes	Liquid	—	Phase 2
Inhale (Pfizer/Aventis)	Pulm	Nektar inhaler (aka, Exubera inhaler)	No	No	Powder	—	Advanced phase 3

Abbreviation: Pulm, pulmonary.

less) and associated with reduced postprandial glycemia, but higher prevalence of hypoglycemia (though rarely severe) and greater weight gain (~2.8 kg). Furthermore, in this study [149], Exubera used as an adjunct with oral hypoglycemic agents was associated with HbA1c improvements of 1.7% compared with 1.2% with Exubera alone. Inhaled insulin or Exubera was also associated with increased titers of insulin antibodies mainly in type 1 diabetes, but this did not appear to have any significant clinical relevance [150]. No significant changes in forced expiratory volume at 1 minute (FEV1) or diffusing lung capacity (DLCo) were noted between the baseline and posttreatment values in this study [149]. Bioequivalence is approximately 1 mg of inhaled insulin for each 3 IU of subcutaneously injected insulin. Exubera is one of the most extensively studied pulmonary insulin products, demonstrating patient satisfaction with the product and efficacy in combination with NPH insulin [149,151–153]. Smoking has been demonstrated to be associated with exaggerated absorption of Exubera [154], similar to findings with other pulmonary insulin delivery systems [155]. In a study [154] of 38 nondiabetic smokers compared with 30 matched nonsmokers, the peak insulin and total insulin exposures following a 2-mg dose of insulin using the Exubera inhaler were found to be three to five times higher in smokers than nonsmokers. As a consequence, hypoglycemia was more prevalent among smokers using Exubera (70% compared with 10% among nonsmokers). Following smoking cessation of approximately 13 weeks, the effect of inhaled insulin had decreased to 49%–59% of the active smoking values suggesting that the smoking related changes are at least partially reversible [154]. There is follow-up data [156] on over 600 patients who have been part of an extended trial comparing Exubera as adjunctive therapy to either metformin or a sulfonylurea or combinations of oral agents. These subjects were followed over 52 weeks and indicate that Exubera therapy was equivalent in efficacy to the standard oral agent combination therapy, was acceptable to subjects and was not associated with any significant change in DLCo over the study period [156]. In a cohort of type 1 and 2 subjects (N = 204) who had been in various open-label studies using Exubera with a mean clinical follow-up of ~4 years, Exubera was found to be associated with extended clinical efficacy, reduced frequency of hypoglycemic episodes, and minimal reductions in FEV1 and DLCo (less than those observed in control diabetic subjects also followed over the same period, but without inhaled insulin use) [157].

The Aradigm insulin system using the AERx inhaler has been studied in subjects who have type 2 diabetes [158]. The AERx inhaled insulin system has been utilized in several trials, which have demonstrated that it was associated with similar pharmacokinetic profiles in elderly and younger patients [159,160]. It has also been evaluated in subjects who have asthma and found to be associated with significantly less absorption in this cohort when compared with nonasthmatics [161]. There were no significant changes in pulmonary function tests observed during these trials [156–161]. There were also no changes in pulmonary function associated with the use of

AERx inhaled insulin in the setting of upper respiratory infections [162]. The AERx inhaled insulin system was studied in comparison with regular subcutaneous insulin in a cohort of 107 subjects who had type 2 diabetes as part of an intensive insulin regimen [163]. There were two groups, 54 subjects in the AERx group and 53 subjects in the subcutaneous insulin–treated group. Both groups were comparable at baseline with mean age of 59 years, mean BMI of 27.7 kg/m^2, and comparable starting HbA1cs of 8.6% (AERx) and 8.5% (subcutaneous insulin) [163]. After 12 weeks of therapy, both groups were associated with HbA1c improvements from 8.6% at study initiation to 7.8% at study end. Fasting blood glucose values, however, were significantly lower in the AERx treated group. While adverse events were similar in both groups, the AERx system was associated with numerically less hypoglycemic episodes (151 versus 211) though this was not statistically different [163]. There were no chest radiograph or pulmonary function test differences observed. The biopotency for this product is ~16% compared with regular subcutaneous insulin.

Reports on Technosphere insulin (using the Medtone inhaler) suggest pharmacokinetics similar to intravenous insulin and thus a much more rapid onset of action than other pulmonary insulin products [140,147,164]. Of note, 100 IU of the Technosphere insulin had a more rapid onset of action than 10 units of regular subcutaneous insulin and similar time to onset of action (~14 minutes) as 5 units of intravenous insulin given to healthy volunteers [140,147,164]. Estimates of its biopotency and bioavailability relative to subcutaneous regular insulin are ~26% [143,144]. It has also been demonstrated to provide early-meal-related insulin akin to the first phase diet-related insulin delivery [160]. Cheatham and colleagues [165] investigated the effects of technosphere insulin on the intact proinsulin release in 24 subjects who had type 2 diabetes. The study subjects each received four different doses of the inhaled insulin product (0, 12, 24, or 48 IU) administered ~5 minutes after commencing a standardized meal on separate study days [165]. Glucose, insulin, and intact proinsulin were then measured at the 0-, 60-, and 120-minute time points following the meal. An expected progressive reduction in postprandial blood glucose was demonstrated with the higher doses of Technosphere insulin, however, of even greater interest was the finding that the higher Technosphere insulin doses (24 and 48 IU) were associated with suppression of intact proinsulin secretion at all measured time points suggesting a potentially protective effect of the agent on postprandial β-cell demands in patients who have type 2 diabetes [165]. The long-term implications of these findings on β-cell health and function in type 2 diabetes are at present unclear, but deserving of further investigation. The dosage format of Technosphere insulin is in increments of 6 IU (equivalent to ~2 IU of subcutaneous insulin).

The Aerodose inhaler from Aerogen is another inhaled insulin delivery system that uses a liquid aerosol insulin [166,167]. The biopotency of this product is ~10% of that of subcutaneous insuline [166,167]. Trials with the

Aerogen inhaler using standard U 500 regular insulin demonstrated faster clinical effects than subcutaneous regular insulin with a shorter time to peak insulin concentration and a shorter time to peak metabolic effect [140,147,166,167]. This product is still in phase 1 evaluation and refinement.

Potential niche

If the issues with bioavailability can be definitively resolved, pulmonary insulin products would have a role in the management of postprandial hyperglycemia and might serve as an alternative to presently available short-acting insulins. It is conceivable that pulmonary insulins may in addition have a place as adjuncts to oral hypoglycemic agents as an alternative means of delaying need for injection-based insulin management regimens in subjects who have type 2 diabetes. The utility of pulmonary insulins as reliable methods of prandial insulin delivery would also suggest a potential niche for providing meal-related bolus insulin (to be combined with long-acting insulins such as glargine and detemir) in subjects who have type 1 and insulinopenic type 2 diabetes.

Adverse reactions, problems, and concerns

For pulmonary insulin, the main concern is long-term safety in terms of potential effects on pulmonary function and potential mitogenic activity or effects on the pulmonary epithelium (especially when administered in high doses over extended durations) [140,147,168]. Other specific concerns include effects of upper respiratory tract infections and airway diseases such as chronic bronchitis and asthma on the delivery of these products. The effects of smoking are also a cause for concern as smoking does increase the permeability of the pulmonary epithelium [169]. Other lingering concerns relate to suggestions that advanced diabetes itself is associated with changes in pulmonary mechanics and function [140,147,168]. Other concerns such as the association of pulmonary insulin with lung irritation and inflammation, allergic reactions, development of insulin antibodies, alterations in pulmonary function including airway function (potential for reversible airway obstruction); and/or diffusion defects (reflected by reductions in measured diffusion lung capacity; DLCo) will require long-term surveillance studies to address them properly and obtain definitive answers [140,147,168].

Oral insulins

Rationale and background

While oral administration of insulin during meals is an attractive idea for controlling meal-related hyperglycemia, the major obstacle remains finding an effective means of insulin delivery that escapes the effects of gut digestive enzymes and maintains therapeutic efficacy. There is no selective insulin transport mechanism within the bowel wall. Thus, even if insulin can be delivered to the bowel wall, high pharmacologic doses need to be administered to enable even a small amount of systemic absorption [140]. To protect orally-administered insulin from enzymatic degradation, various strategies have been used including coating insulin with positively-charged liposomes or impermeable polymers [170–176]. The technology of so-called *nanospheres* and *nanocubicles* as alternative means of oral insulin delivery are still being developed in animal models [177,178]. The variable intestinal transit time and the variable delay in absorption of encapsulated insulin are additional hurdles that any effective oral insulin delivery system will need to overcome [140]. Orally-administered insulin offers the physiologic advantage of insulin delivery in a fashion akin to normal pancreatic insulin, wherein insulin appears first in the portal system (critical for suppression of hepatic glucose output) and then goes out to the systemic bloodstream resulting in lower net insulin levels for maintenance of euglycemia [179–183].

Description of agent

The oral insulin product most extensively studied in human subjects is HIM2, hexyl insulin monoconjugate 2 (also known as insulin Nobex) from the Nobex Corporation. It is an insulin oligomer conjugate formed by covalent bonding of an ampiphilic polymer to the lysine moiety on position 29 of the insulin beta chain [184,185]. It is absorbed from the intestines on oral ingestion because its ampiphilic side chain confers on it resistance to enzymatic degradation and enhances absorption from the bowel wall. It is generally constituted as a semisolid preparation encased in hard gelatinous capsules. In addition, Emisphere Technologies has an oral insulin product for which preliminary data were presented in late breaking abstract form at the 2004 American Diabetes Association meeting [186]. In a 2-week study, 13 well-controlled subjects who have type 2 diabetes (mean age of 59 years with mean BMI of 29 kg/m^2 and mean HbA1c of 6.6%) received either the oral insulin product (300 IU/4×d) or placebo. Overall the product was well tolerated with no reported episodes of hypoglycemia. Though no statistical comparisons were reported, encouraging trends were found in improvements of glycemic control (22% versus 8% reduction in post–OGTT AUCs [oral glucose tolerance test, area under the curve] and 19% versus 11% reduction in poststandard-meal AUCs) [186]. Another oral insulin agent, Oralin, underwent preliminary trials in humans but has had unreliable pharmacokinetics and questionable outcomes. Little has appeared in refereed journals concerning this product thus far [187,188]. The reported data on Oralin (which is a buccal spray insulin) involved a 5-way crossover design in 5 subjects who have type 1 diabetes and involved using between 5 to 20 puffs of the product compared with placebo and 0.1U/kg of regular insulin. Glycemic efficacy was evaluated using a euglycemic clamp. No oral glucose or meal-related glucose data was presented and the only convincing finding demonstrated was an expected dose relationship between increased number of puffs and increased glucose infusion requirement during the clamp study [187,188]. The relevance of these findings to meal-related glycemic control remains unclear.

Available data

Clement and colleagues [184,185] as well as Kipnes and coworkers [189] have studied HIM 2 insulin in preliminary phase 1 and 2 trials restricted to subjects who have type 1 diabetes (30 subjects in two separate studies). In the first study, two doses of the product administered 2 hours apart were found to be associated with good glycemic control over the 2-hour evaluation period in virtually all 16 studied subjects on two separate occasions separated by 1 week. There is now data in humans who have type 2 diabetes indicating that HIM 2 has some efficacy in controlling fasting and postprandial hyperglycemia. Single oral doses of HIM2 between 0.375 mg/kg to 1 mg/kg were found to be equipotent to 8 units of subcutaneous regular insulin, but maintained adequate glycemic control with significantly lower plasma insulin levels [189].

Prospects

The clinical data thus far suggests some promise for HIM 2. However, poor palatability and unpredictable pharmacokinetic properties limit its clinical efficacy.

Potential niche

If HIM 2 and other oral insulins can be demonstrated to have reliable potency and consistent pharmacokinetics, they would likely have a prominent place in future diabetic therapy. The availability of effective oral insulins would likely enable earlier institution of insulin therapy in subjects who have type 2 diabetes and may enable better glycemic control without the hyperinsulinemia accompanying subcutaneous insulin use. It is conceivable that it could become a mainstay of type 2 diabetes management as a whole, either as monotherapy or in combination with other oral agents, but it is too early in their development to make any predictions.

Adverse reactions, problems and concerns

As expected, the major problem with the oral insulin formulations remains their poor bioavailability (1%–4%). The challenge of achieving consistent pharmacodynamic effect while ensuring bioavailability is also a difficult one, which has prevented great progress in this area of research. The oral insulins presently in clinical development only provide an option for prandial replacement. No long-acting oral preparations are presently in development. The potential effects of diarrhea, gastroenteritis, malabsorption syndrome, and other gastrointestinal problems on oral insulin bioavailability also need to clarified.

Stage of development

HIM 2 clinical trials are in early phase 1 and 2 of development for human use, however, formulation issues to improve palatability and dosing flexibility remain critical problems. It is the oral insulin product [184,185,189] that has the largest body of published data from human trials, but still several years removed from potential widespread clinical use. The other products [186–188] for which there is some human data published (Oralin and Emisphere oral insulin) are in preliminary stages of human investigation and it is at present unclear what their ultimate prospects for clinical utility in humans will be.

Other routes of insulin delivery

Although there has been some investigation into the potential of other routes of insulin delivery, none besides those detailed above appear to have clinical potential in the near future [190]. See Table 3 for further details.

Rectal delivery of insulin using suppositories and micro-enemas have been tried [191–194] and found to result in absorption of about 30% of the administered dose into the portal vein. The peak insulin levels are achieved 30 to 45 minutes postadministration, similar to subcutaneous regular insulin [191–194]. Rectal insulin has a bioavailability clearly better than oral with reasonable metabolic control achieved [195,196]. Local side effects such as a diarrhea, rectal discomfort, and the social objection to this route of administration. However, have been major impediments to its translation into clinical utility.

Iontophoresis

Direct skin delivery of large molecules is being investigated as a potential route for insulin delivery [197]. The methodology involves use of low-grade electric current applied to the skin as a means of altering the cutaneous lipophilic barriers to peptides by ionizing the peptide of interest (in this case, monomeric insulin). Early animal studies have been promising [198,199]. Particularly promising is the potential of dermal delivery systems as an alternate route of basal insulin delivery. Dermal implants of insulin placed in synthetic polymers with predictable insulin delivery kinetics are another innovation in preliminary stages of development [200–203].

Insulin delivery as conjuctival drops have been tried in animals but has not shown sufficient promise to justify investigation in humans [204].

Table 3
Insulin delivery routes

Route	Advantages	Disadvantages	Prospects for clinical utility
Intranasal	Physiologic insulin profiles with easy to use nonpainful insulin delivery system	Nasal irritation, low bioavailability and potential for profound alterations in pharmacokinetics by respiratory infections	Prospects for clinical utility in the near future for meal-related insulin delivery appear poor.
Pulmonary	Physiologic insulin profiles, simple nonpainful delivery device. Newer studies suggested improved bioavailabilty	Bioavailability for most products in this group still poor with variable pharmacokinetics. Long-term effects on local insulin on pulmonary function unclear. Some studies raise concerns regarding reduced DLCo.	Phase 3 trials ongoing. Prospects for clinical utility for meal-related insulin delivery appear good.
Oral	Agreeable route of administration, would closely simulate physiologic meal-related insulin delivery	Poor bioavailability with unpredictable pharmacokinetics	Human studies ongoing, but prospects for ultimate clinical utility remain guarded
Dermal	Promising kinetic studies in animals suggest its potential for basal insulin delivery	Local skin side effects including irritation and rashes	Still in early phase of development for utility in humans
Rectal	Good bioavailability, efficacy and acceptable onset of action time	Local rectal side effects and socially disagreeable route of administration	Prospects for wide clinical use poor

Islet neogenesis gene-associated protein

Rationale and background

Recent in vitro studies from animal and human β-cells have demonstrated that β-cells are capable of growth, multiplication, replication, and regeneration [205–211]. During fetal development, pancreatic islets develop predominantly from differentiation from progenitor cells derived from the ductal epithelium [212,213]. Subsequent β-cell growth appears to be the result of differentiation of existing β-cells (~12% of the islets regenerative capacity) and differentiation of progenitor stem cells (~88% of the islets regenerative capacity). A better modulation of these abilities of the β-cell in contrast to the apoptosis typical of type 1 diabetes has recently assumed considerable interest as a strategy for diabetes management and a potential means to achieving a cure for diabetes. β-Cell regeneration and development have been demonstrated in β-cells, ductal epithelial cells of the exocrine pancreas, and adult stem cells [212,213]. Pancreatic islet neogenesis was initially serendipitously observed [214–216] and then subsequently demonstrated to be due to a local paracrine/autocrine factor (not a typical systemic hormone) [204]. This factor was subsequently isolated from regenerating pancreata and shown to stimulate pancreatic neogenesis and reverse streptozotocin-induced diabetes in animal models [204,205,217–219].

INGAP is a 175-amino acid peptide isolated from pancreatic tissue, demonstrated in animal studies to stimulate β-cell growth, multiplication, and regeneration [211,218]. It appears to be the product responsible for the bioactivity of the previously described pancreatic extract [211,218]. It has been demonstrated to reverse streptozotocin-induced diabetes in hamsters similar to the earlier unrefined pancreatic extracts [220,221]. These findings have spurred recent phase 1 and 2 clinical trials in human subjects to investigate its efficacy and safety in type 1 and 2 diabetes cohorts.

Description of agent

INGAP is the endogenous peptide derived from the pancreas with the potential capacity to induce islet neogenesis. Its core biologic activity appears to reside in a 15-amino acid stretch, which has been commercially synthesized. This synthetic peptide is the INGAP peptide [218]. The efficacy of this agent in inducing islet neogenesis (predominantly from pancreatic ductal epithelial derived stem cells) has been documented in several animal models [220,222].

Available data

There is little published data on the use of INGAP or the INGAP peptide in humans as the phase 1 and 2 trials have only recently begun. Animal data, however, is compelling. The INGAP peptide has been demonstrated to stimulate β-cell regeneration in hamsters within 10 days of dosing 5 mg/kg intraperitoneally [207,223–225]. The degree of β-cell growth induced was also found to correlate directly with the dose of peptide administered and duration of use [207,223,224]. Of note, there was no induction of benign or malignant islet neoplastic growth by the administration of the peptide. These findings have been replicated in streptozotocin induced diabetic mice and the neoislets developed have been demonstrated to also include glucagons-producing cells [220,225]. It appears that INGAP plays a critical role in normal fetal development of the pancreatic islets [226,227], thus suggesting a mechanism for its effects in models of apoptotic β-cells and/or islets [119,228,229].

Potential niche

Though still in the early phases of development, INGAP has the potential of adding a new paradigm to diabetes management. If found to have the efficacy suggested by animal studies, INGAP could become a standard addition to all other therapies in type 1 and 2 diabetes with the goal of halting and/or reversing the islet cell damage characteristic of diabetes. There is also the potential of the agent having a place in diabetes prevention strategies among high-risk populations. The potential for *cure* of diabetes, especially in type 1 subjects who have no significant insulin resistance, is another possibility if human studies replicate the exciting findings in animal models.

Adverse reactions, problems, and concerns

The major adverse events and concerns thus far regarding INGAP are related to the need for needle-based administration with the potential for local site reactions similar to those known with insulin (including local pain, lipoatrophy, lipohypertrophy, pruritus, etc). The INGAP peptide as presently constituted is viscid; administration requires using larger bore needles than used for insulin and is significantly more painful, thus potentially leading to poor patient compliance. Other lingering concerns include the possible association of the peptide administration in chronic settings with an anamnestic immune response. Adequate dose response studies are not yet available.

Stage of development

INGAP is presently in the early stages of phase 1 and 2 human trials and no data are yet available to predict that the experimental evidence will be reproduced in humans with diabetes.

Summary

After many decades of relative therapeutic stagnation since the initial discovery of insulin, followed by some modifications on its structure and only having sulfonylureas and biguanides for many years, the last decade has seen a surge in new therapeutic options for the management of diabetes. The results of the United Kingdom Prospective Diabetes Study and Kumamoto study indicate the need for aggressive glycemic control and the slow inexorable clinical deterioration associated with type 2 diabetes over time. The propensity for weight gain and hypoglycemia are the two major limitations that subcutaneous insulin and sulfonylureas have been particularly prone to. The newer antidiabetic medications and those on the horizon attempt to address these limitations. GLP-1 agonists and the DPP-IV inhibitors exploit the innate incretin system to improve glycemia while promoting satiety and weight management. Like GLP-1–related compounds, pramlintide offers the potential to address postprandial hyperglucagonemia associated with type 2 diabetes only limited by the multiple injections and gastrointestinal side effects. The glitazars offer the hope of a new approach to diabetes care addressing not just glycemia, but dyslipidemia and other components of the metabolic syndrome, though the side effect profile remains a major unknown. The INGAP peptide represents the *holy grail* of diabetes care as it offers the potential of a new paradigm: that of islet regeneration and potential for a *cure*. But at this stage, with no human data available, it remains highly speculative.

Beyond these and other novel agents being developed to meet the challenge of the worldwide epidemic of diabetes, the central place of insulin in diabetes care cannot be forgotten. In view of this the continued efforts of improvement in insulin delivery, kinetics and action have spurred such innovations as the various inhaled insulins and new insulin analogues.

There is cause for guarded optimism and excitement about the years ahead. There is reason to expect that despite the growing burden of diabetes worldwide, we will be better equipped to manage it and its comorbidities and prevent its onset and possibly even cure it.

References

[1] Evans AJ, Krentz AJ. Recent developments and emerging therapies for type 2 diabetes mellitus. Drugs R D 1999;2(2):75–94.
[2] Baron AD, Kim D, Weyer C. Novel peptides under development for the treatment of type 1 and type 2 diabetes mellitus. Curr Drug Targets Immune Endocr Metabol Disord 2002; 2(1):63–82.
[3] Kinalski M, Sledziewski A, Telejko B, et al. Postpartum evaluation of amylin levels in gestational diabetes mellitus. American Diabetes Association, 62nd Scientific Sessions, June 2002. San Francisco, California.
[4] Young A, Denaro M. Roles of amylin in diabetes and in regulation of nutrient load. Nutrition 1998;14(6):524–7.
[5] Rachman J, Payne MJ, Levy JC, et al. Changes in amylin and amylin-like peptide concentrations and beta-cell function in response to sulfonylurea or insulin therapy in NIDDM. Diabetes Care 1998;21(5):810–6.
[6] Young AA. Amylin as a neuroendocrine hormone. Scientific World Journal 2001;1(12 Suppl 1):24.
[7] Wang F, Adrian TE, Westermark GT, et al. Islet amyloid polypeptide tonally inhibits beta-, alpha-, and delta-cell secretion in isolated rat pancreatic islets. Am J Physiol 1999;276(1 Pt 1):E19–24.
[8] Gedulin BR, Rink TJ, Young AA. Dose-response for glucagonostatic effect of amylin in rats. Metabolism 1997;46(1):67–70.
[9] Silvestre RA, Rodriguez-Gallardo J, Jodka C, et al. Selective amylin inhibition of the glucagon response to arginine is extrinsic to the pancreas. Am J Physiol Endocrinol Metab 2001;280(3):E443–9.
[10] Kong MF, King P, Macdonald IA, et al. Infusion of pramlintide, a human amylin analogue, delays gastric emptying in men with IDDM. Diabetologia 1997;40(1):82–8.
[11] Kong MF, Stubbs TA, King P, et al. The effect of single doses of pramlintide on gastric emptying of two meals in men with IDDM. Diabetologia 1998;41(5):577–83.
[12] Rushing PA, Hagan MM, Seeley RJ, et al. Amylin: a novel action in the brain to reduce body weight. Endocrinology 2000;141(2):850–3.

[13] Bouali SM, Wimalawansa SJ, Jolicoeur FB. In vivo central actions of rat amylin. Regul Pept 1995;56(2–3):167–74.

[14] Thompson RG, Pearson L, Schoenfeld SL, et al. Pramlintide, a synthetic analog of human amylin, improves the metabolic profile of patients with type 2 diabetes using insulin. The Pramlintide in Type 2 Diabetes Group. Diabetes Care 1998;21(6):987–93.

[15] Kleppinger EL, Vivian EM. Pramlintide for the treatment of diabetes mellitus. Ann Pharmacother 2003;37(7–8):1082–9.

[16] Vella A, Lee JS, Camilleri M, et al. Effects of pramlintide, an amylin analogue, on gastric emptying in type 1 and 2 diabetes mellitus. Neurogastroenterol Motil 2002;14(2):123–31.

[17] Weyer C, Maggs DG, Young AA, et al. Amylin replacement with pramlintide as an adjunct to insulin therapy in type 1 and type 2 diabetes mellitus: a physiological approach toward improved metabolic control. Curr Pharm Des 2001;7(14):1353–73.

[18] Weyer C, Gottlieb A, Kim DD, et al. Pramlintide reduces postprandial glucose excursions when added to regular insulin or insulin lispro in subjects with type 1 diabetes: a dose-timing study. Diabetes Care 2003;26(11):3074–9.

[19] Nyholm B, Brock B, Orskov L, et al. Amylin receptor agonists: a novel pharmacological approach in the management of insulin-treated diabetes mellitus. Expert Opin Investig Drugs 2001;10(9):1641–52.

[20] Nyholm B, Moller N, Gravholt CH, et al. Acute effects of the human amylin analog AC137 on basal and insulin-stimulated euglycemic and hypoglycemic fuel metabolism in patients with insulin-dependent diabetes mellitus. J Clin Endocrinol Metab 1996;81(3):1083–9.

[21] Nyholm B, Orskov L, Hove KY, et al. The amylin analog pramlintide improves glycemic control and reduces postprandial glucagon concentrations in patients with type 1 diabetes mellitus. Metabolism 1999;48(7):935–41.

[22] Fineman M, Weyer C, Maggs DG, et al. The human amylin analog, pramlintide, reduces postprandial hyperglucagonemia in patients with type 2 diabetes mellitus. Horm Metab Res 2002;34(9):504–8.

[23] Vella A, Lee JS, Camilleri M, et al. Effects of pramlintide, an amylin analogue, on gastric emptying in type 1 and type 2 diabetes mellitus. Neurogastroenterol Motil 2002;14(2): 123–31.

[24] Pehling G, Tessari P, Gerich JE, , et alService FJ, Rizza RA. Abnormal meal carbohydrate disposition in insulin-dependent diabetes. Relative contributions of endogenous glucose production and initial splanchnic uptake and effect of intensive insulin therapy. J Clin Invest 1984;74(3):985–91.

[25] Dinneen S, Alzaid A, Turk D, et al. Failure of glucagon suppression contributes to postprandial hyperglycaemia in IDDM. Diabetologia 1995;38(3):337–43.

[26] Gedulin BR, Smith P, Gedulin G, et al. Amylin potently inhibits Ghrelin secretion in rats. American Diabetes Association, 64th Scientific Sessions, 2004. Orlando, Florida.

[27] Hollander P, Ratner R, Fineman M, et al. Addition of pramlintide to insulin therapy lowers HbA1c in conjunction with weight loss in patients with type 2 diabetes approaching glycaemic targets. Diabetes Obes Metab 2003;5(6):408–14.

[28] Hollander PA, Levy P, Fineman MS, et al. Pramlintide as an adjunct to insulin therapy improves long-term glycemic and weight control in patients with type 2 diabetes: a 1-year randomized controlled trial. Diabetes Care 2003;26(3):784–90.

[29] Maggs D, Shen L, Strobel S, et al. Effect of pramlintide on A1C and body weight in insulin-treated African Americans and Hispanics with type 2 diabetes: A pooled post hoc analysis. Metabolism 2003;52(12):1638–42.

[30] Ratner RE, Want LL, Fineman MS, et al. Adjunctive therapy with the amylin analogue pramlintide leads to a combined improvement in glycemic and weight control in insulin-treated subjects with type 2 diabetes. Diabetes Technol Ther 2002;4(1):51–61.

[31] Whitehouse F, Kruger DF, Fineman M, et al. A randomized study and open-label extension evaluating the long-term efficacy of pramlintide as an adjunct to insulin therapy in type 1 diabetes. Diabetes Care 2002;25(4):724–30.

[32] Levetan C, Want LL, Weyer C, et al. Impact of pramlintide on glucose fluctuations and postprandial glucose, glucagon, and triglyceride excursions among patients with type 1 diabetes intensively treated with insulin pumps. Diabetes Care 2003;26(1):1–8.

[33] Heptulla RA, Rodriguez LM, Haymond MW. Post-prandial (PP) glucose homeostasis inpediatric T1 D: Role of Pramlintide as adjunctive therapy. American Diabetes Association, 64th Scientific Sessions, 2004. Orlando, Florida.

[34] Weyer C, Wang Y, Schnabel C, et al. Pramlintide pharmacokinetics in type 1 and type 2 diabetes; effects of injection site, needle length and body size. American Diabetes Association, 64th Scientific Sessions, 2004. Orlando, Florida.

[35] Want LL, Ratner R, Uwaifo GI. Safety and tolerability of long term pramlintide therapy. American Diabetes Association, 64th Scientific Sessions, 2004. Orlando, Florida.

[36] Chapman I, Parker B, Doran S, et al. Effect of pramlintide on Ad-libitum food intake in obese subjects and subjects with type 2 diabetes: A randomized, double blind, placebo controlled, cross-over study. American Diabetes Association, 64th Scientific Sessions, 2004. Orlando, Florida.

[37] Marrero D, Kruger D, Burrell T, et al. Patients with type 1-diabetes: perceptions associated with pramlintide as an adjunctive treatment to insulin. American Diabetes Association, 64th Scientific Sessions, 2004. Orlando, Florida.

[38] Levetan C, Want LL, Weyer C, et al. Reduced glucose fluctuations following 4 weeks of pramlintide treatment in patients with type 1 diabetes intensively treated with insulin pumps. American Diabetes Association, 2002. San Francisco, California.

[39] Want LL, Levetan C, Weyer C, et al. Reduced postprandial glucose, glucagon and triglyceride excursions following 4 weeks of pramlintide treatment in patients with type 1 diabetes treated intensively with insulin pumps. American Diabetes Association, 62nd Scientific Sessions, 2002. San Francisco, California.

[40] Nauck MA, Meier JJ, Creutzfeldt W. Incretins and their analogues as new antidiabetic drugs. Drug News Perspect 2003;16(7):413–22.

[41] Holst JJ, Deacon CF. Inhibition of the activity of dipeptidyl-peptidase IV as a treatment for type 2 diabetes. Diabetes 1998;47(11):1663–70.

[42] Holz GG, Chepurny OG. Glucagon-like peptide-1 synthetic analogs: new therapeutic agents for use in the treatment of diabetes mellitus. Curr Med Chem 2003;10(22):2471–83.

[43] Gefel D, Barg Y, Zimlichman R. Glucagon-like peptide-1 structure, function and potential use for NIDDM. Isr J Med Sci 1997;33(10):690–5.

[44] Doyle ME, Egan JM. Glucagon-like peptide-1. Recent Prog Horm Res 2001;56:377–99.

[45] Thorens B, Waeber G. Glucagon-like peptide-I and the control of insulin secretion in the normal state and in NIDDM. Diabetes 1993;42(9):1219–25.

[46] Thorens B. Glucagon-like peptide-1 and control of insulin secretion. Diabete Metab 1995; 21(5):311–8.

[47] Vilsboll T, Krarup T, Deacon CF, et al. Reduced postprandial concentrations of intact biologically active glucagon-like peptide 1 in type 2 diabetic patients. Diabetes 2001;50(3): 609–13.

[48] Toft-Nielsen MB, Damholt MB, Madsbad S, et al. Determinants of the impaired secretion of glucagon-like peptide-1 in type 2 diabetic patients. J Clin Endocrinol Metab 2001;86(8): 3717–23.

[49] Vilsboll T, Krarup T, Holst JJ. Similar elimination rates of GLP-1 in obese type 2 diabetes patients and matched healthy subjects. American Diabetes Association, 62nd Scientific Sessions, 2002. San Francisco, California.

[50] Perfetti R, Zhou J, Doyle ME, et al. Glucagon-like peptide-1 induces cell proliferation and pancreatic-duodenum homeobox-1 expression and increases endocrine cell mass in the pancreas of old, glucose-intolerant rats. Endocrinology 2000;141(12):4600–5.

[51] Perfetti R, Merkel P. Glucagon-like peptide-1: a major regulator of pancreatic beta-cell function. Eur J Endocrinol 2000;143(6):717–25.

[52] De Leon DD, Deng S, Madani R, et al. Role of endogenous glucagon-like peptide-1 in islet regeneration after partial pancreatectomy. Diabetes 2003;52(2):365–71.

[53] Bregenholt S, Moldrup A, Knudsen LB, et al. The GLP-1 derivative NN2211 inhibits cytokine-induced apoptosis in primary rat bet a cells. Diabetes 2001;50(Suppl 2):A31.

[54] Bregenholt S, Moldrup A, Blume N, et al. The GLP-1 analogue, NN2211, inhibits free fatty acid induced apoptosis in primary rat beta cells. Diabetologia 2001;44(Suppl 1): A19.

[55] Li Y, Hansotia T, Yusta B, et al. Glucagon-like peptide-1 receptor signaling modulates beta cell apoptosis. J Biol Chem 2003;278(1):471–8.

[56] Tourrel C, Bailbe D, Meile MJ, et al. Glucagon-like peptide-1 and exendin-4 stimulate beta-cell neogenesis in streptozotocin-treated newborn rats resulting in persistently improved glucose homeostasis at adult age. Diabetes 2001;50(7):1562–70.

[57] Benthem L, Wei L, Langer KZ, et al. The long acting GLP-1 derivative NN2211 improves glucose tolerance and normalizes body weight in diet induced obese rats. American Diabetes Association, 62nd Scientific Sessions, 2002. San Francisco, California.

[58] Schjoldager BT, Mortensen PE, Christiansen J, et al. GLP-1 (glucagon-like peptide 1) and truncated GLP-1 fragments of human proglucagon, inhibit gatsric acid screetion in humans. Dig Dis Sci 1989;34:703.

[59] Orskov C, Ragenhoj L, Wettergren A, et al. Tissue and plasma concentrations of amidated and glycine-extended glucagon-like peptide 1 in humans. Diabetes 1994;43:535.

[60] Willms B, Werner J, Holst JJ, et al. Gastric emptying, glucose responses, and insulin secretion after a liquid test meal: effects of exogenous glucagon-like peptide-1 (GLP-1)-(7-36) amide in type 2 (noninsulin-dependent) diabetic patients. J Clin Endocrinol Metab 1996;81(1):327–32.

[61] Nauck MA, Kleine N, Orskov C, et al. Normalization of fasting hyperglycaemia by exogenous glucagon-like peptide 1 (7-36 amide) in type 2 (non-insulin-dependent) diabetic patients. Diabetologia 1993;36(8):741–4.

[62] Schirra J, Kuwert P, Wank U, et al. Differential effects of subcutaneous GLP-1 on gastric emptying, antroduodenal motility, and pancreatic function in men. Proc Assoc Am Physicians 1997;109(1):84–97.

[63] Qualmann C, Nauck MA, Holst JJ, et al. Insulinotropic actions of intravenous glucagon-like peptide-1 (GLP-1) [7-36 amide] in the fasting state in healthy subjects. Acta Diabetol 1995;32(1):13–6.

[64] Qualmann C, Nauck MA, Holst JJ, et al. Glucagon-like peptide 1 (7-36 amide) secretion in response to luminal sucrose from the upper and lower gut. A study using alpha-glucosidase inhibition (acarbose). Scand J Gastroenterol 1995;30(9):892–6.

[65] Nauck MA, Holst JJ, Willms B, et al. Glucagon-like peptide 1 (GLP-1) as a new therapeutic approach for type 2-diabetes. Exp Clin Endocrinol Diabetes 1997;105(4):187–95.

[66] Nauck MA, Holst JJ, Willms B. Glucagon-like peptide 1 and its potential in the treatment of non-insulin-dependent diabetes mellitus. Horm Metab Res 1997;29(9):411–6.

[67] Juhl CB, Hollingdal M, Sturis J, et al. Bedtime administration of NN2211, a long-acting GLP-1 derivative, substantially reduces fasting and postprandial glycemia in type 2 diabetes. Diabetes 2002;51(2):424–9.

[68] Elbrond B, Jakobsen G, Larsen S, et al. Pharmacokinetics, pharmacodynamics, safety, and tolerability of a single-dose of NN2211, a long-acting glucagon-like peptide 1 derivative, in healthy male subjects. Diabetes Care 2002;25(8):1398–404.

[69] Agerso H, Jensen LB, Elbrond B, et al. The pharmacokinetics, pharmacodynamics, safety and tolerability of NN2211, a new long-acting GLP-1 derivative, in healthy men. Diabetologia 2002;45(2):195–202.

[70] Matthews D, Madsbad S, Schmitz O, et al. The long acting GLP-1 derivative, NN2211, a new agent for the treatment of type 2 diabetes. American Diabetes Association, 62nd Scientific Sessions, 2002. San Francisco, California.

[71] Nauck MA, Hompesch M, Filipczak R, et al. Liraglutide significantly improves glycemic control and reduces body weight compared with glimeperide as add-on to metformin in type 2 diabetes [abstract]. Diabetes 2004;53(2):A83.

[72] Thorens B, Porret A, Buhler L, et al. Cloning and functional expression of the human islet GLP-1 receptor. Demonstration that exendin-4 is an agonist and exendin-(9-39) an antagonist of the receptor. Diabetes 1993;42(11):1678–82.

[73] Kim D, Taylor K, Bicsak T, et al. Subcutaneous injection of AC 2993 (synthetic exendin-40) lowered fasting glucose concentrations through suppression of glucagon and dose dependent insulinotropism in patients with type 2 diabetes [abstract]. Diabetes 2002; 51(Suppl 2):A104.

[74] Fineman MS, Bicsak T, Shen L, et al. AC 2993 (synthetic exendin-4) added to exisiting metformin (MET) and/or sulfonylurea (SFU) treatment improved glycemic control in patients with type 2 diabetes (DM2) during 28 days of treatment [abstract]. Diabetes 2002; 51(Suppl 2):A85.

[75] Fineman MS, Bicsak TA, Shen LZ, et al. Effect on glycemic control of exenatide (synthetic exendin-4) additive to existing metformin and/or sulfonylurea treatment in patients with type 2 diabetes. Diabetes Care 2003;26(8):2370–7.

[76] Taylor K, et al. The Amigo trials; Exenatide phase 3 trials; (Abstract). Diabetes Metab 2003;29(4):S265.

[77] Taylor K, et al. The Amigo trials; Phase 3 trials of Exenatide-oral presentation. American Diabetes Association Scientific Sessions, 2004. Orlando, Florida.

[78] Kolterman OG, Buse JB, Fineman MS, et al. Synthetic exendin-4 (exenatide) significantly reduces postprandial and fasting plasma glucose in subjects with type 2 diabetes. J Clin Endocrinol Metab 2003;88(7):3082–9.

[79] Hiles R, Carpenter T, Serota D, et al. Exenatide does not cause pancreatic islet cell proliferative leions in rats and mice following 2 year exposure. American Diabetic Association, 64th Scientific Sessions, 2004. Orlando, Florida.

[80] Buse JB, Henry RR, Han J, et al; Exenatide-113 Clinical Study Group. Effects of exenatide (exendin-4) on glycemic control over 30 weeks in sulfonylurea-treated patients with type 2 diabetes. Diabetes Care 2004;27(11):2628–35.

[81] Bridon DP, Thibaudeau K, L'Archeveque BP, et al. The long acting GLP-1 agonist CJC 1131 exhibits high potency and extended pharmacokinetics in vivo [abstract]. Diabetes 2002;51(Suppl 2):A93.

[82] Lawrence B, Wen SY, Jette L, Thibaudeau K, Castaigne JP. CJC-1131, the novel long acting GLP-1 analogue, delays gastric emptying and demonstrates safety and tolerability in preclinical testing [abstract]. Diabetes 2002;51(Suppl 2):A84.

[83] Wen SY, Chatenoud L, Lawrence B, et al. Lack of immunogenicity of CJC-1131, a long acting GLP-1 analog for the treatment of type 2 diabetes. American Diabetes Association, 64th Scientific session, 2004. Orlando, Florida.

[84] Kim J, Baggio L, Drucker DJ. The GLP-1-DAC analogue CJC-1131 upregulates insulin gene expression and exerts a memory effect on glycemic control in db/db mice. American Diabetes Association, 62nd Scientific Sessions, 2002. San Francisco, CA.

[85] Guivarc'h P, Castiagne J, Gagnon C, et al. CJC-1131, a long acting GLP-1 analog safely normalizes post-prandial glucose excursion and fasting glycemia in type 2 diabetes mellitus. Diabetes 2004;53(2):A127.

[86] Kaptiza C, Trautmann M, Heise T, et al. Daily administration of LY307161 (GLP-1 analog) normalizes blood glucose on type 2 diabetes [abstract]. Diabetes 2002;51(Suppl 2): A84.

[87] Trautmann ME, Kapitza C, Mace KF, et al. LY 307161 SR, a sustained release formulation of GLP-1 analog, is suitable for once daily administration in patients with type 2 diabetes [abstract]. Diabetes 2002;51(Suppl 2):A135.

[88] Hoffman J, Chou J, Myers S, et al. LY307161: A fully active DPP-IV resistant analogue of GLP-1 [abstract]. Diabetologia 2000;43(Suppl 1):A145.

[89] Gutniak MK, Larsson H, Heiber SJ, et al. Potential therapeutic levels of glucagon-like peptide I achieved in humans by a buccal tablet. Diabetes Care 1996;19(8):843–8.

[90] Gutniak MK, Larsson H, Sanders SW, et al. GLP-1 tablet in type 2 diabetes in fasting and postprandial conditions. Diabetes Care 1997;20(12):1874–9.

[91] Drucker DJ. Enhancing incretin action for the treatment of type 2 diabetes. Diabetes Care 2003;26(10):2929–40.

[92] Drucker DJ. Therapeutic potential of dipeptidyl peptidase IV inhibitors for the treatment of type 2 diabetes. Expert Opin Investig Drugs 2003;12(1):87–100.

[93] Ryskjaer J, Carr RD, Krarup T, et al. Increased plasma DPP-IV activity in type 2 diabetic patients in the fasting state. American Diabetes Association, 64th Scientific Sessions, 2002. Orlando, Florida.

[94] Conarello SL, Li Z, Shelton B, et al. Dipeptidyl peptidase knockout mice are protected against high fat diet-induced obesity and insulin resistance. American Diabetes Association, 62nd Scientific Sessions, 2002. San Francisco, California.

[95] Tadayyon M, Thomas L, Besenfelder U, et al. Identification of long acting DPP-IV inhibitors and their effect on diabetes prevention and insulin sensitivity in db/db mice. American Diabetes Association, 64th Scientific Sessions, 2004. Orlando, Florida.

[96] Deacon CF, Danielsen P, Klarskov L, et al. Dipeptidyl peptidase IV inhibition reduces the degradation and clearance of GIP and potentiates its insulinotropic and antihyperglycemic effects in anesthetized pigs. Diabetes 2001;50(7):1588–97.

[97] Deacon CF, Hughes TE, Holst JJ. Dipeptidyl peptidase IV inhibition potentiates the insulinotropic effect of glucagon-like peptide 1 in the anesthetized pig. Diabetes 1998;47(5): 764–9.

[98] Knudsen LB, Voss PV, Rolin B, et al. Liraglutide, along acting GLP-1 derivative, reduces body weight and food intake in obese candy fed rats while the DPP-IV inhibitor LAF237 does not. American Diabetes Association, 64th Scientific Sessions, 2004. Orlando, Florida.

[99] Rothenberg P, Kalbag J, Smith H, et al. Treatment with DPP-IV inhibitor, NVP-DPP-728, increases prandial intact GLP-1 levels and reduces glucose exposure in humans [abstract]. Diabetes 2000;49(Suppl 1):A39.

[100] Ahren B, Holst JJ, Martensson H, et al. Improved glucose tolerance and insulin secretion by inhibition of dipeptidyl peptidase IV in mice. Eur J Pharmacol 2000;404(1–2):239–45.

[101] Ahren B, Simonsson E, Larsson H, et al. Inhibition of dipeptidyl peptidase IV improves metabolic control over a 4-week study period in type 2 diabetes. Diabetes Care 2002;25(5): 869–75.

[102] Mitani H, Takimoto M, Kimura M. Dipeptidyl peptidase IV inhibitor NVP-DPP728 ameliorates early insulin response and glucose tolerance in aged rats but not in aged Fischer 344 rats lacking its enzyme activity. Jpn J Pharmacol 2002;88(4):451–8.

[103] Herman GA, Zhao P, Dietrich B, et al. The DPP-IV Inhibitor MK-0431 enhances active GLP-1 and reduces glucose following OGTT in tyoe 2 diabetics [abstract]. Diabetes 2004; 53(Suppl 2):A82.

[104] Ahren B, Landin-Olsson M, Jansson PA, et al. Inhibition of dipeptidyl peptidase-4 reduces glycemia, sustains insulin levels, and reduces glucagon levels in type 2 diabetes. J Clin Endocrinol Metab 2004;89(5):2078–84.

[105] Ahren B, Gomis R, Mills D, et al. The DPP-IV Inhibitor, LAF237, improves glycemic control in patients with type 2 diabetes (T2DM) inadequately treated with metformin [abstract]. Diabetes 2004;53(Suppl 2):A83.

[106] Ahren B, Gomis R, Standl E, et al. Twelve and 52 week efficacy of the dipeptidyl IV inhibitor LAF237 in metformin treated patients who have type 2 diabetes. Diabetes Care 2004;27(12):2874–80.

[107] Pratley R, Galbreath E. Twelve week monotherapy with the DPP-4 Inhibitor, LAF237 improves glycemic control in patients with type 2 diabetes (T2DM). Diabetes 2004; 53(Suppl 2):A83.

[108] Mentlein R. Dipeptidyl-peptidase IV (CD26)—role in the inactivation of regulatory peptides. Regul Pept 1999;85(1):9–24.

[109] Ahren B. Gut peptides and type 2 diabetes mellitus treatment. Curr Diab Rep 2003;3(5): 365–72.

[110] Augustyns K, Bal G, Thonus G, et al. The unique properties of dipeptidyl-peptidase IV (DPP IV / CD26) and the therapeutic potential of DPP IV inhibitors. Curr Med Chem 1999; 6(4):311–27.

[111] Bailey CJ. New pharmacologic agents for diabetes. Curr Diab Rep 2001;1(2):119–26.

[112] Desai RC, Han W, Metzger EJ, et al. 5-aryl thiazolidine-2,4-diones: discovery of PPAR dual alpha/gamma agonists as antidiabetic agents. Bioorg Med Chem Lett 2003;13(16): 2795–8.

[113] Desai RC, Gratale DF, Han W, et al. Aryloxazolidinediones: identification of potent orally active PPAR dual alpha/gamma agonists. Bioorg Med Chem Lett 2003;13(20):3541–4.

[114] Adams AD, Yuen W, Hu Z, et al. Amphipathic 3-phenyl-7-propylbenzisoxazoles; human pPaR gamma, delta and alpha agonists. Bioorg Med Chem Lett 2003;13(5):931–5.

[115] Adams AD, Hu Z, von Langen D, et al. O-arylmandelic acids as highly selective human PPAR alpha/gamma agonists. Bioorg Med Chem Lett 2003;13(19):3185–90.

[116] Schiffrin EL, Amiri F, Benkirane K, et al. Peroxisome proliferator-activated receptors: vascular and cardiac effects in hypertension. Hypertension 2003;42(4):664–8.

[117] Iglarz M, Touyz RM, Viel EC, et al. Peroxisome proliferator-activated receptor-alpha and receptor-gamma activators prevent cardiac fibrosis in mineralocorticoid-dependent hypertension. Hypertension 2003;42(4):737–43.

[118] Iglarz M, Touyz RM, Amiri F, et al. Effect of peroxisome proliferator-activated receptor-alpha and -gamma activators on vascular remodeling in endothelin-dependent hypertension. Arterioscler Thromb Vasc Biol 2003;23(1):45–51.

[119] Wayman NS, Hattori Y, McDonald MC, et al. Ligands of the peroxisome proliferator-activated receptors (PPAR-gamma and PPAR-alpha) reduce myocardial infarct size. FASEB J 2002;16(9):1027–40.

[120] Yajima K, Hirose H, Fujita H, et al. Combination therapy with PPARgamma and PPARalpha agonists increases glucose-stimulated insulin secretion in db/db mice. Am J Physiol Endocrinol Metab 2003;284(5):E966–71.

[121] Ljung B, Bamberg K, Dahllof B, et al. AZ 242, a novel PPARalpha/gamma agonist with beneficial effects on insulin resistance and carbohydrate and lipid metabolism in ob/ob mice and obese Zucker rats. J Lipid Res 2002;43(11):1855–63.

[122] Ye JM, Iglesias MA, Watson DG, et al. PPARalpha/gamma ragaglitazar eliminates fatty liver and enhances insulin action in fat-fed rats in the absence of hepatomegaly. Am J Physiol Endocrinol Metab 2003;284(3):E531–40.

[123] Li L, Beauchamp MC, Renier G. Peroxisome proliferator-activated receptor alpha and gamma agonists upregulate human macrophage lipoprotein lipase expression. Atherosclerosis 2002;165(1):101–10.

[124] Barlocco D. Insulin detemir. Novo Nordisk. Curr Opin Investig Drugs 2003;4(4):449–54.

[125] Dea MK, Hamilton-Wessler M, Ader M, et al. Albumin binding of acylated insulin (NN304) does not deter action to stimulate glucose uptake. Diabetes 2002;51(3):762–9.

[126] Vague P, Selam JL, Skeie S, et al. Insulin detemir is associated with more predictable glycemic control and reduced risk of hypoglycemia than NPH insulin in patients with type 1 diabetes on a basal-bolus regimen with premeal insulin aspart. Diabetes Care 2003;26(3): 590–6.

[127] Hermansen K, Madsbad S, Perrild H, et al. Comparison of the soluble basal insulin analog insulin detemir with NPH insulin: a randomized open crossover trial in type 1 diabetic subjects on basal-bolus therapy. Diabetes Care 2001;24(2):296–301.

[128] Brunner GA, Sendhofer G, Wutte A, et al. Pharmacokinetic and pharmacodynamic properties of long-acting insulin analogue NN304 in comparison to NPH insulin in humans. Exp Clin Endocrinol Diabetes 2000;108(2):100–5.

[129] Hamilton-Wessler M, Ader M, Dea M, et al. Mechanism of protracted metabolic effects of fatty acid acylated insulin, NN304, in dogs: retention of NN304 by albumin. Diabetologia 1999;42(10):1254–63.

[130] Whittingham JL, Havelund S, Jonassen I. Crystal structure of a prolonged-acting insulin with albumin-binding properties. Biochemistry 1997;36(10):2826–31.

[131] Heinemann L, Sinha K, Weyer C, et al. Time-action profile of the soluble, fatty acid acylated, long-acting insulin analogue NN304. Diabet Med 1999;16(4):332–8.

[132] Home P, Bartley P, Russell-Jones D, et al. Insulin detemir offers improved glycemic control compared with NPH insulin in people with type 1 diabetes: a randomized clinical trial. Diabetes Care 2004;27(5):1081–7.

[133] Robertson K, Schonle E, Gucev Z, et al. Benefits of Insulin Detemir over NPH insulin in children and adolescents with type 1 diabetes: Lower and more predictable fastong plasma glucose and lower risk of nocturnal hypoglycemia [abstract]. Diabetes 2004;53(Suppl 2): A144.

[134] Garber AJ, Olsen KJ, Draeger E. Treatment with insulin Detemir provides improved glycemic control and less weight gain compared to NPH insulin in people with diabetes [abstract]. Diabetes 2004;53(Suppl 2):A125.

[135] Rosenstock J, Larsen JJ, Draeger E, et al. Feasibility of improved glycemic control with insulin Detemir and Insulin Glargine in combination with oral agents in insulin naive patients with type 2 diabetes [abstract]. Diabetes 2004;53(2):A145.

[136] Kurtzhals P, Havelund S, Jonassen I, et al. Effect of fatty acids and selected drugs on the albumin binding of a long-acting, acylated insulin analogue. J Pharm Sci 1997;86(12): 1365–8.

[137] Kurtzhals P, Schaffer L, Sorensen A, et al. Correlations of receptor binding and metabolic and mitogenic potencies of insulin analogs designed for clinical use. Diabetes 2000;49(6): 999–1005.

[138] Su M, Testa MA, Turner RR, et al. The relationship between regimen burden and psychological well being in persons with type 1 diabetes: inhaled vs injectable insulin [abstract]. American Diabetes Association, 62nd Scientific session, 2002. San Francisco, California.

[139] Rosenstock J, Cappelleri JC, Bolinder B, et al. Patient satisfaction and glycemic control after 1 year with inhaled insulin (Exubera) in patients with type 1 or type 2 diabetes. Diabetes Care 2004;27(6):1318–23.

[140] Heinemann L, Pfutzner A, Heise T. Alternative routes of administration as an approach to improve insulin therapy: update on dermal, oral, nasal and pulmonary insulin delivery. Curr Pharm Des 2001;7(14):1327–51.

[141] Laube BL, Benedict GW, Dobs AS. The lung as an alternative route of delivery for insulin in controlling postprandial glucose levels in patients with diabetes. Chest 1998;114(6): 1734–9.

[142] Laube BL. Treating diabetes with aerosolized insulin. Chest 2001;120(3 Suppl):99S–106S.

[143] Rave KM, Heise T, Pfutzner A, et al. Results of a dose response study with a new pulmonary insulin formulation and inhaler. Diabetes 2000;49(Suppl 1):A7.

[144] Pfutzner A, Mann A, Steiner S. Technosphere insulin—a new approach for effective delivery of human insulin via the pulmonary route. Diabetes Technol Ther 2002;4:589–93.

[145] Edwards DA, Hanes J, Caponetti G, et al. Large porous particles for pulmonary drug delivery. Science 1997;276(5320):1868–71.

[146] Heinemann L, Klappoth W, Rave K, et al. Intra-individual variability of the metabolic effect of inhaled insulin together with an absorption enhancer. Diabetes Care 2000;23(9): 1343–7.

[147] Heinemann L. Alternative delivery routes: inhaled insulin. Diabetes Nutr Metab 2002; 15(6):417–22.

[148] Heinemann L, Traut T, Heise T. Time-action profile of inhaled insulin. Diabet Med 1997; 14(1):63–72.

[149] Rosenstock J. Mealtime rapid acting inhaled insulin (Exubera) improves glycemic control in patients with type 2 diabetes failing combination oral agents: a 3 month, randomized, comparative trial. American Diabetes Association, 62nd Scientific Sessions, 2002. San Francisco, California.

[150] Heise T, Tusek C, Stephan J, et al. Insulin antibodies with inhaled insulin (Exubera(r)); No evidence for impact on postprandial glucose control. American Diabetes Association, 64th Scientific session, 2004. Orlando, Florida.

[151] Cappelleri JC, Gerber RA, Kourides IA, et al. Development and factor analysis of a questionnaire to measure patient satisfaction with injected and inhaled insulin for type 1 diabetes. Diabetes Care 2000;23(12):1799–803.

[152] Cappelleri JC, Cefalu WT, Rosenstock J, et al. Treatment satisfaction in type 2 diabetes: a comparison between an inhaled insulin regimen and a subcutaneous insulin regimen. Clin Ther 2002;24(4):552–64.

[153] Weiss SR, Cheng SL, Kourides IA, et al. Inhaled insulin provides improved glycemic control in patients with type 2 diabetes mellitus inadequately controlled with oral agents: a randomized controlled trial. Arch Intern Med 2003;163(19):2277–82.

[154] Sha S, Becker RHA, Willavise SA, et al. The effect of smoking cessation on the absorption of inhaled insulin (Exubera(r)). American Diabetes Association, 62nd Scientific Sessions, 2002. San Francisco, California.

[155] Himmelmann A, Jendle J, Mellen A, et al. The impact of smoking on inhaled insulin. Diabetes Care 2003;26(3):677–82.

[156] Barnett AH. Efficacy and one year pulmonary safety of inhaled insulin (Exubera(r)) as adjunctive therapy with metformin or glibenclamide in type 2 diabetes patients poorly controlled on oral agent monotherapy. American Diabetes Association, 64th Scientific Sessions, 2004. Orlando, Florida.

[157] Skyler JS. Sustained long term efficacy and safety of inhaled insulin during 4 years of continuous therapy. American Diabetes Association, 64th Scientific Sessions, 2004. Orlando, Florida.

[158] Hermansen K, Ronnemaa T, Petersen AH, et al. Intensive Therapy With Inhaled Insulin via the AERx Insulin Diabetes Management System: A 12-week proof-of-concept trial in patients with type 2 diabetes. Diabetes Care 2004;27(1):162–7.

[159] Henry RR, Mudaliar S, Chu N, et al. Young and elderly type 2 diabetic patients inhaling insulin with the AERx insulin diabetes management system: a pharmacokinetic and pharmacodynamic comparison. J Clin Pharmacol 2003;43(11):1228–34.

[160] Henry R, Mudaliar S, Chu N, et al. Pharmacokinetics and pharmacodynamics of pulmonary insulin in young and elderly type 2 diabetic patients using the AERx(r) Insulin diabetes management system. American Diabetes Association, 62nd Scientific Sessions, 2002. San Francisco, California.

[161] Henry RR, Mudaliar SR, Howland WC 3rd, et al. Inhaled insulin using the AERx Insulin Diabetes Management System in healthy and asthmatic subjects. Diabetes Care 2003;26(3): 764–9.

[162] McElduff A, Clauson P, Uy C, et al. Pulmonary absorption profiles of insulin during and after an upper respiratory tract infection in healthy volunteers using the AERx(r) insulin diabetes management system. An open labelled cross-over study in healthy volunteers. American Diabetes Association, 62nd Scientific Sessions, 2002. San Francisco, California.

[163] Hermansen K, Ronnemaa T, Petersen AH, et al. Intensive treatment with pulmonary insulin using the AERx(r) Insulin diabetes management system—a proof of concept trial in type 2 diabetic patients. American Diabetes Association, 62nd Scientific Sessions, 2002. San Francisco, California.

[164] Steiner S, Pfutzner A, Wilson BR, et al. Technosphere/Insulin—proof of concept study with a new insulin formulation for pulmonary delivery. Exp Clin Endocrinol Diabetes 2002; 110(1):17–21.

[165] Cheatham WW, Anders BH, Forst T, et al. A novel pulmonary insulin formulation replicates first phase insulin release and reduces s-proinsulin. American Diabetes Association, 64th Scientific Sessions, 2004. Orlando, Florida.

[166] Kim D, Mudaliar S, Plodkowski R, et al. Dose-response relationships of inhaled and subcutaneous insulin in type 2 diabetic patients. American Diabetes Association, 62nd Scientific Sessions, 2002. San Francisico, California.

[167] Kim D, Mudaliar S, Chinnapongse S, et al. Dose-response relationships of inhaled insulin delivered via the Aerodose insulin inhaler and subcutaneously injected insulin in patients with type 2 diabetes. Diabetes Care 2003;26(10):2842–7.

[168] Heinemann L. Variability of insulin absorption and insulin action. Diabetes Technol Ther 2002;4(5):673–82.

[169] Kohler D. Aerosols for systemic treatment. Lung 1990;168(Suppl):677–84.

[170] Cho YW, Flynn M. Oral delivery of insulin. Lancet 1989;2(8678–9):1518–9.

[171] Shenfield GM, Hill JC. Infrequent response by diabetic rats to insulin-liposomes. Clin Exp Pharmacol Physiol 1982;9(4):355–61.

[172] Saffran M, Kumar GS, Savariar C, et al. A new approach to the oral administration of insulin and other peptide drugs. Science 1986;233(4768):1081–4.

[173] Weingarten C, Moufti A, Desjeux JF, et al. Oral ingestion of insulin liposomes: effects of the administration route. Life Sci 1981;28(24):2747–52.

[174] Gwinup G, Elias AN, Domurat ES. Insulin and C-peptide levels following oral administration of insulin in intestinal-enzyme protected capsules. Gen Pharmacol 1991; 22(2):243–6.

[175] Tragl KH, Pohl A, Kinast H. [Oral administration of insulin by means of liposomes in animal experiments (author's translation)]. Wien Klin Wochenschr 1979;91(13): 448–51.

[176] Lowman AM, Morishita M, Kajita M, et al. Oral delivery of insulin using pH-responsive complexation gels. J Pharm Sci 1999;88(9):933–7.

[177] Chung H, Kim J, Um JY, et al. Self-assembled "nanocubicle" as a carrier for peroral insulin delivery. Diabetologia 2002;45(3):448–51.

[178] Radwan MA. Enhancement of absorption of insulin-loaded polyisobutylcyanoacrylate nanospheres by sodium cholate after oral and subcutaneous administration in diabetic rats. Drug Dev Ind Pharm 2001;27(9):981–9.

[179] Shojaee-Moradie F, Powrie JK, Sundermann E, et al. Novel hepatoselective insulin analog: studies with a covalently linked thyroxyl-insulin complex in humans. Diabetes Care 2000; 23(8):1124–9.

[180] Hoffman A, Ziv E. Pharmacokinetic considerations of new insulin formulations and routes of administration. Clin Pharmacokinet 1997;33(4):285–301.

[181] Schade DS, Eaton RP. Insulin delivery: how, when, and where. N Engl J Med 1985;312(17): 1120–1.

[182] Eaton RP, Allen RC, Schade DS, et al. Normal insulin secretion: the goal of artificial insulin delivery systems? Diabetes Care 1980;3(2):270–3.

[183] Eaton RP, Allen RC, Schade DS, et al. Prehepatic insulin production in man: kinetic analysis using peripheral connecting peptide behavior. J Clin Endocrinol Metab 1980;51(3): 520–8.

[184] Clement S, Dandona P, Still JG, et al. Oral modified insulin (HIM2) in patients with type 1 diabetes mellitus: Results from a phase I/II clinical trial. Metabolism 2004;53(1):54–8.

[185] Clement S, Still JG, Kosutic G, et al. Oral insulin product hexyl-insulin monoconjugate 2 (HIM2) in type 1 diabetes mellitus: the glucose stabilization effects of HIM2. Diabetes Technol Ther 2002;4(4):459–66.

[186] Heise T, Kapitza C, Nosek L, et al. Oral insulin as first line therapy in type 2 diabetes: A randomized-controlled pilot study [late-breaking abstract]. American Diabetes Association, 64th Scientific Sessions, 2004. Orlando, Florida.

[187] Raz I, Cernea S, Wohlgelernter J, et al. Pharmacodynamics and pharmcokinetics of dose ranging effects of Oralin s.c. regular insulin in type 1 diabetic subjects. Diabetes 2004; 53(Suppl 2):A114.

[188] Raz I, Cernea S, Wohlgelernter J, et al. Pharmacodymanics and pharmcokinetics of dose ranging effects of Oralin versus S.C. Regular insulin in healthy volunteers [abstract]. Diabetes 2004;53(Suppl 2):A4.

[189] Kipnes M, Dandona P, Tripathy D, et al. Control of postprandial plasma glucose by an oral insulin product (HIM2) in patients with type 2 diabetes. Diabetes Care 2003;26(2):421–6.

[190] Owens DR, Zinman B, Bolli G. Alternative routes of insulin delivery. Diabet Med 2003; 20(11):886–98.

[191] Yamasaki Y, Shichiri M, Kawamori R, et al. The effectiveness of rectal administration of insulin suppository on normal and diabetic subjects. Diabetes Care 1981;4(4):454–8.

[192] Yamasaki Y, Shichiri M, Kawamori R, et al. The effect of rectal administration of insulin on the short-term treatment of alloxan-diabetic dogs. Can J Physiol Pharmacol 1981;59(1): 1–6.

[193] Raz I, Bar-On H, Kidron M, et al. Rectal administration of insulin. Isr J Med Sci 1984; 20(2):173–5.

[194] Ritschel WA, Ritschel GB. Rectal administration of insulin. Methods Find Exp Clin Pharmacol 1984;6(9):513–29.

[195] Aungst BJ, Rogers NJ, Shefter E. Comparison of nasal, rectal, buccal, sublingual and intramuscular insulin efficacy and the effects of a bile salt absorption promoter. J Pharmacol Exp Ther 1988;244(1):23–7.

[196] Nishihata T, Kamada A, Sakai K, et al. Effectiveness of insulin suppositories in diabetic patients. J Pharm Pharmacol 1989;41(11):799–801.

[197] Kennedy FP. Recent developments in insulin delivery techniques. Current status and future potential. Drugs 1991;42(2):213–27.

[198] Kari B. Control of blood glucose levels in alloxan-diabetic rabbits by iontophoresis of insulin. Diabetes 1986;35(2):217–21.

[199] Meyer BR, Katzeff HL, Eschbach JC, et al. Transdermal delivery of human insulin to albino rabbits using electrical current. Am J Med Sci 1989;297(5):321–5.

[200] Wang PY. Prolonged release of insulin by cholesterol-matrix implant. Diabetes 1987;36(9): 1068–72.

[201] Brown L, Munoz C, Siemer L, et al. Controlled release of insulin from polymer matrices. Control of diabetes in rats. Diabetes 1986;35(6):692–7.

[202] Brown L, Siemer L, Munoz C, et al. Controlled release of insulin from polymer matrices. In vitro kinetics. Diabetes 1986;35(6):684–91.

[203] Creque HM, Langer R, Folkman J. One month of sustained release of insulin from a polymer implant. Diabetes 1980;29(1):37–40.

[204] Chiou GC, Chuang CY, Chang MS. Systemic delivery of insulin through eyes to lower the glucose concentration. J Ocul Pharmacol 1989;5(1):81–91.

[205] Hellerstrom C. The life story of the pancreatic B cell. Diabetologia 1984;26(6):393–400.

[206] Rosenberg L, Vinik AI. In vitro stimulation of hamster pancreatic duct growth by an extract derived from the "wrapped" pancreas. Pancreas 1993;8(2):255–60.

[207] Vinik A, Pittenger G, Rafaeloff R, et al. Factors controlling pancreatic islet neogenesis. Tumour Biol 1993;14(3):184–200.

[208] Rosenberg L, Rafaeloff R, Clas D, et al. Induction of islet cell differentiation and new islet formation in the hamster–further support for a ductular origin. Pancreas 1996;13(1):38–46.

[209] Rosenberg L, Vinik AI, Pittenger GL, et al. Islet-cell regeneration in the diabetic hamster pancreas with restoration of normoglycaemia can be induced by a local growth factor(s). Diabetologia 1996;39(3):256–62.

[210] Rosenberg L, Kahlenberg M, Vinik AI, et al. Paracrine/autocrine regulation of pancreatic islet cell proliferation and differentiation in the hamster: studies using parabiosis. Clin Invest Med 1996;19(1):3–12.

[211] Rafaeloff R, Qin XF, Barlow SW, et al. Identification of differentially expressed genes induced in pancreatic islet neogenesis. FEBS Lett 1996;378(3):219–23.
[212] Githens S. The pancreatic duct cell: proliferative capabilities, specific characteristics, metaplasia, isolation, and culture. J Pediatr Gastroenterol Nutr 1988;7(4):486–506.
[213] Dudek RW, Lawrence IE Jr. Morphologic evidence of interactions between adult ductal epithelium of pancreas and fetal foregut mesenchyme. Diabetes 1988;37(7):891–900.
[214] Rosenberg L, Brown RA, Duguid WP. A new approach to the induction of duct epithelial hyperplasia and nesidioblastosis by cellophane wrapping of the hamster pancreas. J Surg Res 1983;35(1):63–72.
[215] Rosenberg L, Vinik AI. Induction of endocrine cell differentiation: a new approach to management of diabetes. J Lab Clin Med 1989;114(1):75–83.
[216] Rosenberg L, Duguid WP, Vinik AI. The effect of cellophane wrapping of the pancreas in the Syrian golden hamster: autoradiographic observations. Pancreas 1989;4(1):31–7.
[217] Vinik A, Rafaeloff R, Pittenger G, et al. Induction of pancreatic islet neogenesis. Horm Metab Res 1997;29(6):278–93.
[218] Rafaeloff R, Pittenger GL, Barlow SW, et al. Cloning and sequencing of the pancreatic islet neogenesis associated protein (INGAP) gene and its expression in islet neogenesis in hamsters. J Clin Invest 1997;99(9):2100–9.
[219] Pittenger GL, Rosenberg L, Vinik AI. Partial purification and characterization of ilotropin, a pancreatic islet specific growth factor. J Cell Biol 1991;115:270A.
[220] Rosenberg L, Wang R, Li J, Pittenger G, et al. INGAP peptide increases B-cell mass and insulin content in adult hamsters and reverses STZ diabetes [abstract]. Diabetes 2000; 49(Suppl 1):A256.
[221] Reifel-Miller A, Borts T, Gerlitz B, et al. Expression, purifcation and characterization of islet neogenesis associated protein (INGAP) [abstract]. Diabetes 1998;47(Suppl 1):A58.
[222] Wang R, Li J, Rosenberg L. Factors mediating the transdifferentiation of islets of Langerhans to duct epithelial-like structures. J Endocrinol 2001;171(2):309–18.
[223] Rosenberg L, Duguid WP, Brown RA, et al. Induction of nesidioblastosis will reverse diabetes in Syrian golden hamster. Diabetes 1988;37(3):334–41.
[224] Rosenberg L, Schwartz R, Dafoe DC, et al. Preparation of islets of Langerhans from the hamster pancreas. J Surg Res 1988;44(3):229–34.
[225] Rosenberg L, Wang R, Li J, et al. INGAP peptide increases B-cell mass and insulin content in adult hamster and reverses STZ diabetes [abstract]. Diabetes 2000;49(Suppl 1):A256.
[226] Camihort G, Del Zotto H, Gomez Dumm CL, et al. Quantitative ultrastructural changes induced by sucrose administration in the pancreatic B cells of normal hamsters. Biocell 2000;24(1):31–7.
[227] Del Zotto H, Massa L, Gomez Dumm CL, et al. Changes induced by sucrose administration upon the morphology and function of pancreatic islets in the normal hamster. Diabetes Metab Res Rev 1999;15(2):106–12.
[228] Flores LE, Garcia ME, Borelli MI, et al. Expression of islet neogenesis-associated protein in islets of normal hamsters. J Endocrinol 2003;177(2):243–8.
[229] Gagliardino JJ, Del Zotto H, Massa L, et al. Pancreatic duodenal homeobox-1 and islet neogenesis-associated protein: a possible combined marker of activateable pancreatic cell precursors. J Endocrinol 2003;177(2):249–59.

ELSEVIER
SAUNDERS

Endocrinol Metab Clin N Am
34 (2005) 199–219

ENDOCRINOLOGY
AND METABOLISM
CLINICS
OF NORTH AMERICA

The Prevention of Type 2 Diabetes Mellitus

Silvio E. Inzucchi, MD*, Robert S. Sherwin, MD*

*Section of Endocrinology/LCI-101, Department of Medicine,
Yale University School of Medicine, 333 Cedar Street,
New Haven, CT 06520-8020, USA*

The scope of the problem

Concurrent with the disturbing increase in the prevalence of obesity in the United States has been a marked increase in the incidence of type 2 diabetes mellitus (T2DM). When last estimated, more than 17 million Americans had diabetes; more than 90% of those had T2DM [1]. The ramifications for our health care system are profound, given the frequent metabolic and vascular complications of this disease which significantly increase mortality and health care–related costs and erode the quality and life expectancy for patients.

Although several, randomized clinical trials definitively related improved glycemic control to a decrease in complication rates [2,3], such reductions are only relative. In addition, the impact of glycemic control on the more common cardiovascular complications remains controversial; the bulk of the evidence suggests that glucose control is insufficient for substantive macrovascular risk reduction [3]. Several intermediate metabolic targets are now published and promoted by professional organizations [4], including those for glycemic, lipid, and blood pressure management. Because of a variety of factors, including systematic issues that are related to current health care delivery in this country, our ability to achieve consistent and sustained glycemic targets outside of clinical trials has been disappointing. Finally, many patients who have newly diagnosed T2DM already have established vascular complications. Diabetes, therefore, is a morbid and costly disease whose frequency is increasing at an alarming rate. Despite increasingly complex approaches that are available for its management, our

---

* Corresponding authors.
E-mail addresses: silvio.inzucchi@yale.edu (S.E. Inzucchi); robert.sherwin@yale.edu (R.S. Sherwin).

0889-8529/05/$ - see front matter © 2005 Elsevier Inc. All rights reserved.
doi:10.1016/j.ecl.2004.11.008
endo.theclinics.com

ability to meet the challenge of optimal control remains, at the least, uncertain. To compound these concerns, such epidemiologic and societal changes are not restricted to the United States. Obesity and T2DM are now global concerns; recent estimates predict that by 2030, 366 million patients will have T2DM, many of whom will live in developing countries [5].

In contrast to these generally discouraging reports, however, have been notable achievements in our understanding of the pathogenesis of this disease over the past several decades. Through a series of elegant investigations, it is now clear that T2DM is the culmination of two key pathophysiologic processes—insulin resistance and relative insulin deficiency (Fig. 1) [6]. Insulin resistance, believed to be a fundamental event by most investigators [7], is manifested initially in skeletal muscle as a reduction in insulin-mediated glucose uptake [8]; in liver by an inadequate suppression of hepatic glucose production; and in the vasculature, by abnormal endothelial function and altered production of inflammatory markers that are believed to be mediators of atherosclerosis [9,10]. In most individuals who are affected, the initial pancreatic β-cell response is to produce more insulin. The resultant hyperinsulinemia serves to maintain glucose levels within the normal range for years to decades. Relative insulin deficiency in a genetically determined subset of the population that is insulin resistant plays a major role in the progression toward diabetes when the pancreatic β cell can no longer compensate adequately for increased peripheral insulin demands [11,12]. As a result, hyperglycemia ensues with progressive insulin deficiency. It is now understood that inherited and environmental factors take part in this complex process.

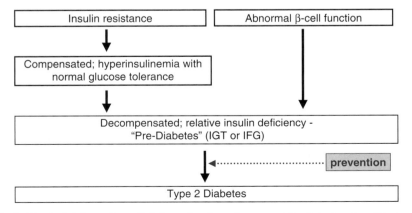

Fig. 1. The dual defects of type 2 diabetes: insulin resistance and β-cell dysfunction. The target for most diabetes prevention trials have been those patients at greatest risk for developing diabetes (ie, those who have "prediabetes"). IFG, impaired fasting glucose; IGT, impaired glucose tolerance.

As β-cell function falters, glucose levels initially increase slightly above the normal, although not into the diabetic range. A fasting plasma glucose (FPG) of between 100 mg/dL and 125 mg/dL now is defined as "impaired fasting glucose" (IFG) [13]. During a 75-g oral glucose tolerance test (OGTT), a 2-hour plasma glucose of 140 mg/dL to 199 mg/dL defines "impaired glucose tolerance" (IGT). Patients who have IFG need not have IGT and vice versa. Both, however, represent stages of "prediabetes"; the progression of patients who have these criteria to a diagnosis of T2DM ranges from 5% to 10% per year, depending on the genetic predisposition. In the third National Health and Nutrition Examination Survey, it was estimated that 15.6 million people have IGT and 13.4 million people have IFG (using the older FPG criterion of 110–125 mg/dL) (Fig. 2) [1]. In a more recent analysis that used the same database, it was estimated that 11.9 million overweight adults, aged 45 to 74 years, have prediabetes and could benefit from diabetes prevention strategies [14]. The number would be substantially higher if the estimation extended to those who are older than 75 years and younger than 45 years and the newer criteria for IFG were used.

Given our understanding of the pathogenesis of T2DM and the significant "incubation phase" between development of the earliest metabolic defects and manifestation of the full expression of the disease, the concept of diabetes prevention emerged. As a result, investigators

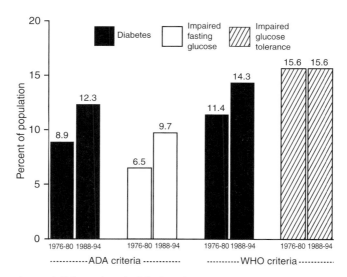

Fig. 2. Prevalence of diabetes, impaired fasting glucose, and impaired glucose tolerance in the U.S. population 40 to 74 years of age, according to National Health and Nutrition Examination Survey (NHANES) II and NHANES III. (*From* Harris MI, Flegal KM, Cowie CC, et al. Prevalence of diabetes, impaired fasting glucose and impaired glucose tolerance in U.S. adults. Diabetes Care 1998;21:523; with permission.)

proposed that lifestyle modification or pharmacologic interventions that reduce mild forms of hyperglycemia by improved insulin sensitivity or improved or preserved β-cell function might have a long-term impact upon the ultimate development of T2DM (either prevention or delay) in at-risk patients (Box 1). Logically, all of the diabetes prevention studies targeted their efforts on patients who had prediabetes (see Fig. 1).

Preventing type 2 diabetes: results of randomized trials

The first published diabetes prevention study was by Sartor and colleagues in 1980 [15]. This nonrandomized investigation suggested that T2DM could be prevented by diet, and to a greater extent, by diet and a sulfonylurea (tolbutamide.) This study's findings were limited by, among other things, its nonrandomized design; however, it deserves mention as a hypothesis-generating work.

The Malmo Feasibility Study

The first randomized study to address the issue of diabetes prevention came from Malmo, Sweden [16]. Eligibility criteria and characteristics of the actual participants are listed in Table 1. This small feasibility study demonstrated normalization of glucose tolerance in 50% of the 181 male

---

Box 1. Risk factors for type 2 diabetes mellitus

Age of at least 45 years
Overweight (body mass index $\geq$ 25 kg/m^2)^a
First-degree relative who has diabetes
Habitual physical inactivity
Member of a high-risk ethnic population (eg, African American, Latino, Native American, Asian American, Pacific Islander)
Previously identified prediabetes (IFG or IGT)
History of gestational diabetes mellitus or delivery of a baby that weighed more than 4.1 kg
Hypertension ($\geq$ 140/90 mm Hg)
High-density lipoprotein level of up to 35 mg/dL or a triglyceride level of at least 250 mg/dl
Polycystic ovarian syndrome
History of vascular disease

---

^{a} May not be correct for all ethnic groups.
Adapted from Sherwin RS, Anderson RM, Buse JB, et al for the American Diabetes Association. The prevention or delay of type 2 diabetes. Diabetes Care 2003;26(Suppl 1):S62.

Table 1
Diabetes prevention trails: eligibility criteria and baseline characteristics of study subjects

Study [Ref.]	Eligibility criteria			Actual participants (mean)		
	Age (y)	BMI	FPG (mg/dL)	Age (y)	BMI	FPG (mg/dL)
Malmo [16]	47–49	NS	NS	47–49	> 25	NG
Da Qing [17]	NS	NS	NS	44	> 25	NG
FDPS [18]	40–65	≥ 25	NS	55	31	110
DPP [19]	≥ 25	≥ 24	95–125	51	34	106
TRIPOD [20]	NS	NS	NS	35	30	94
STOP-NIDDM [21]	40–70	25–40	101–139	55	> 31	101–139

Abbreviations: NG, not given; NS, not specified or relevant to eligibility.

Adapted from Sherwin RS, Anderson RM, Buse JB, et al, for the American Diabetes Association. The prevention or delay of type 2 diabetes. Diabetes Care 2003;26(Suppl 1):S49.

subjects who had IGT after dietary treatment or increase in physical exercise over 6 years. A protective effect on the development of diabetes also was suggested, compared with a group of patients in whom no intervention occurred. Several aspects of this study's design were suboptimal, although the notion of lifestyle intervention to prevent diabetes in high-risk individuals was further supported.

The Da Qing Study

Pan and colleagues [17] in 1997 reported the results of the Da Qing IGT and Diabetes Study. In this multicenter Chinese investigation, 577 patients who had IGT from an industrial city in northern China were randomized to a control group or to one of three active treatment groups that consisted of changes in diet only, exercise only, or diet and exercise. Follow-up was conducted every 3 months for 6 years; 530 subjects were followed systematically until end points had been reached or until study completion at 6 years. During the follow-up visits, a 2-hour postprandial plasma glucose level was measured; patients who had readings of 200 mg/dL or greater were referred for a formal 2-hour OGTT. The diagnosis of diabetes was made on the basis of the OGTT result, or if repeated FPG reached or exceeded 140 mg/dL (using the 1985 World Health Organization [WHO] criteria) or if a "casual" (irrespective of meals) plasma glucose reached or exceeded 200 mg/dl. Thirty-three local health clinics participated the study, with group randomization by clinic rather than by patient. Eligibility criteria and baseline characteristics of the Da Qing subjects are shown (see Table 1).

For the intervention group, a diet of 25 to 30 calories per kg body weight, which consisted of 55% to 65% carbohydrates, 10% to 15% protein, and 25% to 30% fat was designed. Participants were encouraged to increase their daily intake of vegetables, to reduce the consumption of simple sugars, and to control alcohol intake. Those with a body mass index (BMI) of at least 25 kg/m^2 were encouraged to reduce their caloric intake to lose approximately

0.5 kg to 1 kg per month until a BMI of 23 kg/m^2 had been achieved. Patients received individual dietary counseling once weekly for 1 month then monthly for 3 months. For the exercise component of the Da Qing Study [17], participants were asked to increase their leisure activity by one "unit" per day. A "unit" was defined as 30 minutes of mild activity (eg, slow walking), 20 minutes of moderate activity (eg, faster walking), 10 minutes of strenuous activity (eg, slow running), or 5 minutes of very strenuous activity (eg, jumping rope, swimming). Those who were younger than age 50 and no cardiac history were encouraged to increase activity by two units per day. The control group was exposed to general information about diet and exercise but with neither individual recommendations nor counseling sessions.

The cumulative incidence of diabetes at 6 years was 67.7% (95% confidence interval [CI], 59.8%–75.2%) in the control group, and 43.8% (95% CI, 35.5%–52.3%) in the diet group, 41.1% (95% CI, 33.4%–49.4%) in the exercise group, and 46% (95% CI, 37.3%–54.7%) in the diet plus exercise group. In a proportional hazards analysis that was adjusted for differences in baseline BMI and fasting glucose, the diet group experienced a relative risk reduction (RRR) of 31% ($P < .03$); the exercise group experienced a RRR of 46% ($P < .0005$); and the combined group experienced a RRR of 42% ($P < .005$) in the development of diabetes (Fig. 3). The benefits of the interventions did not correlate with changes in body weight.

Although the randomization by clinic in the Da Qing Study [17] may have introduced certain bias, this investigation was the first large, randomized trial to show the impact of diet and exercise on the development of diabetes in high-risk individuals.

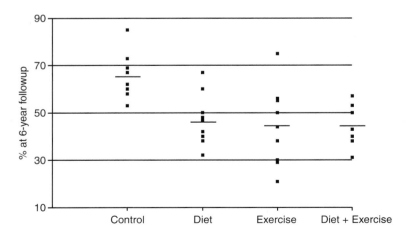

Fig. 3. The Da Qing Study. Mean rates (± SD) of diabetes for each clinic at 6-year follow-up, by intervention group: control, 66% ± 10%; diet, 47% ± 11%; exercise, 45% ± 9%; and diet plus exercise, 44% ± 17%. (*From* Pan XR, Li GW, Hu YH, et al. Effects of diet and exercise in preventing NIDDM in people with impaired glucose tolerance. The Da Qing IGT and Diabetes Study. Diabetes Care 1997;20:537; with permission.)

The Finnish Diabetes Prevention Study

Tuomilehto and colleagues [18] randomly assigned 522 middle-aged, overweight Finnish patients who had IGT to a lifestyle intervention group (n = 265) or to a control group (n = 257) (see Table 1 for eligibility criteria and baseline characteristics) in the Finnish Diabetes Prevention Study (FDPS). Subjects in the intervention group received individualized counseling that targeted five elements: weight reduction (at least 5% of body weight); daily intake of total fat (< 30% of total calories), saturated fat (< 10% of total calories), and dietary fiber (at least 15 g/1000 calories); and the amount of physical activity (at least 30 min/d of moderate exercise). Frequent intake of whole-grain products, fruits, vegetables, low-fat milk and meat products, and vegetable oils that were rich in monounsaturated fats was recommended. Dietary advice was tailored by trained nutritionists for each subject based on 3-day food diaries that were completed quarterly. Each subject in the intervention group underwent dietary counseling seven times during the first year, and then every 3 months for the duration of the study. They also received individualized recommendations on increasing physical activity, and were offered supervised, progressive resistance-training sessions. OGTTs were performed annually, with the diagnosis of diabetes made by conventional fasting or postchallenge criteria (based on the 1985 WHO criteria), and confirmed on repeat testing.

During the first year of the study, the mean body weight decreased in the intervention group by 4.2 ± 5.1 kg, with minimal change (−0.8 ± 3.7 kg) in the control group. Waist circumference, fasting, and 2-hour postchallenge plasma glucose also decreased significantly in the intervention group as compared with controls. At the end of follow-up (mean, 3.2 years), the cumulative incidence of diabetes was lower in the intervention group (11% [95% CI, 6%–15%]) than in the control group (23% [95% CI, 17%–29%]); a statistical difference was apparent by the end of 2 years. According to Cox regression analysis, the cumulative incidence of diabetes was reduced by 58% with intervention (hazard ratio [HR], 0.4; 95% CI, 0.3–0.7; P < .001); the benefit was slightly greater in men (−63%) than in women (−54%) (Fig. 4). When ranked according to their success in achieving the five pre-specified goals, a strong relationship emerged between "success score" and the incidence of diabetes; those subjects in either group who had achieved the greater number of lifestyle goals experienced the greatest protection against diabetes.

The FDPS [18], therefore, was the first optimally randomized study to confirm that lifestyle intervention is highly effective in the prevention of deterioration to diabetes in overweight, middle-aged patients who have IGT. In addition, the relationship between achieving various lifestyle goals and the impact on diabetes risk provides convincing evidence that these individual targets are important alone or in concert. Clearly, the FDPS is notable as a "proof of concept" investigation; however, implementation of

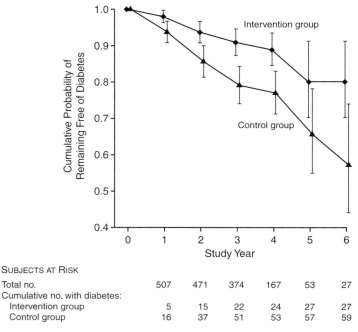

Fig. 4. Proportion of subjects who did not have diabetes during the FDPS. (*From* Tuomilehto J, Lindstrom J, Eriksson JG, et al. Finnish Diabetes Prevention Study Group. Prevention of type 2 diabetes mellitus by changes in lifestyle among subjects with impaired glucose tolerance. N Engl J Med 2001;344:1347; with permission.)

its lifestyle strategy in practice (ie, outside of the clinical trial setting) will be challenging.

The Diabetes Prevention Program

Soon after the publication of the FDPS [18] results, the results of the largest diabetes prevention trial, the Diabetes Prevention Program (DPP), became available [19]. In this 3-year U.S. study, 3234 patients who had IGT were randomly assigned to one of three groups: lifestyle modification; metformin, 850 mg, twice a day; and placebo. The study initially included a fourth arm that used troglitazone, 400 mg/d. This was discontinued in 1998 because of hepatotoxicity that resulted in liver failure and the death of one DPP participant. Eligibility criteria and baseline characteristics of patients are shown (see Table 1).

Patients in the lifestyle intervention group were asked to achieve and maintain a reduction of at least 7% in body weight through a healthy, low-calorie, low-fat diet and to engage in physical activity of moderate intensity (eg, brisk walking) for at least 150 minutes per week. To assist the study participants in achieving these goals, intensive support was required—efforts that are not available to most of our patients in practice. They were provided a flexible, culturally sensitive, and individualized 16-lesson curriculum that covered diet, exercise, and behavior modification [22]. The lessons were conducted on a one-to-one basis by case managers during the first 24 weeks. Subsequently, individual sessions occurred monthly and group sessions were used to reinforce behavioral changes. The end point of diabetes was assessed with semiannual FPG (using 1997 American Diabetes Association [ADA] fasting criteria of FPG $\geq$ 126 mg/dL) and annual OGTTs.

Subjects who were assigned to the lifestyle group experienced much greater weight loss (5.6 kg) and a greater increase in physical activity than other participants (Fig. 5). The crude prevalence of diabetes was 11.0, 7.8, and 4.8 cases per 100 person-years for the placebo, metformin, and lifestyle groups, respectively. The estimated respective cumulative prevalence of diabetes at 3 years were 28.9%, 21.7%, and 14.4%, respectively (Fig. 6). The prevalence of diabetes was reduced by 58% with lifestyle change (95% CI, 48%–66%) and by 31% in the metformin group (95% CI, 17%–43%). When the two intervention groups were compared, the incidence of diabetes was 39% lower (95% CI, 24%–51%) in the lifestyle group than in the metformin group. Translating these findings for potential clinical applications and based on these rates, the estimated number of patients who have prediabetes needed to treat to prevent one case of diabetes during this period was calculated to be approximately 7 using lifestyle changes and 14 using metformin.

On subgroup analysis, several interesting trends were noted. The treatment effects did not differ according to gender or racial or ethnic group. Lifestyle intervention was effective in all subgroups, although it was significantly more effective in those who had lower 2-hour plasma glucose levels during the baseline OGTT. The effect of metformin was reduced in those who had lower BMI and those who had lower FPG levels. The benefit of lifestyle over metformin was more apparent in older individuals and those who had lower BMI. The effect of metformin was insignificant in those who were older than 60 years of age or had a BMI of less than 30 kg/m^2, whereas its effectiveness was essentially equal to lifestyle change in those who were between 25 and 44 years of age or had a BMI of greater than 35 kg/m^2.

One important finding that was reported in a follow-up analysis is that when patients from the DPP who took metformin were reassessed with a repeat OGTT 1 to 2 weeks (average, 11 days) upon discontinuation of the drug, a sizable minority had developed diabetes. This resulted in an overall reduction of the diabetes-preventing effect of metformin from 31% to 25% [23]. This "washout" study suggests that metformin, at least in some patients, may have been "masking" the diabetes and not preventing it. Whether this is a meaningful distinction in patients who are on long-term preventive therapy is not clear.

Adverse effects were greater in the metformin group, particularly gastrointestinal symptoms; however, overall, mortality and hospitalizations were the same in all groups. The study was not powered to assess for

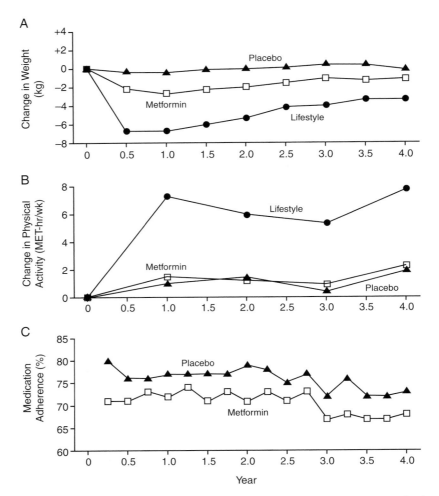

Fig. 5. Changes in body weight (*A*), leisure physical activity (*B*), and adherence to medication regimen (*C*) according to study group in the DPP. Changes in weight and leisure physical activity over time differed significantly among the treatment groups ($P < .001$ for each comparison). (*From* Knowler WC, Barrett-Connor E, Fowler SE, et al. Diabetes Prevention Program Research Group. Reduction in the incidence of type 2 diabetes with lifestyle intervention or metformin. N Engl J Med 2002;346:396; with permission.)

cardiovascular events, although mild reductions in plasma lipids and blood pressure occurred in the lifestyle change group.

The DPP Research Group has also presented, in abstract form only at the time of this writing, provocative results from the study's troglitazone arm, which was aborted because of hepatotoxicity [24]. Three hundred and eighty-seven participants initially were randomized to this thiazolidinedione. When the drug was discontinued, only 10 patients had developed diabetes

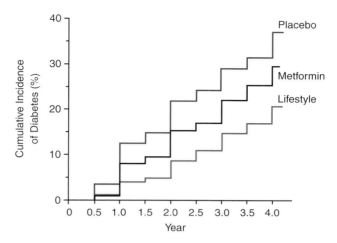

Fig. 6. Cumulative incidence of diabetes according to study group in the DPP. The incidence of diabetes differed significantly among the three groups ($P < .001$ for each comparison). (*From* Knowler WC, Barrett-Connor E, Fowler SE, et al. Diabetes Prevention Program Research Group. Reduction in the incidence of type 2 diabetes with lifestyle intervention or metformin. N Engl J Med 2002;346:397; with permission.)

during their follow-up assessment visits, after a mean of 0.9 years (range, 0.5 to 1.5 years) of therapy. The prevalence was indistinguishable from that seen with lifestyle changes, but was significantly less than that seen with metformin ($P = .02$) and placebo ($P < .001$). The investigators concluded that troglitazone reduced the prevalence of diabetes; however, the short period of use limits the interpretation of these findings.

In a later publication, the DPP Research Group estimated that the costs to the health system from lifestyle and metformin interventions were approximately $750/y per participant [25]. These costs were believed to be modest, and might be reduced with generic metformin and by improving the efficiency of lifestyle intervention staff with the use of group visits.

The ultimate determination of the value of these interventions to health systems and society requires a formal assessment of the costs relative to the actual long-term health benefits that were achieved in the DPP, which may be difficult to quantify.

The Study to Prevent Non Insulin Dependent Diabetes Trial

α-Glucosidase inhibitors, such as acarbose, exert their antihyperglycemic effect by decreasing postprandial glucose concentrations. Therefore, it is logical to assume that this may result in decreased stimulation of pancreatic islets, potentially resulting in "β-cell rest" and a decrease in the conversion to diabetes. The Study to Prevent Non Insulin Dependent Diabetes (STOP-NIDDM) Trial was designed to assess the potential for acarbose to prevent diabetes in patients who had IGT [21]. The study was conducted in several European countries, Israel, and Canada. Entry criteria and baseline characteristics are noted (see Table 1). STOP-NIDDM initially was designed before the change in diagnostic criteria by the ADA and WHO that reclassified the FPG cut-point for the diagnosis of diabetes to 126 mg/dL. In total, 714 patients were assigned randomly to therapy with acarbose, 100 mg, three times a day with meals, and 715 patients were assigned randomly to placebo. Patients were evaluated every 6 months with a measurement of FPG. OGTTs annually or sooner if the FPG increased to greater than 126 mg/dL. The mean daily dosage of acarbose during the study was 194 mg; many patients did not achieve the recommended dosage because of side effects. Twenty-five percent of subjects discontinued their participation early as a result of adverse events that predominantly were gastrointestinal in origin. The mean follow-up was 3.3 years.

Patients who were randomized to acarbose were 25% (HR = 0.75) less likely to develop diabetes than those who were randomized to placebo (Fig. 7). The effect was noted as early as 1 year. Subgroup analysis revealed that the benefit of acarbose applied to all patients, irrespective of age, gender, and BMI. Because the definition of diabetes changed during the trial, the data were reanalyzed to include a diagnosis of diabetes if the FPG reached or exceeded 126 mg/dL on two consecutive visits. Using this criterion, the HR decreased further to 0.68 (RRR = 32%). Using an end

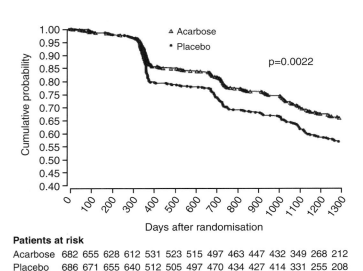

Fig. 7. Effect of acarbose and placebo on the cumulative probability of remaining free of diabetes during the STOP-NIDDM trial. (*From* Chiasson JL, Josse RG, Gomis R, et al. STOP-NIDDM Trial Research Group. Acarbose for prevention of type 2 diabetes mellitus: the STOP-NIDDM randomised trial. Lancet 2002;359:2072; with permission.)

point of diabetes that was diagnosed by any two positive OGTTs, the HR was 0.64 (RRR = 36%). The probability of reverting to normal glucose tolerance over time also was improved significantly with acarbose. Analogous to findings after metformin therapy in the DPP, during a 3-month washout at the conclusion of the study, the conversion to diabetes was greater (15%) in patients who were treated previously with acarbose than in the group that was randomized first to placebo (11%). This suggests some "masking" effect of this pharmacologic approach to diabetes prevention.

In a subsequent report, the development of major cardiovascular events (coronary heart disease, cardiovascular death, congestive heart failure, cerebrovascular event, peripheral vascular disease) and hypertension ($\geq 140/90$ mm Hg) also were assessed by the investigators [26]. Acarbose therapy was associated with an RRR of 49% (2.5% absolute risk reduction) in the development of cardiovascular events (HR, 0.51; 95% CI, 0.28–0.95; $P = .03$). The risk of myocardial infarction was reduced by an impressive 91% (HR, 0.09; 95% CI, 0.01–0.72; $P = .02$). Acarbose also was associated with a 34% RRR in the prevalence of new cases of hypertension (HR, 0.66; 95% CI, 0.49–0.89; $P = .006$). Even after adjusting for other known cardiovascular risk factors, the reduction in the risk of cardiovascular events (HR, 0.47; 95% CI, 0.24–0.90; $P = .02$) and hypertension (HR, 0.62; 95% CI, 0.45–0.86; $P = .004$) associated with acarbose treatment remained statistically significant. Although impressive, these data need to be approached with caution and require confirmation because the study was not designed and powered to assess for cardiovascular outcomes.

The Troglitazone in Prevention of Diabetes Study

Another diabetes prevention study that used a pharmacologic agent was published by Buchanan and colleagues [20] who tested the thiazolidinedione, troglitazone, in a group of predominately Hispanic woman who had a recent history of gestational diabetes. This group of collaborators previously showed that these women convert to diabetes at a rate in excess of 50% over 5 years [27]. They theorized that by improving insulin sensitivity, β-cell function would be preserved, resulting in diabetes prevention. In all, 266 women were enrolled in the Troglitazone in Prevention of Diabetes (TRIPOD) Study and randomized to placebo or troglitazone, 400 mg/d [20]. FPG was measured every 3 months and an OGTT was performed annually. In contrast to other studies, intravenous glucose tolerance tests (IVGTTs) also were performed at baseline and after 3 months of therapy to assess for changes in insulin sensitivity and β-cell response as associated with the risk for diabetes. In addition, 8 months after the conclusion of the trial, those women who did not develop diabetes during TRIPOD returned for OGTT and IVGTT while off study medication.

Baseline characteristics of TRIPOD subjects are listed (see Table 1). With a median follow-up of 30 months, the mean annual prevalence of diabetes was 12.1% and 5.4% in those who were taking placebo or troglitazone ($P < .01$), respectively. This resulted in a 55% RRR with drug therapy (Fig. 8). Protection from diabetes in those women who were randomized to troglitazone seemed to be mediated by a reduction in secretory demands that were placed on the β cell by insulin resistance because it correlated with the degree of reduction in endogenous insulin production during the IVGTT at 3 months. Thus, diabetes prevention seemed to be associated with preservation of β-cell secretion to compensate for insulin resistance. In contrast to the observations after metformin in the DPP and acarbose in STOP-NIDDM, protection persisted 8 months after the cessation of study medication. This continued apparent effect of troglitazone on the development of diabetes suggests a more fundamental effect on the natural history of deterioration to diabetes than the simple masking of hyperglycemia.

Other studies

Additional preliminary reports of apparent diabetes prevention associated with the use of pharmacologic agents have emerged, each involved posthoc secondary analyses of a separate investigation. Heymsfield and colleagues [28] pooled data from 675 obese subjects who were enrolled in three randomized, double-blind, placebo-controlled clinical trials to compare the effects of placebo with the intestinal lipase inhibitor, orlistat; both groups also followed low calorie diets. OGTTs were performed at study initiation and termination. Mean follow-up was 582 days. Subjects

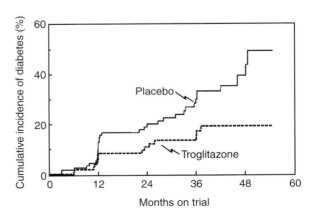

Fig. 8. Cumulative incidence rates of type 2 diabetes in women who were enrolled in TRIPOD study. The rate in the troglitazone group was significantly less than the rate in the placebo group ($P = .009$). (*From* Buchanan TA, Xiang AH, Peters RK, et al. Preservation of pancreatic beta-cell function and prevention of type 2 diabetes by pharmacological treatment of insulin resistance in high-risk Hispanic women. Diabetes 2002;51:2798; with permission.)

who received orlistat lost 6.7 kg compared with 3.8 kg in those who took placebo. Of the 120 subjects who had IGT at baseline, fewer subjects who were treated with orlistat (3.0% versus 7.6% with placebo) progressed to diabetes at the study's conclusion. Of the 67 subjects who had IGT at baseline and were treated with orlistat, 48 (72%) had normal glucose tolerance by the end of the study. Of the 53 patients who were treated with placebo who had IGT at baseline, only 49% had normalized.

Yusuf et al [29] reported a posthoc secondary analysis of the Heart Outcomes Prevention Evaluation trial of 5720 subjects who were older than age 55 and did not have diabetes but had known vascular disease at study entry. The patients were followed for a mean of 4.5 years. Patients were assigned randomly to receive ramipril, up to 10 mg/d, or placebo. A diagnosis of diabetes was determined from self-reports at follow-up visits every 6 months. One hundred and fifty-five individuals (5.4%) who took placebo developed diabetes in contrast to 102 subjects (3.6%) who took ramipril (HR, 0.66; 95% CI, 0.51–0.95).

In the Losartan Intervention for Endpoint Reduction trial, Dahlof and colleagues [30] randomized 9193 subjects who were aged 55 to 80 years and had essential hypertension and left ventricular hypertrophy to a losartan-based or an atenolol-based regimen. After 4 years, despite equal blood pressure control, the losartan group experienced a 13% RRR in the primary end points of death, myocardial infarction, and stroke. Secondary analysis demonstrated that new-onset diabetes also was less frequent with losartan (6%) than with placebo (9%); this represents a 24% risk reduction (95% CI, 12%–36%) that may reflect a mild insulin sensitizing effect of modulation of the renin-angiotensin axis.

In the West of Scotland Coronary Prevention Study, 6595 hypercholes-terolemic men, aged 45 to 64 years were randomized to pravastatin or placebo [31]. After 5 years of follow-up, pravastatin decreased low-density lipoprotein cholesterol levels by 26% and definite coronary events (nonfatal myocardial infarction and coronary death) were reduced by 31%. Pravastatin therapy also was associated with a 30% risk reduction in the development of diabetes (95% CI, 1%–50%). The investigators suggested that this might have been the result of a reduction in circulating triglyceride concentrations or the anti-inflammatory effects or endothelial effects of the drug. Of note, however, no other statin trial, including the large Cholesterol and Recurrent Events study, Scandinavian Simvastatin Survival Study, and the Heart Protection Study, have reported similar posthoc findings.

Several other T2DM prevention trials are underway, including Nateglinide And Valsartan in Impaired Glucose Tolerance Outcomes Research (NAVI-GATOR), Diabetes Reduction Assessment with Ramipril and Rosiglitazone Medication (DREAM), Actos Now for the Prevention of Type 2 Diabetes (ACT NOW; pioglitazone) and Outcome Reduction with Initial Glargine Intervention (ORIGIN; insulin glargine) [32], although results will not be available for several more years.

Questions that remain

Based on the human and financial costs that are associated with the myriad complications of T2DM, disease prevention is a logical, and potentially, a cost-effective strategy, especially if in addition to a reduction in metabolic "events," a reduction of cardiovascular events can be demonstrated. The findings of the diabetes prevention studies reviewed herein (Table 2) are noteworthy and timely, given the extraordinary increase in the prevalence of T2DM. Several key issues are addressed by these investigations, but many important questions remain.

Are the preventive interventions in these studies truly preventive or do they simply delay the inevitable diagnosis of diabetes? The answer can only result from longer-term studies than have been, or are being, performed. It is reasonable to presume that even if the disease is delayed, less overall years of diabetes exposure would translate to deferred morbidity. Therefore, this may be a worthy goal for individual patients, although it might not be cost effective at a societal level.

If we do accept that diabetes prevention (or delay) is an important undertaking, we must clarify the optimal strategy to identify those persons who are at risk and in whom intervention would be warranted. Almost all of the diabetes prevention studies to date targeted patients who had prediabetes (ie, IFG or IGT). The ADA recently decreased its threshold for impaired fasting glucose (100 mg/dL); this will increase the identification of persons who are at risk. Reliance on the fasting glucose alone will fail to detect a substantial proportion of patients who have prediabetes. Therefore, a 2-hour OGTT will be necessary in many patients to demonstrate IGT; however, this may be impractical to implement on a routine basis. Some investigators proposed using other means of identifying those who are at risk for future diabetes based on clinical criteria [33] or more stringent FPG and hemoglobin A1c cut-points [34]. Which is the best approach to screening? Should the formal OGTT be performed in all at-risk individuals? What are the additional cost implications of such a strategy?

In the studies that involved diet and exercise interventions [17–19], significant efforts that were well above the standard of care were required to help patients achieve and sustain lifestyle change. They were not necessarily

Table 2
Summary of diabetes prevention studies

Study, year [Ref.]	Intervention	RRR (%)
Da Qing, 1997 [17]	Diet ± exercise	31–46
FDPS, 2001 [18]	Diet + exercise	58
DPP, 2002 [19]	Diet + exercise	58
	Metformin	31
TRIPOD, 2002 [20]	Troglitazone	55
STOP-NIDDM, 2002 [21]	Acarbose	25

practical within the context of our current health care delivery system. In addition, patients who were recruited to clinical trials may not be representative of the general prediabetic population, in terms of enthusiasm and adherence to lifestyle changes and in the ability to meet target lifestyle goals. Therefore, how do we implement the findings regarding lifestyle modification in our practices, where patients may have neither the commitment nor the ready access to nutritional counseling and exercise programs? National health care policies will need to adapt to these emerging needs.

An important lesson of the metformin arm of the DPP [19], STOP-NIDDM [24], and TRIPOD [26] is that in those patients who cannot or will not initiate lifestyle change, the use of antihyperglycemic pharmacologic agents, particularly those with insulin sensitizing activity, slows the progression to diabetes. Would the combination of lifestyle change plus pharmacotherapy result in even greater risk reduction? Also, with metformin and acarbose, the degree to which prevention occurs is less than with lifestyle modification, and the effect seems to dissipate quickly in many patients upon discontinuation of medication. The more impressive effects of thiazolidinedione therapy in TRIPOD, in terms of RRR and the duration of the effect, must be confirmed in larger trials with a more heterogeneous study population. In this light, the results of the DREAM and ACT NOW trials are awaited anxiously.

Although pharmacotherapy remains a reasonable default strategy, the use of medications to prevent a disease which may be avoided more effectively by adopting a healthy lifestyle has ethical and fiscal considerations. Can our health care system afford the additional expense of providing pharmacologic prevention to the millions of patients who have prediabetes who might qualify? Certainly, cost-effectiveness analyses of any positive study results will be tremendously important (although probably difficult to model).

Finally, how do we place the results of studies that use lifestyle interventions and antihyperglycemic therapies in the context of the preliminary reports that suggest a similar benefit from other drug classes, such as the angiotensin-converting enzyme inhibitors, angiotensin-II receptor blockers, and statins? This question will need to be answered by carefully designed long-term trials.

Guidelines for the clinician

A working group on diabetes prevention, cosponsored by the ADA and the National Institute of Diabetes, Digestive and Kidney Diseases, recently published a position statement, which now serves as a Clinical Practice Recommendation by the ADA [35]. The group believed that there was substantial evidence that T2DM should be prevented and recommended that individuals who are at high risk be identified and treated with at least lifestyle interventions. Its basic recommendations are listed in Box 2. With the data at hand, such recommendations are reasonable. We believe that enough information has accumulated to implement diabetes prevention strategies confidently in all at-risk patients. The identification of individuals who are at greatest risk for developing diabetes (ie, those with prediabetes) seems justifiable, although we continue to prefer the FPG determination as a more practical screen than broad implementation of OGTT. Clearly, lifestyle modification must be the first recommendation to those who have impaired glucose levels. General healthy lifestyle guidelines also could be

---

Box 2. Recommendations of the American Diabetes Association Working Group on the Prevention of Diabetes

- Individuals who are at high risk for developing diabetes should become aware of the benefits of modest weight loss and participation in regular physical activity.
- Screening: based on current screening guidelines for diabetes, men and women who are older than 45 years of age, particularly those who have a BMI of greater than 25 kg/m^2, are candidates for screening to detect prediabetes (IFG or IGT). Screening should be considered in younger individuals who have a BMI that is greater than 25 kg/m^2 and have additional risk factors (see Box 1).
- In individuals who have normoglycemia, rescreening at 3-year intervals seems to be reasonable.
- How to screen: screening should be carried out only as part of a health care office visit. Either an FPG test or a 2-hour OGTT (75-g glucose load) is appropriate. Positive test results should be confirmed on another day.
- Intervention strategy: patients who have prediabetes (IFG or IGT) should be given counseling on weight loss and instruction for increasing physical activity.
- Follow-up counseling seems to be important for success.
- Monitoring for the development of diabetes should be performed every 1 to 2 years.
- Close attention should be given to, and appropriate treatment given for, other cardiovascular disease risk factors (eg, tobacco use, hypertension, dyslipidemia).
- Drug therapy should not be used routinely to prevent diabetes until more information is known about its cost-effectiveness.

Adapted from Sherwin RS, Anderson RM, Buse JB, et al, for the American Diabetes Association. The prevention or delay of type 2 diabetes. Diabetes Care 2003;26(Suppl 1):S62–9; with permission.

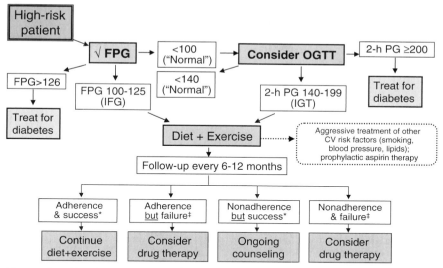

Fig. 9. The prevention of type 2 diabetes: a proposed algorithm. CV, cardiovascular; PG, plasma glucose.

recommended to those who have features of the insulin resistance syndrome, yet who are normoglycemic. Finally, cardiovascular risk factor modification must be considered to be an integral part of any diabetes prevention strategy. A proposed algorithm for the prevention of T2DM, based, in part, on these recommendations, is outlined in Fig. 9.

We are entering an exciting era in the prevention of T2DM. Recently published studies that involved lifestyle and pharmacologic interventions clearly demonstrated their relative effects, at least in the short-term. What is less clear is which intervention will have the greatest acceptance rate by patients who are not participating in clinical trials; which will have the most durable effects; and, which, ultimately, will be the most cost-effective. Furthermore, future implementation of diabetes prevention strategies will depend on whether cardiovascular events can be reduced by those efforts. How we, as clinicians, should implement these strategies optimally in our at-risk patients likely will require years of further study and clinical experience.

References

[1] Harris MI, Flegal KM, Cowie CC, et al. Prevalence of diabetes, impaired fasting glucose, and impaired glucose tolerance in US adults. The Third National Health and Nutrition Examination Survey, 1988–1994. Diabetes Care 1998;21:518–24.
[2] Ohkubo Y, Kishikawa H, Araki E, et al. Intensive insulin therapy prevents the progression of diabetic microvascular complications in Japanese patients with non-insulin-dependent

diabetes mellitus: a randomized prospective 6-year study. Diabetes Res Clin Pract 1995;28: 103–17.

[3] UK Prospective Diabetes Study (UKPDS) Group. Intensive blood-glucose control with sulphonylureas or insulin compared with conventional treatment and risk of complications in patients with type 2 diabetes (UKPDS 33). Lancet 1998;352:837–53.

[4] American Diabetes Association. Standards of medical care for patients with diabetes mellitus. Diabetes Care 2004;27(Suppl 1):S15–35.

[5] Wild S, Roglic G, Green A, et al. Global prevalence of diabetes. Diabetes Care 2004;27: 1047–53.

[6] Ferrannini E. Insulin resistance versus insulin deficiency in non-insulin-dependent diabetes mellitus: problems and prospects. Endocr Rev 1998;19:477–90.

[7] Lillioja S, Mott DM, Spraul M, et al. Insulin resistance and insulin secretory dysfunction as precursors of non-insulin-dependent diabetes mellitus. Prospective studies of Pima Indians. N Engl J Med 1993;329:1988–92.

[8] Henry RR. Insulin resistance: from predisposing factor to therapeutic target in type 2 diabetes. Clin Therap 2003;25(Suppl B):B47–63.

[9] Haffner SM. Insulin resistance, inflammation, and the prediabetic state. Am J Cardiol 2003; 92:18J–26J.

[10] Wheatcroft SB, Williams IL, Shah AM, et al. Pathophysiological implications of insulin resistance on vascular endothelial function. Diabetes Med 2003;20:255–68.

[11] Gerich JE. Contributions of insulin-resistance and insulin-secretory defects to the pathogenesis of type 2 diabetes mellitus. Mayo Clin Proc 2003;78:447–56.

[12] Weyer C, Bogardus C, Mott DM, et al. The natural history of insulin secretory dysfunction and insulin resistance in the pathogenesis of type 2 diabetes mellitus. J Clin Invest 1999;104: 787–94.

[13] Expert Committee on the Diagnosis and Classification of Diabetes Mellitus. Report of the Expert Committee on the Diagnosis and Classification of Diabetes Mellitus. Diabetes Care 2004;27(Suppl 1):S5–S20.

[14] Benjamin SM, Valdez R, Geiss LS, et al. Estimated number of adults with prediabetes in the US in 2000: opportunities for prevention. Diabetes Care 2003;26:645–9.

[15] Sartor G, Schersten B, Carlstrom S, et al. Ten-year follow-up of subjects with impaired glucose tolerance: prevention of diabetes by tolbutamide and diet regulation. Diabetes 1980; 29:41–9.

[16] Eriksson KF, Lindgarde F. Prevention of type 2 (non-insulin-dependent) diabetes mellitus by diet and physical exercise. The 6-year Malmo Feasibility Study. Diabetologia 1991; 34(12):891–8.

[17] Pan XR, Li GW, Hu YH, et al. Effects of diet and exercise in preventing NIDDM in people with impaired glucose tolerance. The Da Qing IGT and Diabetes Study. Diabetes Care 1997; 20:537–44.

[18] Tuomilehto J, Lindstrom J, Eriksson JG, et al. Finnish Diabetes Prevention Study Group. Prevention of type 2 diabetes mellitus by changes in lifestyle among subjects with impaired glucose tolerance. N Engl J Med 2001;344:1343–50.

[19] Knowler WC, Barrett-Connor E, Fowler SE, et al. Diabetes Prevention Program Research Group. Reduction in the incidence of type 2 diabetes with lifestyle intervention or metformin. N Engl J Med 2002;346:393–403.

[20] Buchanan TA, Xiang AH, Peters RK, et al. Preservation of pancreatic beta-cell function and prevention of type 2 diabetes by pharmacological treatment of insulin resistance in high-risk Hispanic women. Diabetes 2002;51:2796–803.

[21] Chiasson JL, Josse RG, Gomis R, et al. STOP-NIDDM Trial Research Group. Acarbose for prevention of type 2 diabetes mellitus: the STOP-NIDDM randomised trial. Lancet 2002; 359:2072–7.

[22] Diabetes Prevention Program (DPP) Research Group. The Diabetes Prevention Program (DPP): description of lifestyle intervention. Diabetes Care 2002;25:2165–71.

[23] Diabetes Prevention Program Research Group. Effects of withdrawal from metformin on the development of diabetes in the diabetes prevention program. Diabetes Care 2003;26: 977–80.

[24] Diabetes Prevention Program Research Group. Prevention of type 2 diabetes with troglitazone in the Diabetes Prevention Program. Diabetes 2003;52(Suppl 1):A58.

[25] Hernan WH, Brandle M, Zhang P, et al. Diabetes Prevention Program Research Group. Costs associated with the primary prevention of type 2 diabetes mellitus in the diabetes prevention program. Diabetes Care 2003;26:36–47.

[26] Chiasson JL, Josse RG, Gomis R, et al and the STOP-NIDDM Trial Research Group. Acarbose treatment and the risk of cardiovascular disease and hypertension in patients with impaired glucose tolerance: the STOP-NIDDM trial. JAMA 2003;290:486–94.

[27] Kjos SL, Peters RK, Kiang A, et al. Predicting future diabetes in Latino women with gestational diabetes: utility of early postpartum glucose tolerance testing. Diabetes 1995;44: 586–91.

[28] Heymsfield SB, Segal KR, Hauptman J, et al. Effects of weight loss with orlistat on glucose tolerance and progression to type 2 diabetes in obese adults. Arch Intern Med 2000;160: 1321–6.

[29] Yusuf S, Gerstein H, Hoogwerf B, et al. HOPE Study Investigators Ramipril and the development of diabetes. JAMA 2001;286:1882–5.

[30] Dahlof B, Devereux RB, Kjeldsen SE, et al. The LIFE Study Group. Cardiovascular morbidity and mortality in the Losartan Intervention For Endpoint reduction in hypertension study (LIFE): a randomised trial against atenolol. Lancet 2002;359:995–1003.

[31] Freeman DJ, Norrie J, Sattar N, et al. Pravastatin and the development of diabetes mellitus: evidence for a protective treatment effect in the West of Scotland Coronary Prevention Study. Circulation 2001;103:357–62.

[32] Simpson RW, Shaw JE, Zimmet PZ. The prevention of type 2 diabetes—lifestyle change or pharmacotherapy? A challenge for the 21st century. Diabetes Res Clin Pract 2003;59:165–80.

[33] Lindstrom J, Tuomilehto J. The diabetes risk score: a practical tool to predict type 2 diabetes risk. Diabetes Care 2003;26:725–31.

[34] Saydah SH, Byrd-Holt D, Harris MI. Projected impact of implementing the results of the diabetes prevention program in the US population. Diabetes Care 2002;25:1940–5.

[35] Sherwin RS, Anderson RM, Buse JB, et al for the American Diabetes Association. The prevention or delay of type 2 diabetes. Diabetes Care 2003;26(Suppl 1):S62–9.

ELSEVIER
SAUNDERS

Endocrinol Metab Clin N Am
34 (2005) 221–235

ENDOCRINOLOGY
AND METABOLISM
CLINICS
OF NORTH AMERICA

Prevention of Cardiovascular Outcomes in Type 2 Diabetes Mellitus: Trials on the Horizon

John B. Buse, MD, PhD[a],*, Julio Rosenstock, MD[b,c]

[a]Divisions of Endocrinology and General Medicine and Clinical Epidemiology,
Diabetes Care Center, University of North Carolina School of Medicine, CB #7110,
5039 Old Clinic Building, Chapel Hill, NC 27599-7110, USA
[b]Dallas Diabetes and Endocrine Center,
7777 Forest Lane, C-618, Dallas, TX 75230, USA
[c]University of Texas Southwestern Medical School, Dallas, TX, USA

Type 2 diabetes mellitus is a clinical syndrome characterized by hyperglycemia in which early cardiovascular (CV) death is the predominant clinical outcome. In the last 20 years several clinical trials have demonstrated unequivocally techniques that reduce the risk for CV events in patients who have diabetes mellitus; these studies form the basis for current guidelines regarding management of patients who have diabetes mellitus, specifically in the areas of lipid modification, blood pressure reduction, modulation of the renin-angiotensin system, antiplatelet therapy, and invasive revascularization procedures.

Despite the many published clinical trials, reviews, and guidelines on diabetes mellitus and cardiovascular disease (CVD), large untested areas of accepted clinical practice remain. Although interventional trials strongly support the notion that more intensive glycemic control is associated with a reduction in microvascular complications, there is only epidemiologic basis for the causal link between glucose control and CVD. Outcomes from the adequately powered clinical trials addressing the relationship between intervention to lower glucose and CV events are awaited with great interest. Furthermore, no outcomes studies have been conducted with insulin analogs or thiazolidinediones. Clinical practice is informed by the best available

Dr. Buse is supported in part by National Institutes of Health Grants RR00046, HC9961, and DK061223.

* Corresponding author.
E-mail address: jbuse@med.unc.edu (J.B. Buse).

0889-8529/05/$ - see front matter © 2005 Elsevier Inc. All rights reserved.
doi:10.1016/j.ecl.2004.11.003

data, but epidemiologic studies can lead one astray, as was the case with hormone replacement therapy as a technique to reduce CVD [1].

This article focuses on the continuing clinical trials in patients who have diabetes mellitus and prediabetes in which CVD outcomes—specifically CV death, myocardial infarction (MI), and stroke—are examined as primary outcomes. These trials were identified using three approaches:

1. Searching www.clinicaltrials.gov, a National Institutes of Health (NIH)–funded website that provides "regularly updated information about federally and privately supported clinical research in human volunteers" with almost 200 diabetes mellitus trials posted [2];
2. Hand-searching titles and abstracts for over 3000 citations identified in the National Library of Medicine PubMed System describing clinical trials in diabetes mellitus cited over the prior 5 years; and
3. Querying thought leaders in diabetes mellitus and CVD as well as representatives of the NIH's National Heart Lung and Blood Institute and National Institute on Diabetes, Digestive and Kidney Diseases.

This is undoubtedly an incomplete representation of the work being conducted in this regard and the authors recognize in advance the potential intellectual risk of any oversights. Many additional studies examine only intermediate surrogate outcomes (eg, intravascular ultrasound, carotid intimal thickness, and CV risk markers), but unfortunately, there is little published information about them. Various search engines were used to identified design details from study websites and press releases, which are referenced to the extent that they provided additional details.

For purposes of discussion these trials have been grouped based on general themes:

- Trials that examine glycemic targets,
- Trials that examine interventional techniques of glucose lowering, and
- Trials that examine nonglycemic interventions.

Some studies involve designs (eg, factorial designs) in which more than one intervention is examined. In those cases, the theme of the study will be introduced in the earlier section and additional details regarding other interventions in subsequent sections.

Trials examining glycemic targets

The most hotly debated clinical questions in diabetes mellitus are whether glycemic control is associated with a reduction in CVD outcomes and how low a glycemic target should be pursued. Because the risk for severe hypoglycemia increases as lower targets are achieved, there is a floor below which benefits will be counterbalanced by risk. Guidelines suggest that hemoglobin A1c (HbA1c) targets of less than 7% [3], 6.5% [4], or 6.1% [5] are appropriate. These goals have been imputed by examining epidemiologic studies because there are no CVD outcomes studies in diabetes mellitus that have provided clear-cut, statistically significant reductions in endpoints. Indeed, no reported interventional outcome study has yet achieved the above recommended A1c targets. The clinical trial that comes closest to meeting such criteria is the United Kingdom Prospective Diabetes Study (UKPDS) [6], which suggests that the method of glucose lowering may be more important than the target or the average level of glycemia achieved [7]. Three current clinical trials are testing directly the hypothesis that glucose lowering in the setting of type 2 diabetes mellitus is associated with a reduction in CVD events (Table 1).

ADVANCE

In the ADVANCE trial (Action in Diabetes and Vascular Disease: Preterax and Diamicron MR Controlled Evaluation), 11,140 patients who have type 2 diabetes mellitus were recruited in 200 centers in Australia, Asia, Europe, and North America. The eligibility criteria are broad: diagnosis of type 2 diabetes mellitus after 30 years of age, age 55 or more years, and high risk for CVD. Patients are randomized in a 2 × 2 factorial design to an open-label, modified-release (MR) sulfonylurea (gliclazide MR)–based intensive treatment with a goal of achieving a HbA1c level of 6.5% or less versus standard care for glycemia as well as a blood pressure intervention (see later discussion). There are two primary endpoints: (1) the composite of stroke, MI, and CV death, and (2) the composite of new or worsening nephropathy or microvascular eye disease. The scheduled postrandomization follow-up is 4.5 years. The study is designed to provide 90% power to detect a 16% reduction in the relative risk of each of the primary endpoints for each of the randomized comparisons. More design details are published [8,9] and available on the website for the coordinating center, the George Institute for International Health in Sydney, Australia. In particular, 11,140 patients have been randomized and final results are

Table 1
Studies of glycemic control and its relationship to cardiovascular disease outcomes

Study [Ref.]	No. of participants	Follow-up, years	A1c target, %		Expected results
			Intensive	Standard	
ADVANCE [8–10]	11,140	~4.5	≤ 6.5	~7.5 (usual care)	2006
VADT [11]	~1700	5–7	≤ 6.0	8–9	2007
ACCORD [12]	~10,000	4–8 (average 5.6)	< 6.0	7.0–7.9 (expected mean 7.5)	2010
ORIGIN[a] [17]	~10,000	4–8	FPG < 95 mg/dL (glargine)	< 7 A1c (standard care with no insulin)	2008

[a] This study's glycemic target in the intervention group is FPG.

expected in 2006, with an expected difference in HbA1c levels between randomized arms of 1%. Discussion on the website suggests that the difference between arms remains a challenge for the study [10].

VADT

The VADT (Veterans Affairs Diabetes Trial) started in December of 2000 with the goal of enrolling 1700 men and women 41 years of age or older with HbA1c level of 7.5% or higher despite therapy with oral agents or insulin. Volunteers are randomized to an intensive or standard treatment program and followed for 5 to 7 years for major CV events (MI, stroke, new or worsening congestive heart failure [CHF], amputation for ischemic diabetic gangrene, invasive intervention for coronary or peripheral arterial disease, and CV death). The study is designed to have 86% power to detect a 21% relative reduction in major CV events. In the intensive arm, the goal is to achieve an HbA1c level of 6% or less by sequential addition and titration of metformin, rosiglitazone, or evening intermediate NPH insulin or long-acting insulin glargine to achieve near-normal fasting glucose levels, and subsequent morning or multiple daily injections of short-acting insulins or other therapies as needed (eg, glimepiride and α-glucosidase inhibitors). In the standard arm, the goal is to avoid deterioration in HbA1c, keeping levels at 8% to 9%. The treatment algorithm for the standard group is less rigid and generally uses submaximal doses of oral agents. The investigators expect a difference between arms of 1.5% to 2% in HbA1c level. All patients receive an identical program of individualized diabetes mellitus education, medical nutrition therapy, blood pressure management, lipid management, aspirin therapy, and smoking cessation counseling per American Diabetes Association guidelines. Further details are available in a published methods paper [11].

ACCORD

The ACCORD trial (Action to Control Cardiovascular Risk in Diabetes) examines three independent medical treatment strategies for patients who have type 2 diabetes mellitus. At approximately 70 centers in the United States and Canada, 10,000 patients who have type 2 diabetes mellitus will be randomized in a double 2 × 2 design. All participants will be in the overarching trial that examines glycemic targets. Two subtrials will examine lipid and blood pressure hypotheses (see later discussion). The clinical question tested by the glycemia trial is: "in middle-aged or older people with type 2 diabetes who are at high risk for having a CVD event because of existing clinical or subclinical CVD or CVD risk factors, does a therapeutic strategy that targets a HbA1c level of < 6% reduce the rate of CVD events more than a strategy that targets a HbA1c level of 7% to 7.9% (with the expectation of achieving a median level of 7.5%)" [12]. Participants will be treated for 4 to 8 years (mean approximately 5.6 years) with main study results to be reported in 2010. The primary outcome measure of the trial is time to the first occurrence of a major CVD event (MI, stroke, or CV death), with the study designed to have 89% power to detect a 15% treatment effect of intensive glycemic control compared with standard glycemic control.

These three trials should answer definitively the clinical question of whether intensive glucose management will reduce the risk for CVD. Each seeks to achieve glycemic targets below levels reported in large clinical trials, and should inform the discussion about the appropriate targets for glycemic control and the magnitude of the risk of hypoglycemia involved. They also will examine effects on microvascular complications, quality of life, and cost-effectiveness. Because each uses different strategies to achieve different target levels of glycemic control in different populations, they will provide a rich set of data to drive future clinical recommendations. Although it is assumed widely that the hypotheses they seek to test are correct, there is substantial doubt as to the outcomes of these studies. Positive results will put tremendous pressure on health care systems to achieve even more stringent levels of control. Negative results will suggest the need to achieve HbA1c levels of approximately 7% to prevent microvascular complications, and that the attention vis-à-vis CV risk management should be on blood pressure, lipid, and thrombotic risk in diabetes mellitus.

Trials examining glycemic management techniques

The second fundamental question in diabetes management is whether particular glucose-lowering approaches, and more specifically insulin sensitizers, provide benefits beyond glucose lowering in managing CV risk. The possibility first was suggested based on the notion that insulin resistance is linked epidemiologically with components of the metabolic syndrome including dyslipidemia, dysglycemia, hypertension, a procoagulant state, vascular inflammation, endothelial dysfunction, and premature vascular disease (see articles by Reaven and Kunhiraman et al elsewhere in this issue). Several small and medium-sized studies have supported the idea that insulin-sensitizing approaches could be superior to approaches that supplement deficient insulin secretion, suggesting improvements in markers of CV risk during treatment with metformin and thiazolidinediones when compared with other therapies. Furthermore, in the UKPDS, among overweight subjects, those randomly assigned to initial therapy with metformin (but not to insulin or sulfonylurea) demonstrated a reduction in diabetes mellitus–related deaths and MI compared with those treated with lifestyle intervention; the validity of this observation has been challenged because of the relatively limited sample size and the unusual responses in a subsequent subrandomization [7].

BARI 2D

Arguably the BARI 2D study (Bypass Angioplasty Revascularization Investigation in Type 2 Diabetes) will offer the most straightforward assessment of this controversy. This multicenter study will recruit 2800 patients who have type 2 diabetes mellitus. Important inclusion criteria include age over 25 years and a coronary arteriogram showing one or more vessels amenable to revascularization with at least a 50% or greater stenosis and either objective documentation of ischemia or typical angina with at least a 70% coronary stenosis. Patients will be randomized in a 2 × 2 factorial design to examine two treatment strategies: one cardiac-related (coronary revascularization plus aggressive medical therapy versus aggressive medical therapy alone) and one diabetes-related (comparing insulin-providing versus insulin-sensitizing therapy). The diabetes treatment randomization will be to treatment focusing on providing more insulin, either endogenously, stimulated through the use of insulin secretagogues, or exogenously, administered through subcutaneous insulin injections, versus a strategy of increasing sensitivity to insulin by using metformin and/or one of the commercially available thiazolidinediones, pioglitazone or rosiglitazone. All patients will be treated with a target HbA1c level of < 7%. For those unable to achieve an HbA1c level less than 8% with one treatment strategy, crossover to combined treatment approaches will be used. The other randomization will examine two approaches to manage CVD: elective revascularization using surgery or catheter-based therapies combined with aggressive medical therapy versus aggressive medical therapy alone. The primary outcome for this trial is CV mortality. Additional outcomes include MI, angina, quality of life, employment, cost, and cost-effectiveness. Recruitment is expected to be complete in 2004, with results reporting in 2007 [13,14].

PROactive

Several pharmaceutical industry–sponsored clinical trials will examine the effect of various specific agents on CV outcomes. Little published information on these trials is available. One exception is the PROactive study (Prospective Pioglitazone Clinical Trial in Macrovascular Events), which has reported its design and baseline characteristics. PROactive has randomized 5238 patients from 19 countries who have type 2 diabetes mellitus and a history of macrovascular disease to the addition of pioglitazone versus placebo onto existing baseline antidiabetic therapy. The primary endpoint is the time from randomization to occurrence of a new macrovascular event or death. The study was expected to reach its prespecified follow-up period depending on the rate of accrual of events in 2005 [15].

RECORD

The RECORD study (Rosiglitazone Evaluated for Cardiac Outcomes and Regulation of Glycaemia in Diabetes) will randomize 6000 patients who have type 2 diabetes mellitus failing either sulfonylurea or metformin.

Patients entering the study on metformin will be randomized to combination with sulfonylurea or rosiglitazone and patients entering the study on sulfonylurea will be randomized to combination with metformin or rosiglitazone. At 18 months, an interim analysis will examine glycemic control between arms. Patients will be followed for 6 years on rosiglitazone plus metformin or sulfonylurea versus metformin plus sulfonylurea or acarbose for combined CV endpoints [16].

ORIGIN

The ORIGIN trial (Outcome Reduction with Initial Glargine Intervention) is a multicenter international study that will randomize in a 2 × 2 factorial design 10,000 people 50 years of age or older at high risk for CVD who have early type 2 diabetes mellitus as defined by an HbA1c level less than 9% if drug naïve or a lower A1c if treated with one oral antidiabetic agent. Persons who have prediabetes with either impaired fasting glucose (IFG) or with impaired glucose tolerance (IGT) will also be included. For the first randomization, patients will be assigned to treatment with insulin glargine titrated to normalize fasting glucose to < 95 mg/dL versus standard care, which generally will involve metformin or sulfonylurea therapy, at least in patients who have fasting hyperglycemia with sequential conventional tactics aiming at achieving A1c < 7%. Patients also will be randomized to a supplement of omega-3 polyunsaturated fatty acids versus placebo. The primary endpoint is combined CV morbidity and mortality outcomes, with projected study completion in late 2008 [17].

NAVIGATOR

The NAVIGATOR trial (Nateglinide and Valsartan in Impaired Glucose Tolerance Outcomes Research) has randomized over 8000 individuals 55 years of age or older who have IGT in over 30 countries in a 2 × 2 factorial design to valsartan versus placebo and to the insulin secretagogue nateglinide versus placebo. Rate of progression from IGT to diabetes mellitus as an endpoint, will be examined 3 years after the last participant is randomized. After 1000 CV events have accrued, estimated to occur with 5 to 6 years of follow-up, composite CV morbidity and mortality outcomes will be examined as an endpoint [18,19].

DREAM

The DREAM study (Diabetes Reduction Assessment with Ramipril and Rosiglitazone Medication) is similar in design to NAVIGATOR, but only examines CVD endpoints and surrogate CV risk markers as secondary endpoints. It also uses a 2 × 2 factorial design to examine the primary outcome if treatment with an angiotensin-converting enzyme (ACE) inhibitor (ramipril) or a thiazolidinedione (rosiglitazone) versus matched placebo can delay or prevent the development of type 2 diabetes mellitus in people who have IGT or impaired fasting glucose (IFG). Follow-up is planned until 2006 in the 5269 patients who have been recruited; further details are published [20].

Table 2 provides an overview of these six studies. In particular, the BARI 2D study should answer the question of whether sensitizer-based therapy is superior to insulin-supplementing therapy. The others likely will be confounded somewhat by differences in levels of glycemic control. To the extent that the studies involving patients who have prediabetes and early diabetes unlikely will exhibit much in the way of elevated glucose, even in the placebo or usual care groups, the effect of differences in glycemia on CVD risk should be minimized, isolating nonglycemic effects of these therapies to some extent. As a body of work, these studies will provide substantial new guidance for optimal treatment strategies in approaching glycemic targets in type 2 diabetes mellitus.

Studies examining nonglycemic therapies

Revascularization interventions

Table 3 details other interventions under investigation. In the initial BARI trial, among the diabetic subgroup a dramatic advantage of coronary artery bypass graft surgery (CABG) was observed compared with percutaneous coronary intervention (PCI) with angioplasty; the benefit was seen primarily in the more than 80% of patients who had an internal mammary artery graft [21]. Since then, several advances have been made in the management of the acute coronary syndrome [22,23], the medical

Table 2
Studies of techniques of glycemic control and effects on cardiovascular disease

Study [Ref.]	Population	No. of participants	Estimated completion	Randomized treatments 1	2
BAR1 2D [13,14]	DM and coronary lesion	2800	2007	Insulin sensitizing	Insulin providing
PROACTIVE [15]	DM	5238	2005	Pioglitazone:	Placebo:
RECORD [16]	DM	6000		metformin + rosiglitazone ± sulfonylurea	metformin + sulfonylurea ± acarbose
ORIGIN [17]	DM and prediabetes	10,000	2008	Glargine	Standard care
NAVIGATOR [18]	Prediabetes	8000	2006	Nateglinide	Placebo
DREAM [20]	Prediabetes	5269	2006	Rosiglitazone	Placebo

management of coronary disease [24], and the techniques of PCI (eg, stents and, most promisingly, drug-eluting stents) [25–28].

This leaves questions regarding the appropriate management of the patient who has diabetes mellitus and flow-limiting coronary disease. Two trials will explore these issues robustly. The BARI 2D trial will explore whether intensive medical management or intensive medical management plus bypass surgery or PCI improves survival in patients who have type 2 diabetes mellitus [13,14]. The FREEDOM trial (Future Revascularization Evaluation in Patients with Diabetes Mellitus: Optimal Management of Multivessel Disease) will compare CABG to PCI using the drug-eluting stents in diabetic patients who have multivessel disease, following the patients for 5 years to examine mortality as the primary endpoint. Investigators at 100 sites will recruit 2300 patients who have diabetes mellitus and at least two stenotic lesions in at least two major epicardial coronary arteries amenable to either PCI or surgical revascularization over 18 months. Intermediate endpoints, quality of life, neurocognitive function, and cost-effectiveness also will be examined. FREEDOM is planned to be complete in 2010 [29]. The CARDia trial (Coronary Artery Revascularization in Diabetes) is a smaller study of 600 individuals in the UK and Ireland that began recruitment in 2002 and is similar in intent to FREEDOM. CARDia addresses the hypothesis that optimal PCI is not inferior to modern CABG in patients who have diabetes with multivessel or complex

Table 3
Other interventions under study

| Study [Ref.] | Randomized treatments | |
	1	2
BAR1 2D [13,14]	CABG or PCI + medical management	Medical management
FREEDOM [29]	CABG	Sirolimus-eluting stent
HPS II, SEARCH [33,34]	High-dose simvastatin	Lower-dose simvastatin
TNT [35]	High-dose atorvastatin	Lower-dose atorvastatin
IDEAL [33]	High-dose atorvastatin	Moderate-dose simvastatin
FIELD [36]	Fenofibrate	Placebo
ACCORD–Lipid [12]	Simvastatin + fenofibrate	Simvastatin + placebo
ACCORD–BP [12]	SBP < 120 mmHg	SBP < 140 mmHg
NAVIGATOR [18,19]	Valsartan	Placebo
DREAM [20]	Ramipril	Placebo
SPARCL (stroke) [37]	High-dose atorvastatin	Placebo
SHARP [38]	Simvastatin + ezetimibe	Simvastatin
ADVANCE [8,9]	ACE + thiazide	Placebo
Look AHEAD [40]	Lifestyle management for weight loss	Diabetes support and education
ORIGIN, ASCEND [17,44]	Omega fatty acid supplement	Placebo
SEARCH, HPS II [33,34]	Vitamins	Placebo
ASCEND [44]	Aspirin	Placebo
CARDia [30]	CABG	PCI

single-vessel coronary disease assuming that the PCI 1-year event rate is 9%. The primary endpoint of death, nonfatal MI, and nonfatal stroke will be assessed at 1 year and the population followed for a total of 5 years for a broad range of secondary endpoints [30].

Lipid interventions

No area of CVD research in diabetes has received more attention than lipid management. Numerous studies in primary prevention and secondary intervention with statins and fibrate lipid-lowering agents are underway [31]. The guidelines regarding lipid management are in flux based on the rapidly evolving landscape of clinical trials that have recently and soon will be reported. Recent guidelines discussed elsewhere in this issue reinforce prior recommendations that in high-risk patients like those who have type 2 diabetes mellitus, the low-density lipoprotein cholesterol (LDL-C) goal is less than 100 mg/dL, but suggest that in the highest risk patients, such as those who have acute coronary syndrome or diabetes mellitus and clinical CVD, further lowering to an LDL-C level of 70 mg/dL or less is "a therapeutic option, ie, a reasonable clinical strategy" [32].

A remaining question is how low should one go in managing lower risk patients who have diabetes mellitus? Several trials addressing this will report in the near future: HPS II (Heart Protection Study II), IDEAL (Incremental Decrease in Endpoints through Aggressive Cholesterol Lowering) [33], SEARCH (Study of the Effectiveness of Additional Reductions in Cholesterol and Homocysteine) [34], and TNT (Treating to New Targets) [35]. Each examines the effect of different levels of low-density lipoprotein (LDL) control with high and moderate doses of one agent (HPS II, SEARCH, and TNT) or different levels of control obtained in comparisons of two agents (IDEAL). Approximately 40,000 patients are randomized in those studies, which will report starting in 2005.

Despite fairly robust demonstration of the role of gemfibrozil in the management of CV risk, issues have arisen regarding the safety of combining statins and fibrates. Thus, with many statin trials documenting the usefulness of statins to reduce CVD in virtually every clinical situation, questions exist regarding the appropriate role of fibrates in the management of CVD risk in diabetes mellitus. The FIELD trial (Fenofibrate Intervention and Event Lowering in Diabetes) randomized 9795 people who had type 2 diabetes with average total cholesterol (115–250 mg/dL) and elevated triglyceride to high-density lipoprotein cholesterol (HDL-C) ratio (> 9.2) or triglyceride level greater than 88 mg/dL to fenofibrate or placebo. FIELD is expected to report on the primary endpoint, CVD death and nonfatal MI, in 2005 [36]. FIELD should establish the role of fenofibrate, a newer fibrate with fewer issues regarding drug interactions with statins.

The ACCORD study has a lipid substudy in which approximately 5800 participants also will be randomized to fenofibrate or placebo in the context of therapy with simvastatin to achieve LDL levels of approximately 100 mg/dL or lower. The ACCORD lipid study will answer whether a treatment strategy that uses a fibrate to raise HDL-C and lower triglycerides and a statin to treat LDL reduces the rate of CVD events compared with a strategy that uses only a statin for treatment of LDL-C, establishing the safety and efficacy of statin-fibrate combination therapy [12].

Finally, several studies will examine the role of lipid management in particular clinical situations common in patients who have diabetes mellitus, such as the SPARCL study (Stroke Prevention by Aggressive Reduction in Cholesterol Levels), which will evaluate the effects of atorvastatin in the setting of transient ischemic attack [37], and SHARP (Study of Heart and Renal Protection), which will examine the effect of simvastatin versus simvastatin/ezetimibe combination therapy in dialysis patients [38].

Blood pressure interventions

Many have argued that blood pressure management is the most important aspect of diabetes care because it has tremendous impact on the risk for microvascular and macrovascular complications [39]. Strictly speaking, the current systolic blood pressure goal of less than 130 mm Hg has not been tested formally in clinical trials because that level has not been achieved and sustained in studies; the diastolic goal of less than 80 mm Hg is better studied.

ACCORD's second substudy will randomize 4200 participants to two levels of blood pressure control to answer whether, in the context of good glycemic control, a therapeutic strategy that targets a systolic blood pressure (SBP) of < 120 mm Hg reduces the rate of CVD events compared with a strategy that targets a SBP of < 140 mm Hg. The ADVANCE trial also has a blood pressure substudy in which patients will be randomized to a fixed low-dose combination of the ACE inhibitor perindopril and the thiazide diuretic indapamide or matching placebo to produce a difference in blood pressure between arms. NAVIGATOR and DREAM will examine the roles of valsartan, an angiotensin-receptor blocker, and ramipril, an ACE inhibitor, on CVD.

Lifestyle interventions

Another crucial question in diabetes management is whether lifestyle intervention can affect CVD outcomes. Lifestyle management is a critical component of all diabetes management. Short-term studies of medical nutrition therapy, physical activity, and comprehensive lifestyle approaches have improved the control of classic CVD risk factors as well as intermediate markers of CVD risk, such as C-reactive protein. However, no long-term large-scale study of intentional weight loss has been powered to examine CVD endpoints.

Look AHEAD (Action for Health in Diabetes) will examine CVD events for up to 11.5 years in patients 45 to 74 years of age who have type 2 diabetes mellitus and a body mass index $\geq 25 \text{ kg/m}^2$ [40]. Patients will be randomized to a 4-year intensive weight-loss program (calorie restriction and physical activity) or to "diabetes support and education." With planned recruitment of 5000 patients at 16 centers over 2.5 years, the study is designed to provide a 0.90 probability of detecting an 18% difference in major CVD event rates between arms.

Miscellaneous interventions

Finally, a related topic is whether antioxidant vitamins, B-vitamin supplementation to lower homocysteine, or various fatty acids can promote CV health in diabetes mellitus. All have been associated with lower risk in epidemiologic analysis, although no consistent findings have emerged from large-scale randomized trials in people who have diabetes mellitus [41–43]. The ORIGIN trial will evaluate the effect of omega fatty acids in patients who have diabetes mellitus and prediabetes and CVD risk factors; ASCEND (A Study of Cardiovascular Events in Diabetes) also will do so in patients who have diabetes mellitus in the setting of primary prevention in a 2 × 2 factorial design in which the second randomization will be to aspirin, 100 mg/d, versus placebo [44]. SEARCH and HPS II will randomize subjects to various vitamin supplements or placebo to examine whether these relatively inexpensive interventions provide clinical benefit to reduce CVD as well.

Summary

There has been an explosion of interest in CVD and diabetes mellitus because of the epidemic nature of the diseases and their tight epidemiologic link. Clinical trials over the past decade have built substantial evidence for the role of lipid management, blood pressure control, and antiplatelet therapy in managing risk for CVD in patients who have diabetes mellitus. The many clinical trials underway will not only hone existing recommendations by establishing appropriate targets and techniques for lipid and blood pressure management, but also should demonstrate the role and most appropriate techniques for management of glycemia, flow-limiting coronary lesions, and obesity.

Acknowledgments

The authors wish to thank the Council for the Advancement of Diabetes Research and Education (CADRE) for assistance in gathering information for this study.

References

[1] Buse J, Raftery L. What we think and what we know. Diabetes Care 2002;25:1876–8.

[2] ClinicalTrials.gov. Available at: http://clinicaltrials.gov/ct. Accessed on August 8, 2004.

[3] American Diabetes Association. Standards of medical care in diabetes. Diabetes Care 2004; 27(Suppl 1):S15–35.

[4] American Association of Clinical Endocrinologists and the American College of Endocrinology. The American Association of Clinical Endocrinologists medical guidelines for the management of diabetes mellitus: the AACE system of intensive diabetes self-management—2002 update. Endocr Pract 2002;8(Suppl 1):40–82.

[5] Third Joint Task Force of European and Other Societies on Cardiovascular Disease Prevention in Clinical Practice. European guidelines in cardiovascular disease prevention in clinical practice. Eur J Cardiovasc Prev Rehabil 2003;10(Suppl 1):S1–78.

[6] UK Prospective Diabetes Study Group. Intensive blood-glucose control with sulphonylureas or insulin compared with conventional treatment and risk of complications in patients with type 2 diabetes (UKPDS 33). Lancet 1998;352(9131):837–53.

[7] UK Prospective Diabetes Study Group. Effect of intensive blood-glucose control with metformin on complications in overweight patients with type 2 diabetes (UKPDS 34). Lancet 1998;352(9131):854–65.

[8] ADVANCE Management Committee. Study rationale and design of ADVANCE: action in diabetes and vascular disease—preterax and diamicron MR controlled evaluation. Diabetologia 2001;44(9):1118–20.

[9] Rationale and design of the ADVANCE study: a randomised trial of blood pressure lowering and intensive glucose control in high-risk individuals with type 2 diabetes mellitus. Action in diabetes and vascular disease: preterax and diamicron modified-release controlled evaluation. J Hypertens Suppl 2001;19(Suppl 4):S21–8.

[10] The George Institute for International Health. Available at: http://www.iih.org. Accessed March 12, 2004.

[11] Abraira C, Duckworth W, McCarren M, et al for the participants of the VA Cooperative Study of Glycemic Control and Complications in Diabetes Mellitus Type 2. Design of the cooperative study on glycemic control and complications in diabetes mellitus type 2. Veterans Affairs Diabetes Trial. J Diabetes Complications 2003;17(6):314–22.

[12] ACCORD purpose. Available at: http://www.accordtrial.org/public/purpose.cfm. Accessed August 8, 2004.

[13] Sobel BE, Frye R, Detre KM. Burgeoning dilemmas in the management of diabetes and cardiovascular disease. Rationale for the Bypass Angioplasty Revascularization Investigation 2 Diabetes (BARI 2D) Trial. Circulation 2003;107(4):636–42.

[14] Bypass Angioplasty Revascularization Investigation in Type 2 Diabetics (BARI 2D). Available at: http://www.clinicaltrials.gov/ct/show/NCT00006305?&order = 1. Accessed August 8, 2004.

[15] Charbonnel B, Dormandy J, Erdmann E, et al on behalf of the PROactive Study Group. The prospective pioglitazone clinical trial in macrovascular events (PROactive): can pioglitazone reduce cardiovascular events in diabetes? Study design and baseline characteristics of 5238 patients. Diabetes Care 2004;27(7):1647–53.

[16] Homan R. Shifting the paradigm from stepwise to early combination therapy. Available at: http://www.cmeondiabetes.com/pub/shifting.the.paradigm..from.stepwise.to.early. combination.therapy..php. Accessed August 8, 2004.

[17] The ORIGIN Trial (Outcome Reduction with Initial Glargine Intervention). Available at: http://www.clinicaltrials.gov/ct/show/NCT00069784?&order = 1. Accessed August 8, 2004.

[18] Pratley R. NAVIGATOR: nateglinide and valsartan in impaired glucose tolerance outcomes research. Available at: http://www.novartis.se/products/diabetes/Pratleypermissions.ppt. Accessed August 8, 2004.

[19] Novartis Pharmaceuticals USA. Novartis announces largest diabetes and cardiovascular disease prevention trial with starlix and diovan. Available at: http://www.pharma.us. novartis.com/newsroom/pressReleases/releaseDetail.jsp?PRID = 141&checked = y. Accessed August 8, 2004.

[20] Gerstein HC, Yusuf S, Holman R, et al. Rationale, design and recruitment characteristics of a large, simple international trial of diabetes prevention: the DREAM trial. Diabetologia 2004;47(9):1519–27.

[21] The BARI investigators. Influence of diabetes on 5-year mortality and morbidity in a randomized trial comparing CABG and PTCA in patients with multivessel disease: the Bypass Angioplasty Revascularization Investigation (BARI). Circulation 1997;96: 1761–9.

[22] Fox KA. Management of acute coronary syndromes: an update. Heart 2004;90(6):698–706.

[23] Schwartz GG, Olsson AG, Ezekowitz MD, et al. Myocardial Ischemia Reduction with Aggressive Cholesterol Lowering (MIRACL) Study Investigators. Effects of atorvastatin on early recurrent ischemic events in acute coronary syndromes: the MIRACL study: a randomized controlled trial. JAMA 2001;285(13):1711–8.

[24] Pitt B, Waters D, Brown WV, et al. Aggressive lipid-lowering therapy compared with angioplasty in stable coronary artery disease. Atorvastatin versus Revascularization Treatment Investigators. N Engl J Med 1999;341(2):70–6.

[25] Levine GN, Kern MJ, Berger PB, et al. American Heart Association Diagnostic and Interventional Catheterization Committee and Council on Clinical Cardiology. Management of patients undergoing percutaneous coronary revascularization. Ann Intern Med 2003;139(2):123–36.

[26] Beyar R. Novel approaches to reduce restenosis. Ann N Y Acad Sci 2004;1015:367–78.

[27] Kokolis S, Cavusoglu E, Clark LT, et al. Anticoagulation strategies for patients undergoing percutaneous coronary intervention: unfractionated heparin, low-molecular-weight heparins, and direct thrombin inhibitors. Prog Cardiovasc Dis 2004;46(6):506–23.

[28] Bavry AA, Kumbhani DJ, Quiroz R, et al. Invasive therapy along with glycoprotein IIb/IIIa inhibitors and intracoronary stents improves survival in non-ST-segment elevation acute coronary syndromes: a meta-analysis and review of the literature. Am J Cardiol 2004;93(7): 830–5.

[29] FREEDOM Trial: Future Revascularization Evaluation in Patients with Diabetes Mellitus: Optimal Management of Multivessel Disease. Available at: http://www.clinicaltrials.gov/ct/show/NCT00086450. Accessed August 15, 2004.

[30] Kapur A, Malik IS, Bagger JP, et al. The Coronary Artery Revascularisation in Diabetes (CARDia) trial: background, aims, and design. Am Heart J 2005;149:13–9.

[31] Deedwania PC, Hunninghake DB, Bays H. Effects of lipid-altering treatment in diabetes mellitus and the metabolic syndrome. Am J Cardiol 2004;93(11A):18C–26C.

[32] Grundy SM, Cleeman JI, Merz CN, et al. Coordinating Committee of the National Cholesterol Education Program; National Heart, Lung, and Blood Institute; American College of Cardiology Foundation; American Heart Association. Implications of recent clinical trials for the National Cholesterol Education Program Adult Treatment Panel III guidelines. Arterioscler Thromb Vasc Biol 2004;24(8):e149–61.

[33] Deanfield JE. Clinical trials: evidence and unanswered questions—hyperlipidaemia. Cerebrovasc Dis 2003;16(Suppl 3):25–32.

[34] MacMahon M, Kirkpatrick C, Cummings CE, et al. A pilot study with simvastatin and folic acid/vitamin B12 in preparation for the Study of the Effectiveness of Additional Reductions in Cholesterol and Homocysteine (SEARCH). Nutr Metab Cardiovasc Dis 2000;10(4): 195–203.

[35] Waters DD, Guyton JR, Herrington DM, et al. TNT Steering Committee Members and Investigators. Treating to New Targets (TNT) Study: does lowering low-density lipoprotein cholesterol levels below currently recommended guidelines yield incremental clinical benefit? Am J Cardiol 2004;93(2):154–8.

[36] FIELD. Available at: http://www.ctc.usyd.edu.au/trials/cardiovascular/field.htm. Accessed August 15, 2004.

[37] Amarenco P, Bogousslavsky J, Callahan AS, et al. SPARCL Investigators. Design and baseline characteristics of the stroke prevention by aggressive reduction in cholesterol levels (SPARCL) study. Cerebrovasc Dis 2003;16(4):389–95.

[38] Study of Heart and Renal Protection (SHARP): study summary. Available at: http://www.ctsu.ox.ac.uk/~jobs/SHARPsummary.doc. Accessed August 12, 2004.

[39] Snow V, Weiss KB, Mottur-Pilson C. Clinical Efficacy Assessment Subcommittee of the American College of Physicians. The evidence base for tight blood pressure control in the management of type 2 diabetes mellitus. Ann Intern Med 2003;138(7):587–92.

[40] Ryan DH, Espeland MA, Foster GD, et al. Look AHEAD (Action for Health in Diabetes): design and methods for a clinical trial of weight loss for the prevention of cardiovascular disease in type 2 diabetes. Control Clin Trials 2003;24(5):610–28.

[41] Stanger O, Herrmann W, Pietrzik K, et al. Clinical use and rational management of homocysteine, folic acid, and B vitamins in cardiovascular and thrombotic diseases. Z Kardiol 2004;93(6):439–53.

[42] Jha P, Flather M, Lonn E, et al. The antioxidant vitamins and cardiovascular disease. A critical review of epidemiologic and clinical trial data. Ann Intern Med 1995;123(11):860–72.

[43] Montori VM, Farmer A, Wollan PC, et al. Fish oil supplementation in type 2 diabetes: a quantitative systematic review. Diabetes Care 2000;23(9):1407–15.

[44] ASCEND: a randomised study of aspirin and of omega-3 fatty acid supplementation for the primary prevention of cardiovascular events in diabetes. Available at: http://www.ctsu.ox.ac.uk/ascend/. Accessed September 6, 2004.

ELSEVIER
SAUNDERS

Endocrinol Metab Clin N Am
34 (2005) 237–255

ENDOCRINOLOGY
AND METABOLISM
CLINICS
OF NORTH AMERICA

Index

Note: Page numbers of article titles are in **boldface** type.

A

A Study of Cardiovascular Events in Diabetes (ASCEND), 227, 229

A1c level. See *Hemoglobin A1c level.*

Absolute insulin deficiency, 140

Acarbose, antihyperglycemic mechanisms of, 77
for type 2 diabetes mellitus, 207–209
medical benefit evidence, 82

ACCORD (Action to Control Cardiovascular Risk in Diabetes) Trials, 32, 39, 221–223, 227–229

ACT NOW (Actos Now for the Prevention of Type 2 Diabetes), 211, 213

Action for Health in Diabetes (Look AHEAD) Study, 227, 229

Action in Diabetes and Vascular Disease (ADVANCE) Trial, 221–222, 227, 229

Action to Control Cardiovascular Risk in Diabetes (ACCORD) Trial, 32, 39, 221–223, 227–229

Activity level, for type 2 diabetes mellitus prevention, 214–215
dyslipidemia and, 11
hypertension and, 65–66

Actos Now for the Prevention of Type 2 Diabetes (ACT NOW), 211, 213

Adiponectin, insulin sensitizers and, 124

Adipose tissue, insulin sensitivity of, 49, 54

ADOPT Study, of thiazolidinediones, 118

ADVANCE (Action in Diabetes and Vascular Disease) Trial, 221–222, 227, 229

Aerodose inhaler, for insulin delivery, 174

Aerosolized insulins, for type 2 diabetes mellitus, 171–175, 180

AERx inhaler, for insulin delivery, 172–174

AFCAPS-TexCAPS (Air Force Coronary Atherosclerosis Prevention Study-Texas Coronary Atherosclerosis Prevention) Trial, 28–30

Air Force Coronary Atherosclerosis Prevention Study-Texas Coronary Atherosclerosis Prevention (AFCAPS-TexCAPS) Trial, 28–30

Albumin:creatinine ratio, insulin sensitizers and, 122, 125

Albuminuria, in diabetic hypertension, 63–64, 68
insulin sensitizers and, 124–125

Alcohol consumption, diabetic hypertension and, 65

ALLHAT (Antihypertensive and Lipid-Lowering treatment to prevent Heart Attack Trial), 68–69

α and γ-Peroxisome proliferator activator receptor agonists, for type 2 diabetes mellitus, 166–168

α-Antagonists, for diabetic hypertension, 62, 70

α-Glucosidase inhibitors (AGIs), adverse effects of, 81
antihyperglycemic mechanisms of, 75, 77–79
contraindications to, 90
effects on A1c, 80–81
for type 2 diabetes mellitus, 207–209
individualized regimens, 89–92
medical benefit evidence, 82

American Diabetes Association (ADA), diabetes diagnostic criteria, 205, 208, 212–213
diabetes prevention recommendations, 213–215
diabetes treatment recommendations, dyslipidemia and, 8–9, 11–12, 14, 16, 33–35
hypertension and, 61

0889-8529/05/$ - see front matter © 2005 Elsevier Inc. All rights reserved.
doi:10.1016/S0889-8529(05)00027-7

β-Blockers (BB), for diabetic hypertension, 62, 68–69

β-Cell dysfunction/loss, antihyperglycemic agents action on, 76, 78, 80, 84, 92
  elevated glucose impact on, 138
  Homeostasis Model Assessment of, 145
  in compensatory hyperinsulinemia, 47–48
  in diabetes mellitus, 144–147
    early insulin preservation of function, 145–146
    evidence for progressive, 144–145
    insulin replacement strategies, 146–147
    insulin sensitizers and, 128
    insulin therapy specific for, 181–183
    type 2 pathophysiology, 198–200, 210

Bezafibrate Infarction Prevention (BIP) Trial, 6, 13

Biguanides, antihyperglycemic mechanisms of, 77

Bile acid sequestrants, for diabetic dyslipidemia, 14

BIP (Bezafibrate Infarction Prevention) Trial, 6, 13

Blood glucose level, elevated. See also *Hyperglycemia.*
    consequences of, 138–140
    metabolism pathways for, 138–139
    type 2 diabetes pathophysiology, 198–200
  in-hospital control parameters for. See *Glycemic management; Hospital management.*

Blood pressure, evaluation methods for, 64–66
  nocturnal dipping of, 64–66

Blood pressure interventions, for cardiovascular disease prevention, with type 2 diabetes mellitus, 227–229

Body mass index (BMI), in type 2 diabetes prevention trials, 201–202, 205, 208, 214
  insulin therapy based on. See *specific agent.*

Bypass Angioplasty Revascularization Investigation in Type 2 Diabetes (BARI 2D) Study, 118, 223–224, 226–227

C

C-reactive protein (CRP), insulin sensitizers and, 119, 123–124

Calcium antagonists, for diabetic hypertension, 62, 69

Captopril Prevention Project, 67

Cardiac surgery outcome, with hyperglycemia, and intravenous insulin therapy, 101

Cardiovascular (CV) disease, insulin sensitizer benefits for, 117–135
    adiponectin and, 124
    albuminuria and, 124–125
    coagulation and, 123
    combination therapy, 128
    congestive heart failure and, 125–128
    endothelial function and, 121–122
    fibrinolysis and, 123
    hypertension and, 121
    inflammation and, 123–124
    insulin resistance pathology, 115–117, 119
    left ventricular mass and, 125–128
    lipid metabolism and, 119–121
    metabolic syndrome risk determinants, 116–117
    modes and sites of action, 117, 154–155
    ongoing thiazolidinediones studies, 117–118
    potential risk reduction, 117, 119
    risk factor effects, 115–117, 120
    type 2 diabetes and, 40–41, 125–128
    vascular reactivity and, 121–122
    vascular wall abnormalities and, 122–123
  with compensatory hyperinsulinemia, 48, 58
  dyslipidemia mechanisms, 50–57
  with diabetes mellitus, 137–154
    ambulatory clinical trials, 147–148
    of dyslipidemia, 3–7
    dyslipidemia management and, 1–25. See also *Dyslipidemia.*
    elevated glucose level consequences, 138–140
    explanation for, 1–3, 137–141
    insulin-based approaches to reduction of, 147–148
    insulin deficiency consequences, 140

Cardiovascular (*continued*)
    insulin resistance factor, 115–117,
      119, 140–141
    insulin therapy benefits for, 82,
      141
    insulin therapy clinical trial
      results, 141–144
      safety in large trials, 144
      type 1 diabetes mellitus, 143
      type 2 diabetes mellitus,
        141–143
      without diabetes mellitus,
        143
    prevention trials for, **221–235**
      examining glycemic
        management
        techniques, 223–226
      examining glycemic targets,
        220–223
      examining nonglycemic
        therapies, 226–230
      identification approaches,
        220
      interest in, 219–220, 230
    public health implications of,
      136–137
    risk factor assessment, 1,
      135–136

CARDS (Collaborative Atorsastatin
  Diabetes Study), 4–5, 14, 31, 34

CARE (Cholesterol and Recurrent Events)
  Trial, 3–4, 14, 211

Carvedilol, for diabetic hypertension, 69

CDP (Coronary Drug Project), 7, 29, 31

Chlorpropamide, antihyperglycemic
  mechanisms of, 77, 87

Cholesterol-absorption inhibitors, 39–40

Cholesterol and Recurrent Events (CARE)
  Trial, 3–4, 14, 211

Cholesterol ester transfer protein (CETP),
  in lipoprotein metabolism, 3, 27

Cholesterol levels, with type 2 diabetes,
  cardiovascular disease and, 3–7,
  227–229. See also *Diabetic
  dyslipidemia.*

Chronic kidney disease (CKD), in diabetic
  hypertension, 63
    drug therapy for, 67–68

CJC-1131, for type 2 diabetes mellitus,
  161–162

Coagulation, insulin sensitizers and, 123

Colesevolam, 39

Collaborative Atorsastatin Diabetes Study
  (CARDS), 4–5, 14, 31, 34

Combination therapy, for type 2 diabetes
  mellitus, with dyslipidemia, insulin
  sensitizers, 128
    pioglitazone, 41
    statins, 16–19, 38–40
      with fibrates, 18–19
      with niacin, 17–18
    with hypertension, 62, 69
    with antihyperglycemic agents,
      advancing strategies, 84–85
      standard oral methods, 87

Combined α and γ-peroxisome proliferator
  activator receptor agonists, for type 2
  diabetes mellitus, 166–168

Combined dyslipidemia, with compensatory
  hyperinsulinemia, 54–55

Compensatory hyperinsulinemia, **49–62**
  β-cell role, 47–48
  cardiovascular disease risks with, 48,
    58
    dyslipidemia mechanisms, 50–57
  clinical syndromes associated with,
    48–49
  combined dyslipidemia with, 54–55
  differential tissue insulin sensitivity
    and, 48–49
  dyslipidemia risks with, 48, 50–58
  high-density lipoprotein cholesterol,
    57
  hypertriglyceridemia with, 50–53
  insulin-resistance pathophysiology,
    11–12, 47–48, 50
  insulin suppression test for, 47, 51,
    54–55
  low-density lipoprotein particle
    diameter with, 56–57
  postprandial lipemia with, 55–56
  steady-state plasma glucose
    distributions, 47–48, 51

Congestive heart failure (CHF), insulin
  sensitizers and, 125–128

Coronary artery bypass graft (CABG)
  outcomes, with hyperglycemia, clinical
  trials on, 226–227
    intravenous insulin therapy and,
      101

Coronary Drug Project (CDP), 7, 29, 31

Coronary heart disease (CHD), with
  diabetic dyslipidemia, 1
    ACP guidelines for, 9–10
    ADA guidelines for, 8–9, 11–12,
      14, 16, 33–35
    clinical trial results, 3–7

examining nonglycemic
therapies, 226–230
examining targets, 220–223
for hyperglycemia, 102, 178
insulin-based trials on,
147–148

Stroke Prevention by Aggressive Reduction
in Cholesterol Levels (SPARCL)
Study, 227–229

Study of Heart and Renal Protection
(SHARP), 227, 229

Study of the Effectiveness of Additional
Reductions in Cholesterol and
Homocysteine (SEARCH), 227–228,
230

Study to Prevent Non Insulin Dependent
Diabetes Trial (STOP-NIDDM),
207–210, 212–213

Subcutaneous (SC) insulin therapy, for
in-hospital hyperglycemia, 105–106
standardized orders example,
109–111

Sulfonylurea secretagogues,
antihyperglycemic mechanisms of,
75–79, 83
when adding oral agents, 88
with monotherapy, 84, 86–87
contraindications to, 90
effect on A1c, 80–81
medical benefit evidence, 82

"Survival skills," for diabetic patients, 105

T

Technosphere insulin delivery system, for
type 2 diabetes mellitus, 172, 174

Tesaglitazars, for type 2 diabetes mellitus,
168

TG-rich remnant lipoproteins, in
compensatory hyperinsulinemia,
55–56

Thiazide diuretics, for diabetic
hypertension, 62, 68–69

Thiazolidinediones (TZDs), adverse effects
of, 81
antihyperglycemic mechanisms of, 75,
77–79, 84
when adding insulin, 87–89, 91
cardiovascular benefits of, **117–135**
adiponectin and, 124
albuminuria and, 124–125
coagulation and, 123
combination therapy, 128

congestive heart failure and,
125–128
endothelial function and,
121–122
fibrinolysis and, 123
hypertension and, 121
inflammation and, 123–124
insulin resistance pathology,
115–117, 119
left ventricular mass and,
125–128
lipid metabolism and, 40–41,
119–121
metabolic syndrome risk
determinants, 116–117
modes and sites of action, 117,
154–155
ongoing thiazolidinediones
studies, 117–118
potential risk reduction, 117, 119
risk factors review, 115–117, 120
type 2 diabetes and, 40–41,
125–128, 166
vascular reactivity and, 121–122
vascular wall abnormalities and,
122–123
contraindications to, 90
effect on A1c, 80–81
individualized regimens, 89–92
medical benefit evidence, 82
time-course of action, 82

Tissue insulin sensitivity, differential, in
compensatory hyperinsulinemia, 48–49

TNT (Treating to New Targets), 227–228

Tolazamide, antihyperglycemic mechanisms
of, 77

Treat-to-Target Trial, 84, 88

Treating to New Targets (TNT), 227–228

Tricarboxylic acid cycle, mitochondrial, for
elevated intracellular glucose, 138–139

Triglycerides (TGs), in compensatory
hyperinsulinemia, 50–53, 57
rich remnant lipoproteins and,
55–56
in diabetic dyslipidemia, current
therapy guidelines for, 25–26
dyslipidemia pathogenesis, 1–3,
26–28
insulin resistance and metabolism
of, 26–28
insulin sensitizers and, 116,
119–121
interventions for cardiovascular
disease prevention, 227–229
management approaches, 32–35

Changing Your Address?

Make sure your subscription changes too! When you notify us of your new address, you can help make our job easier by including an exact copy of your Clinics label number with your old address (see illustration below.) This number identifies you to our computer system and will speed the processing of your address change. Please be sure this label number accompanies your old address and your corrected address—you can send an old Clinics label with your number on it or just copy it exactly and send it to the address listed below.

We appreciate your help in our attempt to give you continuous coverage. Thank you.

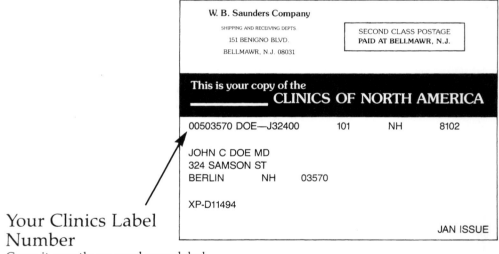

Your Clinics Label Number

Copy it exactly or send your label along with your address to:
W.B. Saunders Company, Customer Service
Orlando, FL 32887-4800
Call Toll Free 1-800-654-2452

Please allow four to six weeks for delivery of new subscriptions and for processing address changes.